METHODS IN MOLECULAR BIOLOGY

Series Editor
John M. Walker
School of Life and Medical Sciences
University of Hertfordshire
Hatfield, Hertfordshire, AL10 9AB, UK

For further volumes:
http://www.springer.com/series/7651

Food Allergens

Methods and Protocols

Edited by

Jing Lin

*Bioinformatics Institute, A*STAR, Singapore; Institute of High Performance Computing, A*STAR, Singapore; Pediatric Allergy and Immunology, Icahn School of Medicine at Mount Sinai, New York, NY, USA*

Marcos Alcocer

School of Biosciences, University of Nottingham, Sutton Bonington Campus, Leicestershire, UK

Humana Press

Editors
Jing Lin
Bioinformatics Institute
A*STAR
Singapore

Institute of High Performance Computing
A*STAR
Singapore

Pediatric Allergy and Immunology
Icahn School of Medicine at Mount Sinai
New York, NY, USA

Marcos Alcocer
School of Biosciences
University of Nottingham
Sutton Bonington Campus
Leicestershire, UK

ISSN 1064-3745 ISSN 1940-6029 (electronic)
Methods in Molecular Biology
ISBN 978-1-4939-6923-4 ISBN 978-1-4939-6925-8 (eBook)
DOI 10.1007/978-1-4939-6925-8

Library of Congress Control Number: 2017936062

Printed on acid-free paper

This Humana Press imprint is published by Springer Nature
The registered company is Springer Science+Business Media LLC
The registered company address is: 233 Spring Street, New York, NY 10013, U.S.A.

Preface

Food allergies, which are abnormal immune responses to food proteins (known as food allergens), have become a major public health problem due to their increasing prevalence, life-threatening potential, and enormous medical and economic impact. So far, the most common food allergens are described in few food products such as cow's milk, eggs, tree nuts, peanuts, soy, wheat, fish, and shellfish. With the recent advances in genomics, molecular biology, and immunology techniques, a complex network of interactions and cross-reactivities becomes apparent. While improved versions of traditional methods (e.g., ELISA) are still widely applied in many laboratories for food allergen studies and allergy diagnostics, novel techniques (e.g., microarray, flow cytometry, mass spectrometry) have led to new methods in the food allergy field.

Food Allergens: Methods and Protocols provides a collection of methodologies for both basic research and clinical diagnosis/treatment relevant to food allergens, including food allergen production, purification, characterization, detection, and quantification, together with bioinformatics approaches applied to modern food allergen studies. In addition, current developments and future trends in food allergen-related laboratory techniques are also covered.

Chapter 1 is an introductory overview chapter describing commonly used methods for food allergen production, detection, and epitope mapping. The remaining 19 chapters are divided into four parts:

Part I, Food Allergen Purification and Production, provides methods of producing recombinant food allergens in bacterial and yeast expression systems, the two most commonly used system for protein production, and the chromatographic methods in protein purification.

Part II, Food Allergen Discovery, Detection, and Quantification, can be classified into three types of methods including DNA-based methods, protein-based methods (e.g., Western blotting, ELISA), and cell-based methods (e.g., basophil activation assay). Many of these methods are also useful for food diagnostics.

Part III, Allergenic Epitope Mapping, comprises experimental methods used for mapping of B-cell epitopes (IgE epitopes) or T-cell epitopes, in silico epitope prediction method, and an overview of bioinformatics resources/tools in epitope/allergen prediction.

Part IV, Methods Currently Being Developed and Future Development, deals mainly with the new concepts of allergenicity as an outcome of protein and food matrix interaction. The particular search for NKT bioactive lipids is described as well as a review on the novel techniques in development for food allergen detection.

Over the past decades, the development of new innovations and technologies has led to great improvements in many aspects of food allergen studies (e.g., reproducibility, sensitivity, specificity, and high throughput capacity). These methods greatly facilitate identification, characterization, and quantification of food allergen and are slowly leading to a better understanding of food allergic diseases and their diagnosis and pointing toward specific therapeutics. We have tried to include in this book a set of important protocols highly relevant to food allergens studies. We hope that the protocols provided here would be valuable resources not only to immunologists, biochemists, molecular biologists, and medical doctors/students working in the food allergy area but also useful for the food industry, legislators, food standard agencies, allergologists, pediatricians, and clinicians/biologists working in the general field of allergic diseases and immunology.

We would like to take this opportunity to express our gratitude to all the authors for sharing their valuable expertise through the contribution of detailed protocols and notes for this book. We also want to thank Professor John Walker and the editorial staff of Springer for continuous assistance and encouragement.

Singapore *Jing Lin*
Sutton Bonington, Leicestershire, UK *Marcos Alcocer*

Contents

PART III ALLERGENIC EPITOPE MAPPING

PART IV METHODS CURRENTLY BEING DEVELOPED AND FUTURE DEVELOPMENT

Contributors

MARCOS ALCOCER • *School of Biosciences, University of Nottingham, Sutton Bonington Campus, Leicestershire, UK*

EMAN ALI ALI • *Division of Molecular Therapeutics and Formulation, School of Pharmacy, University of Nottingham, Nottingham, UK*

GLORIA ALVAREZ-LLAMAS • *Laboratorio de Inmunoalergia y Proteomica, Departamento de Inmunologia, IIS-Fundacion Jimenez Diaz, Madrid, Spain*

LUIS L. DIEGO ARCHILA • *Benaroya Research Institute at Virginia Mason, Seattle, WA, USA*

MARIA G. BARDERAS • *Department of Vascular Physiopathology, Hospital Nacional de Parapléjicos, Toledo, Spain*

LUDA BARDINA • *Elliot and Roslyn Jaffe Food Allergy Institute, Division of Allergy and Immunology, Department of Pediatrics, Icahn School of Medicine at Mount Sinai, New York, NY, USA*

SARA BENEDÉ • *Instituto de Investigación en Ciencias de la Alimentación (CIAL, CSIC-UAM), Madrid, Spain; Pediatric Allergy and Immunology, Icahn School of Medicine at Mount Sinai, New York, NY, USA*

BARBARA CASES • *Research and Development Department, Inmunotek S.L., Madrid, Spain*

SILVIA DE LA CRUZ • *Departamento de Nutrición, Bromatología y Tecnología de los Alimentos, Facultad de Veterinaria, Universidad Complutense de Madrid, Madrid, Spain*

FERNANDO DE LA CUESTA • *Centre for Cardiovascular Science, Queen's Medical Research Institute, University of Edinburgh, Edinburgh, UK*

FRANCO H. FALCONE • *Division of Molecular Therapeutics and Formulation, School of Pharmacy, University of Nottingham, Nottingham, UK*

ZHIYAN FU • *Genome Institute of Singapore, A*STAR, Singapore*

AINA GARCÍA • *Departamento de Nutrición, Bromatología y Tecnología de los Alimentos, Facultad de Veterinaria, Universidad Complutense de Madrid, Madrid, Spain*

TERESA GARCÍA • *Departamento de Nutrición, Bromatología y Tecnología de los Alimentos, Facultad de Veterinaria, Universidad Complutense de Madrid, Madrid, Spain*

ASHFAQ GHUMRA • *School of Biosciences, University of Nottingham, Sutton Bonington, Loughborough, UK*

ISABEL GONZÁLEZ • *Departamento de Nutrición, Bromatología y Tecnología de los Alimentos, Facultad de Veterinaria, Universidad Complutense de Madrid, Madrid, Spain*

ALEXANDER GRISHIN • *Elliot and Roslyn Jaffe Food Allergy Institute, Division of Allergy and Immunology, Department of Pediatrics, Icahn School of Medicine at Mount Sinai, New York, NY, USA*

GALINA GRISHINA • *Elliot and Roslyn Jaffe Food Allergy Institute, Division of Allergy and Immunology, Department of Pediatrics, Icahn School of Medicine at Mount Sinai, New York, NY, USA*

NUZUL N. JAMBARI • *Department of Food Sciences, Faculty of Food Sciences and Technology, University of Putra Malaysia, Serdang, Selangor, Malaysia*

MOHANAPRIYA KAMALAKANNAN • *Division of Allergy and Immunology, Department of Pediatrics, The Jaffe Food Allergy Institute, Icahn School of Medicine at Mount Sinai, New York, NY, USA*

GEORGE N. KONSTANTINOU • *Department of Allergy and Clinical Immunology, General Military Training Hospital, Thessaloniki, Greece; Division of Allergy and Immunology, Jaffe Food Allergy Institute, Icahn School of Medicine at Mount Sinai, New York, NY, USA*

WILLIAM W. KWOK • *Benaroya Research Institute at Virginia Mason, Seattle, WA, USA; Department of Medicine, University of Washington, Seattle, WA, USA*

JING LIN • *Bioinformatics Institute, A*STAR, Singapore; Institute of High Performance Computing, A*STAR, Singapore; Pediatric Allergy and Immunology, Icahn School of Medicine at Mount Sinai, New York, NY, USA*

CHANGQI LIU • *School of Exercise and Nutritional Sciences, San Diego State University, San Diego, CA, USA*

INÉS LÓPEZ-CALLEJA • *Departamento de Nutrición, Bromatología y Tecnología de los Alimentos, Facultad de Veterinaria, Universidad Complutense de Madrid, Madrid, Spain*

ROSINA LÓPEZ-FANDIÑO • *Instituto de Investigación en Ciencias de la Alimentación (CIAL, CSIC-UAM), Madrid, Spain*

RAQUEL MADRID • *Departamento de Nutrición, Bromatología y Tecnología de los Alimentos, Facultad de Veterinaria, Universidad Complutense de Madrid, Madrid, Spain*

ROSARIO MARTÍN • *Departamento de Nutrición, Bromatología y Tecnología de los Alimentos, Facultad de Veterinaria, Universidad Complutense de Madrid, Madrid, Spain*

MADHAN MASILAMANI • *Division of Allergy and Immunology, Department of Pediatrics, The Jaffe Food Allergy Institute, Icahn School of Medicine at Mount Sinai, New York, NY, USA; Immunology Institute and The Mindich Child Health and Development Institute, Mount Sinai School of Medicine, New York, NY, USA*

ELENA MOLINA • *Instituto de Investigación en Ciencias de la Alimentación (CIAL, CSIC-UAM), Madrid, Spain*

RYOSUKE NAKAMURA • *Division of Medicinal Safety Science, National Institute of Health Sciences, Setagaya-ku, Tokyo, Japan*

MARIA NEOPHYTOU • *School of Biosciences, University of Nottingham, Sutton Bonington, Loughborough, UK*

MARIONA PASCAL • *Immunology Department, CDB, Hospital Clinic de Barcelona, Universitat de Barcelona, Barcelona, Spain*

CARLOS PASTOR-VARGAS • *Department of Immunology, IIS Fundación Jiménez Diaz-UAM, Madrid, Spain*

MARINA PEREZ-GORDO • *Institute for Applied Molecular Medicine (IMMA), School of Medicine, Universidad CEU San Pablo, Madrid, Spain*

HUGH A. SAMPSON • *Pediatric Allergy and Immunology, Icahn School of Medicine at Mount Sinai, New York, NY, USA; The Jaffe Food Allergy Institute, Icahn School of Medicine at Mount Sinai, New York, NY, USA*

SHRIDHAR K. SATHE • *Department of Nutrition, Food and Exercise Sciences, Florida State University, Tallahassee, FL, USA*

XIAOWEI WANG • *School of Biosciences, University of Nottingham, Sutton Bonington, UK*

LEANNA N. WILLISON • *School of Science, Mathematics and Computing, Albany State University, Albany, GA, USA*

Chapter 1

Overview of the Commonly Used Methods for Food Allergens

Jing Lin and Marcos Alcocer

Abstract

Food allergy has become a major public health problem worldwide. In the past two decades, development in molecular biology and immunology has led to many new techniques that had improved traditional methods in the food allergy field. These methods greatly facilitate identification, characterization, and quantification of food allergen and are certainly leading to better diagnostics and therapeutics for food allergic diseases. Here we review methods commonly used for food allergens.

Key words Food allergens, Allergen quantification, Recombinant allergen, Epitope mapping, Allergy diagnostics

1 Introduction

Food allergy, an adverse immune response to food components (food allergens), has become an emerging major public health problem worldwide [1]. So far more than 170 foods have been reported to provoke allergic reactions. Of these, the most common foods which account for 90% of all reported food allergies are peanuts, soybeans, crustacea, fish, cows' milk, eggs, tree nuts, and wheat [2]. With the development of genomics, molecular biology, and immunology, many other allergens and allergenic sources are now reported. New techniques, such as microarray, flow cytometry, and mass spectrometry, have been applied in food allergy field, which greatly facilitate food allergen identification, characterization, and quantification and lead to better diagnostics and therapeutics for food allergic diseases. In this chapter, we review methods commonly used for food allergens. Further details regarding these methods are described within the individual chapters in this book.

Jing Lin and Marcos Alcocer (eds.), *Food Allergens: Methods and Protocols*, Methods in Molecular Biology, vol. 1592, DOI 10.1007/978-1-4939-6925-8_1, © Springer Science+Business Media LLC 2017

2 Methods for Allergen Purification and Production

2.1 Recombinant Allergen Production

For accurate food allergy diagnostics and quantification of food allergens, a large quantity of purified allergens is required. However, purification of the native food allergens from their natural sources is usually difficult due to their low abundance and existence of multiple isoforms, a natural genotype abundantly found in the plant kingdom. Therefore recombinant allergens produced using heterologous systems have been widely used as alternatives to their native counterparts in food allergy field. The recombinant proteins can also be used as allergen vaccines by using molecular cloning technique to modify the amino acid sequence in order to reduce or abolished IgE binding activity for safer allergy immunotherapy.

Currently the great majority of available recombinant allergens are produced in bacterial or yeast expression systems. *E. coli* bacterial expression systems are the most convenient and cost-effective platforms for the production of recombinant allergens. But the expressed recombinant proteins may not be properly folded lacking critical posttranslational processings such as glycosylation, disulphide bridges, and all the folding check points contained in a eukaryotic system. To overcome those limitations yeast expression systems have been used. The yeast *P. pastoris* for instance can yield high levels of recombinant allergens and is capable of generating properly folded and secreted protein allergens. However as a lower eukaryote, its pattern of glycosylation differs from higher eukaryotes (such as plants and animals) and may lead to glycosylation problems that can restrict its usage.

Both mammalian and plant expression systems [3] have also been applied for the production of recombinant allergens with the advantage of offering higher eukaryotic posttranslational modifications. The plant expression system, in particular, is attractive considering that most allergens are of plant origin and may carry plant-specific posttranslational modifications which are important for IgE recognition. However, they are expensive and more difficult to manipulate than bacterial and yeast systems and therefore not widely used.

2.2 Allergen Purification

For both native and recombinant allergens, it is necessary to purify the allergens with high level of purity for research or clinical purposes. Usually one or more chromatographic steps are included in a protein purification protocol. Allergens can be isolated from other components using different chromatographic techniques based on their difference in size (size exclusion chromatography), charge (anion-exchange and cation-exchange chromatography), binding affinity (affinity chromatography), and hydrophobicity (hydrophobic interaction and reverse phase chromatography). A well-designed selection and combination of different chromatographic techniques can significantly increase the yield and purity of the purified allergens. The ability to generate in vivo biotinylated proteins, as described in the yeast expression system in the following chapters of this book, will certainly help many critical steps from this procedure.

3 Methods for Allergen Discovery/Identification

Historically food allergens have been identified by antibody-based assays, using serum samples from allergic patients. In these immunoassays, IgE antibodies present in the serum samples are the primary detection reagents that specifically recognize the allergens. The bound IgE antibodies are then detected using labeled anti-IgE antibodies. The labeling can be an enzyme (e.g. horseradish peroxidase, alkaline phosphatase) which interact with the added substrate to induce colour change or emit light, a radioactive isotope (e.g. ^{125}I), or a fluorescent tag.

Immunoblotting is a commonly used immunoassay for detecting protein allergens. A simple immunoblotting technique is dot blotting in which proteins are spotted directly on a membrane (nitrocellulose or PVDF) and probed with IgE antibodies. Several other immunoassays, such as radio-allergosorbent test (RAST) and enzyme-linked immunosorbent assay (ELISA), are similar in principle to dot blotting, although proteins are immobilized and analyzed in microplate wells instead of membrane. The secondary antibody used in RAST is labeled with a radioactive isotope, while enzyme (such as horseradish peroxidase) labeled secondary antibody is used in ELISA.

Most food allergens however are members of large protein families with high sequence similarity that cannot be easily distinguished by antibodies. Dot blotting methods cannot fractionate proteins and only have limited applications in food allergen discovery. Protein separation techniques such as one-dimensional and two-dimensional gel electrophoresis (2DGE) can aid in the allergen discovery and identification processes by resolving isoforms for immunodetection and providing certain discriminating characteristics such as isoelectric points or molecular mass. Using 2DGE, proteins are fractionated according to their isoelectric points in the first dimension and molecular mass in the second dimension. When combined with immunoblotting (also known as western blotting), separated proteins are transferred from the gel to a membrane and probed with enzyme or isotope labeled antibodies. 2DGE coupled with western blotting is a sensitive method that has been extensively used to identify new allergens [4].

Gel electrophoresis however is a time-consuming procedure and immunoblotting provides mostly qualitative analysis rather than quantitative measurement, and therefore are not very well-adapted techniques for routine allergen analysis. Recent development in proteomics has greatly improved allergen identification and quantification. For example, mass spectrometry, when coupled with 2DGE and immunoblotting, can distinguish different allergen isoforms and provide an accurate determination of their amino acid sequence.

4 Methods for Food Allergen Detection/Quantification

Currently methods for allergen quantifications can be classified into three types: methods measuring allergen coding genes, methods measuring allergenic protein levels, and methods measuring effector cell activation levels. The choice of method is dependent on the food concerned (e.g. availability of specific antibodies/DNA primers and the achievable detection limit). There are several major advantages of using DNA methods, explored in the PCR methods in this book; one of them is the use of a nonprotein probe so the specificity of the putative antibody will not affect its performance. Nevertheless, methods based on protein or cell reaction have their roles and additional applications. They can be used in food allergy diagnostics by detecting/quantifying IgE antibodies or cell responses from patients, and are powerful tool on the establishment of allergenicity of proteins which is not measurable by the DNA-based method.

4.1 DNA-Based Method

Methods measuring allergen coding genes are based on amplification of a specific DNA fragment within the allergen gene by PCR using specific primers. With real-time PCR, quantitative results can be obtained. There are controversies regarding the use of DNA analysis in allergen detection/quantification since proteins rather than DNA are the component causing allergic reactions and the proportion of nucleic acids and proteins may be differentially affected during processing.

4.2 Protein-Based Method

Many of the immunoassays used for food allergen discovery/detection can be adapted for quantification of food allergenic protein. Due to the limited amount of patients' sera and variability in specificity and avidity between different donors, most of the antibodies used in routine analytical labs are raised in animals such as rabbit, rat, or goat. So far ELISA is the most commonly used method in laboratories for allergen detection and quantification due to its simple handling, high precision, and good potential for standardization. Two sensitive ELISA approaches, competitive ELISA and sandwich ELISA are often used for the quantification of allergens/proteins and numerous ELISA test kits are commercially available to quantify specific allergens from various food sources [5].

A more recently developed method, the protein microarray-based immunoassay, also known as component resolved diagnostics when referring to pure proteins, allows thousands of immobilized proteins/protein extracts to be screened simultaneously by a small amount of patient's serum. Protein microarray is similar in principle to dot blotting, but in a high-throughput format and providing highly quantitative data. It has great potential to be used for food allergy diagnosis due to its ability to measure IgE antibodies to thousands of allergens using a small quantity of patient's serum in one single assay.

The recent progress in mass spectrometry equipments and techniques has turned this methodology into quite an attractive technique for detection and quantification of food allergens [6]. Once the allergen has been identified and characterized, mass spectrometry can be used to quantify traces of allergenic proteins in complex mixture, or determine the presence of multiple allergens in a single analysis. Mass spectrometric method directly targets the allergens instead of indirect measurement relying on antibody, and therefore independent of the individual sensitivity of each allergic patient or the specificity of the detecting antibody.

4.3 Cell-Based Method

Cell-based method (also known as basophil activation test (BAT) or basophil degranulation assay) is based on the principle that cross-linking of the surface bound IgE antibodies by specific allergens activate allergen effector cells (i.e. basophils) and lead to cell surface marker (e.g. CD63) expression and mediators (e.g. histamine) release. Cells collected from patients and cell lines which are passively sensitized by patient's serum may be used and measurement monitored by either the expression of the cell activation marker or the amount of released mediator. BAT can be used for allergen quantification, and also as a complementary diagnostic tool for food allergy when using fresh blood samples from patients. However, cell-based methods are highly dependent on the blood/serum samples from human donors which cannot be replaced by antibodies raised in animals. Due to the broad variability in basophil activity or IgE sensitivity between different donors, this method is difficult to be standardized and has so far not been employed for routine analysis of food allergens.

5 Methods for Mapping Allergenic Epitopes

Epitopes are the groups of amino acids within allergens that are recognized and bound to IgE antibodies (B cell epitopes) or T cells (T cell epitopes). There are two types of epitopes: A linear (or continuous) epitope is a sequence of contiguous amino acids, while a conformational epitope is comprised of amino acids that line up because of the tertiary structure of an allergen. Studies of epitopes are critically important for food allergens characterization, food allergy diagnosis/prognosis, and the design of immunotherapeutic reagent. For example, the current trends in allergy immunotherapy are to modify B cell epitopes to prevent IgE binding while preserving T cell epitopes, or peptide-based immunotherapy using T cell epitope-containing peptides (too short to effectively cross-link allergen-specific IgE on mast cells and basophils) as an alternative strategy [7] for efficacious desensitization without significant reactions.

Bioinformatic resources and tools are very useful not only in the analyses of the data from in vitro epitope mapping experiments, but also in in silico epitope prediction using sequence and structural information of proteins. Many free database and analysis resources are available online, for example, the IEDB database (immune epitope databases and analysis resources) which is a commonly used database containing a wide range of epitopes, including both B- and T cell epitopes, and provide various tools for predicting both B cell and T cell epitopes.

5.1 B Cell Epitope Mapping

B cell epitopes (also known as IgE epitopes) can be either linear or conformational. Linear epitopes have been suggested to be more important in food allergens because food proteins are usually cooked and digested, leading to alteration and break-up of the tertiary structure before reacting with the immune system.

Methods to determine IgE linear epitopes have been developed over the last few years. The conventional method to localize B cell epitopes involved protein digestion using proteolytic enzyme (such as pepsin), followed by western blotting using patients' sera and mass spectrometry analysis or sequencing to determine the amino acid sequence of the IgE binding fragments. Another traditional method is SPOT membrane-based immunoassay [8] which involves in situ synthesis of overlapping peptides covering the primary amino acid sequence of food allergens on the membrane and probing with the patients' sera. This technique can be easily set up in most laboratories. However, it has several limitations: a large volume of patient's serum is required to probe the membrane with only a limited number of peptides spots, and its peptide synthesis procedure is time-consuming and involves many cycles of coupling, blocking, and deprotection reactions resulting in high percentage of peptide byproducts affecting the specificity.

Recently peptide microarray immunoassay has been widely applied for mapping the linear IgE epitopes of many food sources [9]. It uses the high-throughput microarray platform which allows screening of thousands of commercially synthesized peptides in parallel using microliter quantities of serum, remarkably reducing the biological sample cost of individual assays. As the purity of the peptides undergoes strict QC control, its data is more reliable than SPOT membrane immunoassay. One major problem of peptide microarray immunoassay is that it requires microarray printer and scanners which may be only available in centralized technology-based laboratories.

Conformational epitopes are important for allergens involved in oral allergy syndrome and allergens with compact folding and high stability that enables them to survive gastric digestion [10]. Due to the limitation of available three-dimensional structures of food allergens and the difficulty of maintaining protein stability, studies of conformational epitopes are far behind those of sequential epitopes. Mimotope mapping technique is one option for mapping conformational epitopes [11]. Using random peptide phage display libraries, peptides are generated and screened based on their binding affinity with allergen-specific IgE. The selected peptides are known as mimotopes as they mimic the binding sites of the allergens and the resulting mimotope can be mapped onto the structure of the allergen using computational techniques.

Epitopes can be also predicted using bioinformatics tools, such as ElliPro [12], which is available on the IEDB analysis resource website and predicts both linear and discontinuous epitopes based on protein's 3D structure. Another option is meta-servers, such as EPMeta [13], which combines several other web tools and show relatively higher accuracy. But due to the difficulty in predicting protein 3D structures, currently available bioinformatic tools show low accuracy in general in predicting B cell epitopes, especially conformational B cell epitopes.

5.2 T Cell Epitope Mapping

The majority of T cell epitopes are linear because antigens must be processed into peptide fragments or epitopes by proteasomes prior to MHC binding and presentation to T cells. Similar to the methods for mapping linear B cell epitope, traditional T-cell epitope discovery uses short synthetic peptides spanning the entire length of the allergen in T-cell proliferation assays. This assay is based on the principle that CD4+ T cells undergo massive proliferation when stimulated with the specific peptides loaded on MHC class II molecules on the antigen presenting cells. In this assay, peripheral blood mononuclear cells (PBMCs) are stimulated with the peptides, and the proliferative responses can be evaluated by thymidine incorporation assay. Tritiated thymidine is a radioactive nucleoside commonly used to determine the extent of cell division due to its incorporation in newly synthesized DNA during cell division.

Two flow cytometry-based mapping methods have been recently developed for mapping allergen T-cell epitopes. One analyzes T-cell proliferation by measuring the decrease of proliferation dyes, such as carboxyfluorescein diacetate succinimidyl ester (CFSE), to detect proliferating cells by their reduced staining intensity. The advantage of this method is the use of nonradioactive reagents and the versatility of simultaneous detection of multiple markers for phenotypic characterization of T cells. However, in conditions where the frequency of individual peptide-specific T cells is very low, this method may not be applicable due to the poor resolution of proliferating T cells.

The other flow cytometry-based method identifies T cell epitopes through a novel technique known as "tetramer-guided epitope mapping". In this assay, fluorochrome-labeled peptide MHC class II tetramers are generated by loading peptide pools or individual peptide onto MHC class II molecules and used to stain PBMCs that have been previously stimulated with the corresponding peptide mixture. Positive staining is then identified by flow cytometry. Tetramer assays are very specific and sensitive, but knowing the HLA type of the subject is a prerequisite to apply this assay.

For the above epitope mapping methods, a large number of overlapping peptides are required to cover the full protein sequence of allergens, but their screening is restricted by a small number of PBMCs from patients. As peptide binding to MHC class II molecules is required for interaction with T cells, the sequence of the allergen can be pre-screened to identify sequence with higher potential to bind to MHC class II molecules and exclude the ones with no MHC binding potential from synthesis and further analysis. Both in silico approaches, such as the various tools for predicting MHC II binders provided by IEDB, and in vitro assays, such as ELISA assays measuring the binding between synthetic peptides and recombinant human MHC II molecules, can provide rapid preliminary selection on T cell epitopes [14]. Commercial peptide-MHC binding assays are also available, such as ProImmune REVEAL assays which identify MHC class II binding peptides based on their ability to stabilize the MHC complex. The advantage of these binding assays is their cell-free system to save patient samples from testing peptides that are unlikely to contain T cell epitopes.

6 Methods for Food Allergy Diagnostics

The gold standard for food allergy diagnosis is the double-blind, placebo-controlled oral food challenge (DBPCFC), but it is expensive, difficult to run, and carries a risk of life-threatening allergic reactions. Despite its many limitations, skin prick test (SPT) is still one of the most widely used methods in allergy clinics. In vitro measurements of allergen-specific serum IgE, along with the patient's clinical history, are used to predict the clinical reactivity of food allergic patients. As mentioned earlier, methods for allergen detection/quantification (e.g. RAST, ELISA, basophil activation tests) can be used to measure the amount of IgE antibodies and effector cell responses, and applied for allergy diagnostics. Currently the most commonly used laboratory test for allergy diagnosis is ImmunoCAP, which was developed by Phadia more than three decades ago and utilizes a "sandwich" ELISA technique. The solid phase used in ImmunoCAP consists of an encapsulated cellulose polymer with high protein binding capacity to allergens and thus produces sensitive and reproducible results.

In addition to the measurement of allergen-specific IgE, recent studies have found a positive relationship between patients' IgE epitope recognition and allergy severity/persistence, with several informative epitopes identified as candidate biomarkers to predict the development of tolerance [15]. Therefore methods used for IgE epitope mapping (e.g. peptide microarray) may provide an additional tool for allergy diagnosis and prognosis.

Over the past decades, the development of novel technologies has led to great improvements in many aspects of food allergen studies. These methods greatly facilitate identification, characterization, and quantification of food allergen and are slowly leading to a better understanding of food allergic diseases, their diagnosis and pointing towards specific therapeutics.

Within the following chapters we have tried to address many of the techniques described above and include important protocols highly relevant to the work with food allergens.

References

1. Sicherer SH, Sampson HA (2014) Food allergy: epidemiology, pathogenesis, diagnosis, and treatment. J Allergy Clin Immunol 133(2):291–307
2. Hefle SL, Nordlee JA, Taylor SL (1996) Allergenic foods. Crit Rev Food Sci Nutr 36:S69–S89
3. Schmidt G, Gadermaier G, Pertl H et al (2008) Production of recombinant allergens in plants. Phytochem Rev 7(3):539–552
4. Westermeier R (2014) Looking at proteins from two dimensions: a review on five decades of 2D electrophoresis. Arch Physiol Biochem 120(5):168–172
5. Jayasena S, Smits M, Fiechter D et al Comparison of six commercial ELISA kits for their specificity and sensitivity in detecting different major peanut allergens. J Agric Food Chem 63(6):1849–1855
6. Di Girolamo F, Muraca M, Mazzina O et al (2015) Proteomic applications in food allergy: food allergenomics. Curr Opin Allergy Clin Immunol 15(3):259–266
7. Tanabe S (2007) Epitope peptides and immunotherapy. Curr Protein Pept Sci 8(1):109–118
8. Frank R (2002) The SPOT synthesis technique—synthetic peptide arrays on membrane supports—principles and applications. J Immunol Methods 267(1):13–26
9. Lin J, Bardina L, Shreffler WG et al (2009) Development of a novel peptide microarray for large-scale epitope mapping of food allergens. J Allergy Clin Immunol 124(2):315–322 322. e1–3
10. Sathe SK, Teuber SS, Roux KH (2005) Effects of food processing on the stability of food allergens. Biotechnol Adv 23(6):423–429
11. Riemer A, Scheiner O, Jensen-Jarolim E (2004) Allergen mimotopes. Methods 32(3):321–327
12. Ponomarenko J, Bui HH, Li W et al (2008) ElliPro: a new structure-based tool for the prediction of antibody epitopes. BMC Bioinformatics 9:514
13. Liang S, Zheng D, Standley DM et al (2010) EPSVR and EPMeta: prediction of antigenic epitopes using support vector regression and multiple server results. BMC Bioinformatics 11:381
14. Salvat R, Moise L, Bailey-Kellogg C et al (2014) A high throughput MHC II binding assay for quantitative analysis of peptide epitopes. J Vis Exp (85), e51308, doi:10.3791/51308
15. Lin J, Sampson HA (2009) The role of immunoglobulin E-binding epitopes in the characterization of food allergy. Curr Opin Allergy Clin Immunol 9(4):357–363

Part I

Food Allergen Purification and Production

Chapter 2

Allergen Extraction and Purification from Natural Products: Main Chromatographic Techniques

Barbara Cases, Carlos Pastor-Vargas, and Marina Perez-Gordo

Abstract

The development of techniques and methods for allergen purification is essential for diagnosis and the development of safe immunotherapeutic agents. The most common purification techniques include chromatographic methodologies. In this chapter, we review and describe the details of the methodologies of using ion-exchange, gel-filtration, and affinity chromatography to purify two well-known panallergens, profilin and parvalbumin.

Key words Allergy, Allergen extraction, Allergen purification, Chromatography, Chromatographic techniques, Profilin, Parvalbumin

1 Introduction

Allergy is becoming a serious health problem [1]. The improvement of allergy prevention and therapy depends mainly on the reliability of the diagnosis. The development of techniques and methods for allergen purification is an essential requisite for many of the advancements made in allergy diagnosis. For this reason, the extraction and purification of allergens for diagnostic and therapeutic purposes is an expanding field [2].

Allergen extracts are prepared from different source materials such as food, pollens, dander animal, arthropods, fungi, or dusts. The composition of allergen extracts can vary depending on the source, processing, and storage conditions. Allergen extracts are a heterogeneous mixture of proteins, glycoproteins, carbohydrates, nucleic acids, lipids, and other substances. From this complex sample, the allergens must be purified to be used for diagnostic purposes. Different methods have been described to achieve higher allergen yields and a removal of host contaminants, such as lipids, nucleic acids, polyphenols, and polysaccharides [3]. However, a standard protocol for allergen purification from any source is not available.

Jing Lin and Marcos Alcocer (eds.), *Food Allergens: Methods and Protocols*, Methods in Molecular Biology, vol. 1592, DOI 10.1007/978-1-4939-6925-8_2, © Springer Science+Business Media LLC 2017

The most common purification techniques undoubtedly include chromatographic techniques [4]. The main chromatographic techniques utilize the intrinsic properties of allergens to separate from other extract components. The different types of chromatography include [5]:

- **Ion-exchange chromatography**: based on the reversible adsorption of charged solute molecules to immobilized ion-exchange groups of opposite charge. Ion-exchange chromatography includes Anion-exchange chromatography and Cation-exchange chromatography.
- **Gel-filtration chromatography or size-exclusion chromatography**: based on the possibility of parting molecules in solution on the basis of their size as they pass through a column packed with a gel.
- **Hydrophobic Interaction and Reversed-Phase Chromatography**: These techniques separate biomolecules according to differences in their hydrophobicity.
- **Affinity chromatography**: separates proteins on the basis of a reversible interaction between a protein (or group of proteins) and a specific ligand coupled to a chromatography matrix.

In this chapter, we review and describe the methodologies of using ion-exchange, gel-filtration, and affinity chromatography to purify profilin and parvalbumin, two well-known panallergens (proteins ubiquitous in nature, that share highly conserved sequence regions, structure, and function and responsible for many IgE cross-reactions between unrelated allergen sources) [6, 7].

2 Materials

Prepare all solutions using ultrapure water (prepared by purifying deionized water to attain a sensitivity of 18 MΩ cm at 25 °C). Store all reagents at 4 °C. To prevent clogging, always filter the sample through a 0.45 μm filter prior to loading the columns.

2.1 Chromatography Columns and Buffers

2.1.1 HiPrep Q XL 16/10 (GE Healthcare): Anionic-Exchange Column

1. Binding buffer: 50 mM Tris–HCl, pH 8.8. Weigh 6.05 g Tris-HCl and transfer to a 1 L cylinder. Add 900 mL of water, mix and adjust pH with HCl (6 N). Make up to 1 L with water. Store at 4 °C.
2. Elution buffer: Elution is achieved with 2 M NaCl. To prepare 1 M solution, weigh 116.88 g of NaCl in 1 L of water.

2.1.2 HiPrep DEAE FF 16/10 (GE Healthcare): Anionic-Exchange Column

1. Binding buffer: 50 mM Tris–HCl, pH 7.4. Weigh 6.05 g Tris and transfer to a 1 L cylinder. Add 900 mL of water, mix and adjust pH with HCl (6 N). Make up to 1 L with water. Store at 4 °C.

2. Elution buffer: Elution is achieved with a linear gradient from 0 to 1 M NaCl. To prepare 1 M solution, weigh 58.44 g of NaCl in 1 L of water.

2.1.3 Superdex 75 10/300 (GE Healthcare): Size-Exclusion Column

1. Equilibration Buffer: Buffered-phosphate saline (PBS), pH 7.9. Weigh 2.39 g NaH_2PO_4 (20 mM), 2.84 g NaH_2PO_4 (20 mM) and 8.76 g NaCl (150 mM) and transfer to a 1 L cylinder, add 900 mL of water, mix and adjust to a pH required with a 6 N HCl solution. Make up to 1 L with water. Store at 4 °C.

2.1.4 Mono-Q 5/50 GL (GE Healthcare): Anionic-Exchange Column

For Profilin Purification

1. Binding buffer: 20 mM Tris–HCl, pH 7.9. Weigh 2.42 g Tris and transfer to a 1 L cylinder. Add 900 mL of water, mix and adjust pH with HCl (6 N). Make up to 1 L with water. Store at 4 °C.
2. Elution buffer: Elution is achieved with a linear gradient from 0 to 0.5 M NaCl. To prepare 0.5 M solution NaCl, weigh 29.22 g of NaCl in 1 L of water.

For Parvalbumin Purification

3. Binding buffer: 10 mM Tris–HCl, pH 7.5. Tris 10 mM, pH 7.5. Weigh 1.21 g Tris and transfer to a 1 L cylinder. Add 900 mL of water, mix and adjust pH with HCl (6 N). Make up to 1 L with water. Store at 4 °C.
4. Elusion buffer: Elution is achieved with a linear gradient from 0 to 1 M NaCl. To prepare 1 M solution, weigh 58.44 g of NaCl in 1 L of water.

2.1.5 Sepharose Poly-Proline: Affinity Chromatography Column

1. Binding buffer (Buffer A): 100 mM KCl, 100 mM Gly, 10 mM Tris–HCl, 0.5 mM dithiothreitol (DTT); pH 7.8. Weigh 7.45 g KCl, 7.5 g Gly, 1.21 g Tris, and 77 mg 0.5 DTT. Transfer to a 1 L cylinder, add 900 mL of water, and adjust pH with HCl (6 N). Make up to 1 L with water. Store at 4 °C.
2. Elution buffer (Buffer B): 100 mM KCl, 100 mM Gly, 10 mM Tris–HCl, 0.5 mM dithiothreitol (DTT), 3 M urea; pH 7.8. Weigh 7.45 g KCl, 7.5 g Gly, 1.21 g Tris, 77 mg 0.5 DTT, and 180.18 g urea. Transfer to a 1 L cylinder, add 900 mL of water, and adjust pH with HCl (6 N). Make up to 1 L with water. Store at 4 °C.
3. Elution buffer (Buffer C): 100 mM KCl, 100 mM Gly, 10 mM Tris–HCl, 0.5 mM dithiothreitol (DTT), 8 M urea; pH 7.8. Weigh 7.45 g KCl, 7.5 g Gly, 1.21 g Tris, 77 mg 0.5 DTT, and 480.48 g urea. Transfer to a 1 L cylinder, add 900 mL of water, and adjust pH with HCl (6 N). Make up to 1 L with water. Store at 4 °C.

2.2 Other Buffers and Components

1. 0.1 M ammonium bicarbonate buffer. Weigh 0.79 g ammonium bicarbonate and transfer to a 1 L cylinder, add make up to 1 L with water. Rinse the dialysis membrane (Spectra/Por 6 RC Dialysis Membranes, 32 mm wide, Spectrum Chemical Corp) into deionized water for 10 min. Store at 4 °C (*see* **Note 1**).
2. Affinity chromatography activation buffer: 0.1 M $NaHCO_3$, pH 8.3 buffer with 0.5 M NaCl. Weigh 0.84 g $NaHCO_3$, and transfer to a 1 L cylinder, add 900 mL of water and adjust pH with HCl (6 N). Make up to 1 L with water. Store at 4 °C. Affinity chromatography blocking buffer: 1 M Tris–HCl, pH 8. Weigh 121.14 g Tris, and transfer to a 1 L cylinder, add 900 mL of water and adjust pH with HCl (6 N). Make up to 1 L with water. Store at 4 °C.
3. Amicon stirred cell system (Millipore) (*see* **Note 2**).

2.3 Components for Watermelon Extract Preparation

1. Extraction buffer: 10 mM K_2HPO_4 pH 7, 2% (p/v) PVPP (Polyvinyl poly-pyrrolidone) and 2 mM EDTA (Ethylene diamine tetra acetic acid) buffer. Weigh 1.74 g K_2HPO_4 and transfer to a 1 L cylinder, add 500 mL of water weigh 20 g PVPP and 5.84 g EDTA and adjust pH with HCl (6 N). Make up to 1 L with water (*see* **Note 3**).
2. Cellulose acetate 0.22 μm pore filter (Corning, New York).

2.4 Components for Fish Extract Preparation

1. Extraction buffer: Phosphate-buffered saline (PBS), pH 7.2 with 1 mM PMSF (phenylmethylsulfonyl fluoride). To prepare 100 mM of PMSF weigh 17.4 mg of PMSF per milliliter of isopropanol and store at −20 °C. Add 10% volume of 100 mM PMSF to PBS pH 7.2 buffer.
2. Delipidation buffer: Diethyl ether 98% (Sigma) (*see* **Note 4**).

3 Methods

3.1 Production of the Watermelon Extracts

1. Homogenize watermelon pulp in extraction buffer 1/20 (w/v).
2. Extract proteins overnight (12 h), at 4 °C under magnetic stirring.
3. Centrifuge at 15,000 × *g* at 4 °C for 30 min.
4. Discard the pellet, consisting of non-soluble material, and clarify supernatant by filtration through a cellulose acetate 0.22 μm pore filter.

3.2 Pre-purification

In order to enrich the protein content in the extract, carbohydrates are removed using an anionic-exchange chromatography column HiPrep Q XL 16/10 (GE Healthcare):

1. Dialyze the watermelon extract against Tris–HCl 50 mM, pH 8.8 buffer.
2. Load the column with 200 mL of watermelon extract.
3. Wash the column with three volumes of binding buffer.
4. Elute with 2 M NaCl in binding buffer in ten column volumes (200 mL).
5. Restore column conditions following the instructions provided by the manufacturer.
6. Concentrate the eluted fraction using the Amicon system (Millipore) and cellulose membranes.
7. Dialyze against 0.1 M ammonium bicarbonate, adjust protein concentration to 1 mg/mL and freeze dry for storage.

3.3 Isolation of Native Profilin

We present two chromatographic methods to isolate watermelon profilin as described before [8].

After each chromatographic step, eluted fractions should be dialyzed against 0.1 M ammonium bicarbonate and freeze dried for storage if necessary.

3.3.1 Conventional Chromatography-Based Method

This method is based on conventional chromatography using a FPLC AKTA Purifier (GE Healthcare).

HiPrep DEAE FF 16/10

1. Dialyze the watermelon extract, previously prepurified by the HiPrep Q XL 16/10 (GE Healthcare), against 50 mM Tris–HCl 50 mM, pH 7 (binding buffer).
2. Load 25 mL of watermelon extract in the chromatography column.
3. Wash the column with three column volumes of binding buffer (60 mL).
4. Elute with a linear gradient from 0 to 1 M NaCl in binding buffer in 15 column volumes (300 mL). Fraction with profilin, together with other proteins, should elute in the range of 40–170 mM NaCl.
5. Dialyze the fraction (or fractions) of interest against ammonium bicarbonate and freeze dry.
6. Restore column conditions following the instructions provided by the manufacturer.

Superdex 75 10/300

1. Resuspend the sample in 100 μL of PBS and filter through a 0.22 μm filter.
2. Inject the sample onto the Superdex 75 10/300 chromatography column.

3. Wash with PBS and collect the fraction containing the profilin. This should appear approximately after 12–14 mL.
4. Dialyze the fractions of interest against 0.1 M ammonium bicarbonate.
5. Restore column conditions following the instructions provided by the manufacturer.

Mono-Q 5/50 GL

1. Dialyze the fractions collected in the previous step against 20 mM Tris–HCl pH 7.9.
2. Inject the sample onto the Mono-Q 5/50 GL chromatography column (*see* **Note 5**).
3. Wash the column with five volumes of binding buffer (5 mL) at a flow rate of 2 mL/min.
4. Elute with a linear gradient from 0 to 0.5 M NaCl in binding buffer in 15 column volumes (15 mL). Fraction containing purified profilin should be eluted approximately at 60 mM NaCl.
5. Dialyze against 0.1 M ammonium bicarbonate and freeze dry.
6. Restore column conditions following the instructions provided by the manufacturer.

3.3.2 Affinity Chromatography-Based Method

This method is based on affinity chromatography using a non-commercial Poly-L-Proline coupled to a Sepharose 4B (GE Healthcare) column.

Column Preparation

Use a glass column of 1 cm diameter and 25 cm height (column volume: 19.7 mL) to package the slurry (*see* **Note 6**).

1. Weigh 6 g Sepharose 4B (GE Healthcare)
2. To activate the Sepharose 4B (GE Healthcare), wash with 1 mM HCl (1/200 w/v) using a glass funnel fitted with Whatman filter.
3. Add 0.5% Poly-proline ligand in activation buffer: weigh 100 mg Poly-proline and resuspend in 20 mL of activation buffer.
4. Incubate the activated Sepharose 4B with the Poly-proline in activation buffer overnight at 4 °C under magnetic stirring conditions.
5. Centrifuge 5 min at 14,000 × *g* and discard supernatant containing the excess of Poly-Proline.
6. Wash with three column volumes (60 mL) of blocking buffer to avoid unspecific binding to the reactive groups, 2 h at 4 °C under magnetic stirring conditions.
7. Centrifuge 1 min at 14,000 × *g* and discard supernatant.

8. Perform three consecutive washes of 30 min each with five column volumes of alternative pH buffer, using 0.1 M acetic acid pH 4 and the binding buffer (*see* **Note 7**).
9. Mount the packaging reservoir with end piece and rinse with water.
10. Mount the column in the packaging reservoir vertically and pour the slurry taking care of no air bubbles are trapped and close with a top closing piece connected to a peristaltic pump.
11. After slurry packaging, load 500 μL of human serum, wash with five column volumes of buffer A (100 mL) and elute with buffer B, followed by buffer C (five column volumes each).
12. Equilibrate column in buffer A by washing with five column volumes (100 mL) of buffer A.

Profilin Purification

1. Dialyze the watermelon extract against buffer A.
2. Load 25 mL of the extract into the column.
3. Wash with three column volumes of buffer A (60 mL) to wash off the excess of proteins that do not bind to the poly-proline residues.
4. Elute with three column volumes (60 mL) of buffer B to elute the actin-profilin complexes.
5. Elute with three column volumes (60 mL) of buffer C to elute purified profilins.
6. Dialyze the fractions of interest against 0.1 M ammonium bicarbonate.

3.4 Preparation of Fish Extracts

1. 30 g of cooked muscle filets (100 °C for 30 min) is extracted in 10% (w/v) of PBS, pH 7.2, with 1mM PMSF at 4 °C undergoing constant stirring for 24 h (*see* **Note 3**).
2. After centrifugation at 12,000 × *g* for 30 min at 4 °C, lipids from supernatants are extracted using diethyl ether 98% (delipidation buffer) (*see* **Note 4**).
3. The delipidated extract is dialyzed against 0.1 M ammonium bicarbonate.
4. Protein extracts are lyophilized and stored at 4 °C.

3.5 Purification of Parvalbumins

Purification protocol is based on the protocol described by Bugajska-Schretter et al. [9] with some modifications [10].

1. The parvalbumin-enriched fraction was redissolved in Tris 10 mM, pH 7.5.
2. Inject the sample onto the Mono-Q 5/50 GL chromatography column (*see* **Note 5**).
3. Wash the column with five volumes of binding buffer (5 mL) at a flow rate of 2 mL/min.

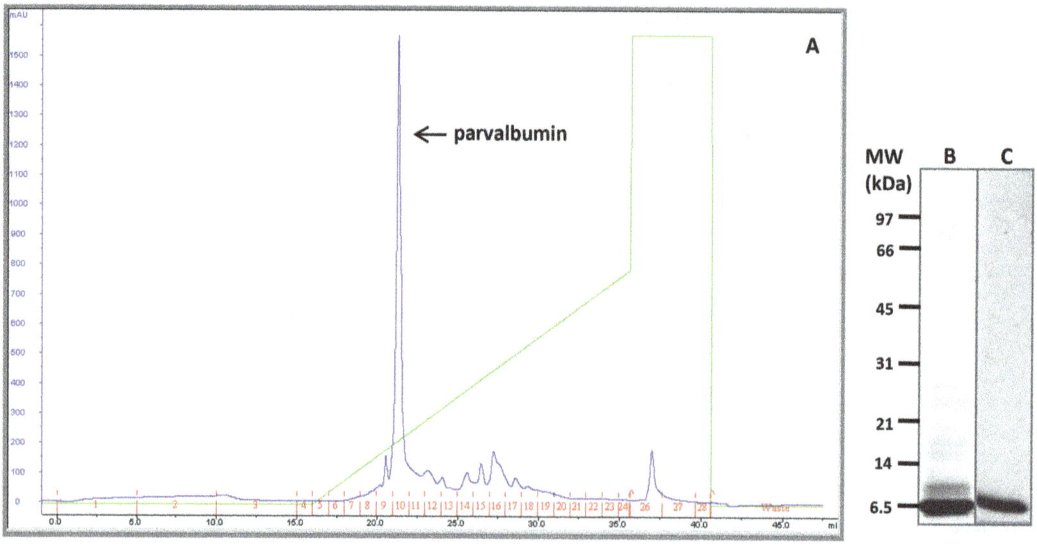

Fig. 1 Parvalbumin purification from whiff complete fish extract. (**a**) MonoQ 5/50 GL chromatogram showing A_{280nm} (*dark blue*) and elution buffer (*green*). (**b**) SDS-PAGE (14%) of eluted fraction. (**c**) Immunodetection obtained by incubation with sera from fish allergic patients

4. Elute with a linear salt gradient from 0 to 1 M NaCl in binding buffer in 15 column volumes (15 mL). Fraction containing purified parvalbumin should be eluted approximately at 140 mM NaCl (*see* Fig. 1).
5. Dialyze against 0.1 M ammonium bicarbonate and freeze dry.
6. Restore column conditions following the instructions provided by the manufacturer.

3.6 Purity and Reactivity Confirmation Tests

To confirm purity, fractions obtained after chromatography will be run in 14% Sodium Dodecyl Sulfate Polyacrylamide Gel Electrophoresis (SDS-PAGE) as described elsewhere [13] and analyzed by mass spectrometry (MS). To confirm allergenic potential, immunodetection analysis must be performed using allergic serum pool [10].

Fractions containing more than 90% of purified protein can be used for further experiments. An example of these studies performed with purified parvalbumin is given in Fig. 1.

4 Notes

1. Attach one end of the membrane with the tubing closure provided by the kit and add the extract with a pipette. Attach the other end and put the membrane into the cylinder with a magnetic stir bar. Keep it O/N in constant stirring at 4 °C. Change the dialysis buffer twice for three days.

2. This system allows rapid concentration without the need of purification by applying nitrogen gas pressure (not exceeding a pressure limit of 75 psi). The cut-off will determine the solutes to be retained in the cell or be passing through the pore of the membrane. In this case a 3 kDa cellulose membrane was selected, to eliminate salts and water. Fill the cell with the extract to concentrate, after pressurization, put the system in a magnetic stirring table and concentrate up to the desirable volume.
3. The use of the water-insoluble PVPP is for the removal of phenolic compounds present in vegetable tissues that could interact with proteins [10, 12]. EDTA is a chelating agent frequently used as a protease inhibitor in protein extraction buffers [11].
4. Delipidation technique consists of forming a biphasic system by adding diethyl ether to the extracted fish extracts. 100 mL of extract is shaken vigorously with 50 mL of diethyl ether. After 5 min the lower layer is removed and mixed with another 50 mL of diethyl ether per each 100 mL. This cycle is repeated two times more.
5. Manufacturer recommends loading up to 45 mg.
6. To determine the volume of a packaging reservoir apply the formula:

$$\text{Volume} = \pi \times \text{reservoir height} \times \text{radius}^2$$

7. To change from one buffer to the other, centrifuge a few second at 15,000 × g and discard supernatant. Then add the new buffer.

Acknowledgement

This work was supported by grants from the Instituto de Salud Carlos III (PI 13/00477, PI 13/00928), co-supported by FONDOS FEDER and the Institute of Applied Molecular Medicine of CEU San Pablo University of Madrid.

References

1. Platts-Mills TA (2015) The allergy epidemics: 1870-2010. J Allergy Clin Immunol 136(1): 3–13
2. Sastre J (2013) Molecular diagnosis and immunotherapy. Curr Opin Allergy Clin Immunol 13(6):646–650
3. Pastorello EA, Trambaioli C (2001) Isolation of food allergens. J Chromatogr B Biomed Sci Appl 756(1–2):71–84
4. Huang JX, Guiochon G (1989) Applications of preparative high-performance liquid chromatography to the separation and purification of peptides and proteins. J Chromatogr 492:431–469
5. Richard RB, Murray PD (2009) Guide to protein purification. Methods Enzymol. doi:10.1016/S0076-6879(09)63049-4
6. Breiteneder H, Radauer C (2004) A classification of plant food allergens. J Allergy Clin Immunol 113(5):821–830
7. Van Do T, Elsayed S, Florvaag E, Hordvik I, Endersen C (2005) Allergy to fish parvalbumins: studies on the cross-reactivity of allergens from 9 commonly consumed fish. J Allergy Clin Immunol 116(6):1314–1320
8. Pastor C, Cuesta-Herranz J, Cases B, Pérez-Gordo M, Figueredo E, de las Heras M,

Vivanco F (2009) Identification of major allergens in watermelon. Int Arch Allergy Immunol 149(4):291–298

9. Bugajska-Schretter A, Grote M, Vangelista L, Valent P, Sperr WR, Rumpold H et al (2000) Purification, biochemical and immunological characterisation of a major food allergen: different immunoglobulin E recognition of the apo- and calcium-bound forms of carp parvalbumin. Gut 46(5):661–669
10. Perez-Gordo M, Cuesta-Herranz J, Maroto AS, Cases B, Ibáñez MD, Vivanco F, Pastor-Vargas C (2011) Identification of sole parvalbumin as a major allergen: study of cross-reactivity between parvalbumin in a Spanish fish-allergic population. Clin Exp Allergy 41(5):750–758
11. Landa-Pineda CM, Guidos-Fogelbach G, Marchat-Marchau L et al (2013) Profilins: allergens with clinical relevance. Rev Alerg Mex 60(3):129–143
12. Kondratiuk AS, Savchuk OM, Hur JS (2015) Optimization of protein extraction for lichen thalli. Mycobiology 43(2):157–162
13. Laemmli UK (1970) Cleavage of structural proteins during the assembly of the head of bacteriophage T4. Nature 227(5259):680–685

Chapter 3

Recombinant Allergen Production in *E. coli*

Changqi Liu, LeAnna N. Willison, and Shridhar K. Sathe

Abstract

Recombinant protein allergens have been used in allergy studies, allergy diagnosis, and epitope mapping. Messenger RNAs (mRNAs) are isolated from tissues of interest for complementary DNA (cDNA) library construction. Subsequently, the allergen gene is amplified by polymerase chain reaction (PCR) and sequenced. The amplified gene is then cloned into an expression vector, expressed in *Escherichia coli* cells, and purified from the cell lysate. This chapter describes the protocols for recombinant allergen production.

Key words Allergy, Food allergen, Recombinant allergen

1 Introduction

Type I food allergies are induced by food proteins (allergens) through cross-linking immunoglobulin E (IgE) molecules on the surface of mast cells and basophils [1]. Approximately 400 proteins in >170 foods have been reported to cause type I allergic reactions [2]. In the US, milk, eggs, fish, Crustacean shellfish, tree nuts, peanuts, wheat, and soybean are the most common offending foods, accounting for over 90% of food allergies [3]. Considerable research has been conducted to identify and characterize the specific allergens in these foods. Although native allergens are the optimum choice for analysis, they are difficult to isolate and their properties may vary between samples due to presence of multiple isoforms, cultivar variations, different developmental stages, and environmental influences. Alternatively, molecular cloning techniques are useful in producing large quantities of molecularly defined homogenous allergens of consistent purity and quality. Therefore, recombinant allergens have been widely used in food allergy diagnosis, assessing cross-reactivity, epitope mapping, and analyzing the effects of food matrix, food processing, and digestion on allergen immunoreactivity [4]. A comparison between the immunoreactivity of native and recombinant almond major allergen amandin is illustrated in Fig. 1. Detailed information on

Jing Lin and Marcos Alcocer (eds.), *Food Allergens: Methods and Protocols*, Methods in Molecular Biology, vol. 1592,
DOI 10.1007/978-1-4939-6925-8_3, © Springer Science+Business Media LLC 2017

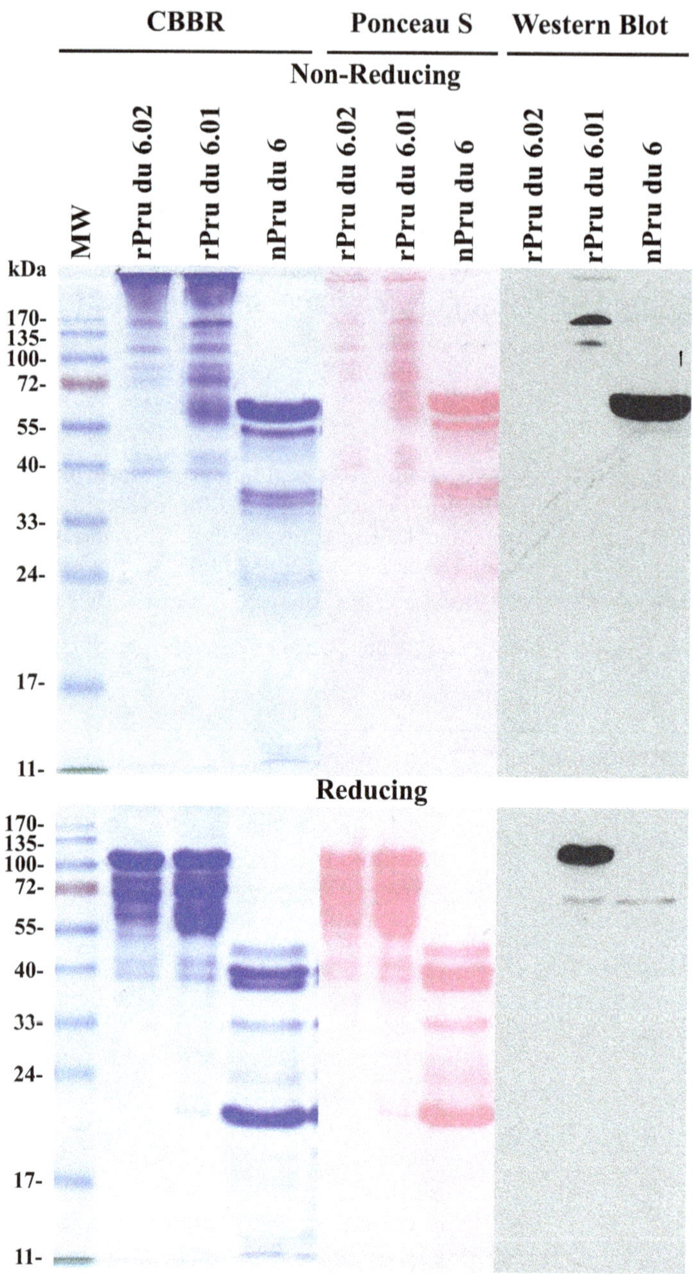

Fig. 1 Comparison of the native and recombinant almond major allergen amandin (Pru du 6). Proteins on polyacrylamide gel and nitrocellulose membrane were stained by Coomassie Brilliant Blue R (CBBR) and Ponceau S, respectively. Immunoreactive polypeptides were recognized by murine anti-amandin monoclonal antibody 4C10 in Western blot. MW: molecular weight standards; rPru du 6.01: recombinant Pru du 6.01-maltose binding protein (MBP) fusion protein; rPru du 6.02: recombinant Pru du 6.02-MBP fusion protein; nPru du 6: native amandin purified by column chromatography

production of recombinant food allergens is available in references [5, 6] and specific kit manuals. Protocols we used to produce recombinant allergens of almond [7, 8], cashew [9–11], pecan [12, 13], and pistachio [14] are described in this chapter.

2 Materials

2.1 RNA Extraction Reagents

1. Liquid nitrogen.
2. Denaturing solution (solution D): 4 M guanidinium thiocyanate, 25 mM sodium citrate, pH 7.0, 0.5% (w/v) *N*-lauroylsarcosine (Sarkosyl), and 0.1 M β-mercaptoethanol. Prepare stock solution by dissolving 250 g guanidinium thiocyanate in 293 mL deionized water at 65 °C, then adding 17.6 mL 0.75 M sodium citrate (pH 7.0) and 26.4 mL 10% (w/v) Sarkosyl. Prepare working solution by adding 0.36 mL 98% β-mercaptoethanol to 50 mL stock solution. The stock and working solutions can be stored at room temperature (RT, 25 °C) for 3 and 1 months, respectively. Solution D is also commercially available as TRIzol (Thermo Fisher Scientific) and TRI reagents (Sigma-Aldrich).
3. Diethylpyrocarbonate (DEPC)-treated water: Add 0.2 mL DEPC to 100 mL deionized water and shake vigorously. Autoclave the solution to inactivate DEPC. DEPC is used to inactivate RNase and prevent RNA degradation. DEPC-treated water should always be used when handling RNA.
4. Sodium acetate buffer (2 M, pH 4.0): Add 16.42 g anhydrous sodium acetate to 40 mL deionized water and 35 mL glacial acetic acid. Adjust to pH 4.0 with glacial acetic acid and bring the final volume to 100 mL with DEPC-treated water. Store up to 1 year at RT.
5. Water-saturated phenol: Dissolve 100 g phenol crystals in deionized water at 65 °C. Aspire the upper water phase and store at 4 °C for 1 month.
6. Chloroform:isoamyl alcohol (49:1, v/v).
7. Isopropanol.
8. Ethanol (75%, v/v): Add 75 mL absolute ethanol to 25 mL DEPC-treated water.

2.2 mRNA Isolation Reagents

PolyATtract mRNA isolation kit (Promega Corporation). This kit includes biotinylated Oligo(dT) probe solution (50 pmol/μL), saline-sodium citrate (SSC) buffer 20× concentrate, streptavidin MagneSphere paramagnetic particles (SA-PMPs), nuclease-free water, mRNA user tubes, and a MagneSphere magnetic separation stand.

2.3 cDNA Production Reagents

ZAP Express cDNA Gigapack III Gold cloning kit (Agilent Technologies). This kit includes ZAP Express vector, pBR322 test insert, XL1-Blue MRF' strain, Gigapack III Gold packaging extract, VCS257 host strain, AccuScript reverse transcriptase (AccuScript RT), RNase block ribonuclease inhibitor, first-strand methyl nucleotide mixture, 10× first-strand buffer, linker-primer, test mRNA, DEPC-treated water, 10× second-strand buffer, second-strand dNTP mixture, *E. coli* RNase H, *E. coli* DNA polymerase, 3 M sodium acetate, blunting dNTP mixture, cloned *Pfu* DNA polymerase, *Eco*R I adapters, 10× ligase buffer, 10 mM rATP, T4 DNA ligase, T4 polynucleotide kinase, *Xho* I, *Xho* I buffer, Sepharose CL-2B gel filtration medium, column-loading dye, and STE buffer (10×). Additional reagents and media required include:

1. SM buffer: Add 5.8 g NaCl, 2.0 g $MgSO_4{\bullet}7H_2O$, and 5.0 mL 2% (w/v) gelatin to 50 mL 1 M Tris–HCl (pH 7.5), add deionized water to a final volume of 1 L.
2. 20× SSC buffer: Add 175.3 g NaCl and 88.2 g sodium citrate to 800 mL deionized water, adjust pH to 7.0, add deionized water to a final volume of 1 L.
3. LB broth: Add 10 g NaCl, 10 g tryptone, and 5 g yeast extract to 800 mL deionized water, adjust pH to 7.0, add deionized water to a final volume of 1 L. Autoclave the broth.
4. LB agar: Add 10 g NaCl, 10 g tryptone, 5 g yeast extract, and 20 g agar to 800 mL deionized water, adjust pH to 7.0, add deionized water to a final volume of 1 L. Autoclave and pour into petri dishes. Let solidify at RT, then store at 4 °C until use.
5. LB broth with supplements: Add 10 mL 1 M $MgSO_4$, 3 mL 2 M maltose solution in 1 L of LB broth. Store at 4 °C until use.
6. NZY agar: Add 5 g NaCl, 2 g $MgSO_4{\bullet}7H_2O$, 5 g yeast extract, 10 g NZ amine, and 15 g agar to 800 mL deionized water, adjust pH to 7.5, add deionized water to a final volume of 1 L. Autoclave and pour into petri dishes. Let solidify at RT, then store at 4 °C until use.
7. NYZ broth: Add 5 g NaCl, 2 g $MgSO_4{\bullet}7H_2O$, 5 g yeast extract, and 10 g NZ amine to 800 mL deionized water, adjust pH to 7.5, add deionized water to a final volume of 1 L. Autoclave, allow to cool, and store at 4 °C until use.
8. NYZ top agar: Add 0.7% (w/v) agarose to 1 L NZY broth. Autoclave and store at 4 °C until use.
   See **Note 1** concerning media storage.

2.4 Rapid Amplification of cDNA Ends (RACE) Reagents

SMARTer RACE cDNA Amplification kit (Clontech Laboratories). This kit includes SMARTer II A oligonucleotide (oligo), 3′ and 5′ RACE CDS Primer A, 5× first-strand buffer (250 mM Tris–HCl, 375 mM KCl, 30 mM $MgCl_2$, pH 8.3), 20 mM dithiothreitol

(DTT), deionized water, RNase inhibitor, SMARTScribe reverse transcriptase, 10× universal primer A mix, dNTP mix, and Tricine EDTA buffer (10 mM Tricine-KOH, 1.0 mM EDTA, pH 8.5). Prepare enough of the following reagents:

1. Buffer Mix (for each 10 μL cDNA synthesis reaction): Mix 2.0 μL 5× first-strand buffer, 1.0 μL 20 mM DTT, and 1.0 μL 10 mM dNTP mix.
2. Master Mix (for each 10 μL cDNA synthesis reaction): Mix 4.0 μL Buffer Mix, 0.2 μL RNase inhibitor, and 1.0 μL SMARTScribe reverse transcriptase.
3. RACE Mix (for each 50 μL PCR reaction): Mix 34.5 μL PCR-grade water, 5.0 μL 10× Advantage 2 PCR buffer, 1.0 μL dNTP mix, and 1.0 μL 50× Advantage 2 polymerase mix.

2.5 TA Cloning Reagent

TOPO TA Cloning Kit (Invitrogen). This kit includes: pCR 2.1-TOPO vector (10 ng/μL plasmid DNA in 50% glycerol, 50 mM Tris–HCl, pH 7.4, 1 mM EDTA, 1 mM DTT, 0.1% Triton X-100, 100 μg/mL BSA, phenol red), salt solution (1.2 M NaCl, 0.06 M $MgCl_2$), and One Shot competent cells.

2.6 pMAL Protein Fusion and Purification Reagent

pMAL Protein Fusion and Purification System (New England BioLabs). This kit includes: pMAL-c5X vector, amylose resin, Factor Xa, anti-maltose binding protein (MBP) monoclonal antibody, MBP5 protein, and NEB Express *E. coli* ER2523. Additional solutions and media are required:

1. Rich medium: 10 g tryptone, 5 g yeast extract, 5 g NaCl, 2 g glucose in 1 L, autoclave and add sterile ampicillin to 100 μg/mL.
2. Isopropyl β-D-1-thiogalactopyranoside (IPTG, 0.1 M) stock: 1.19 g IPTG, add deionized water to 50 mL, filter sterilize, store at −20 °C.
3. Column buffer: 20 mM Tris–HCl, 200 mM NaCl, 1 mM EDTA, 1 mM sodium azide, 10 mM β-mercaptoethanol, pH 7.4.
4. Sodium phosphate buffer: 20 mM sodium phosphate, 25 mM NaCl, pH 5.5.
5. Elution buffer (10 mM maltose): dissolve 0.0342 g maltose in 10 mL column buffer. Store at −20 °C until use.

3 Methods

An overall flow of the recombinant allergen production procedures is illustrated in Fig. 2.

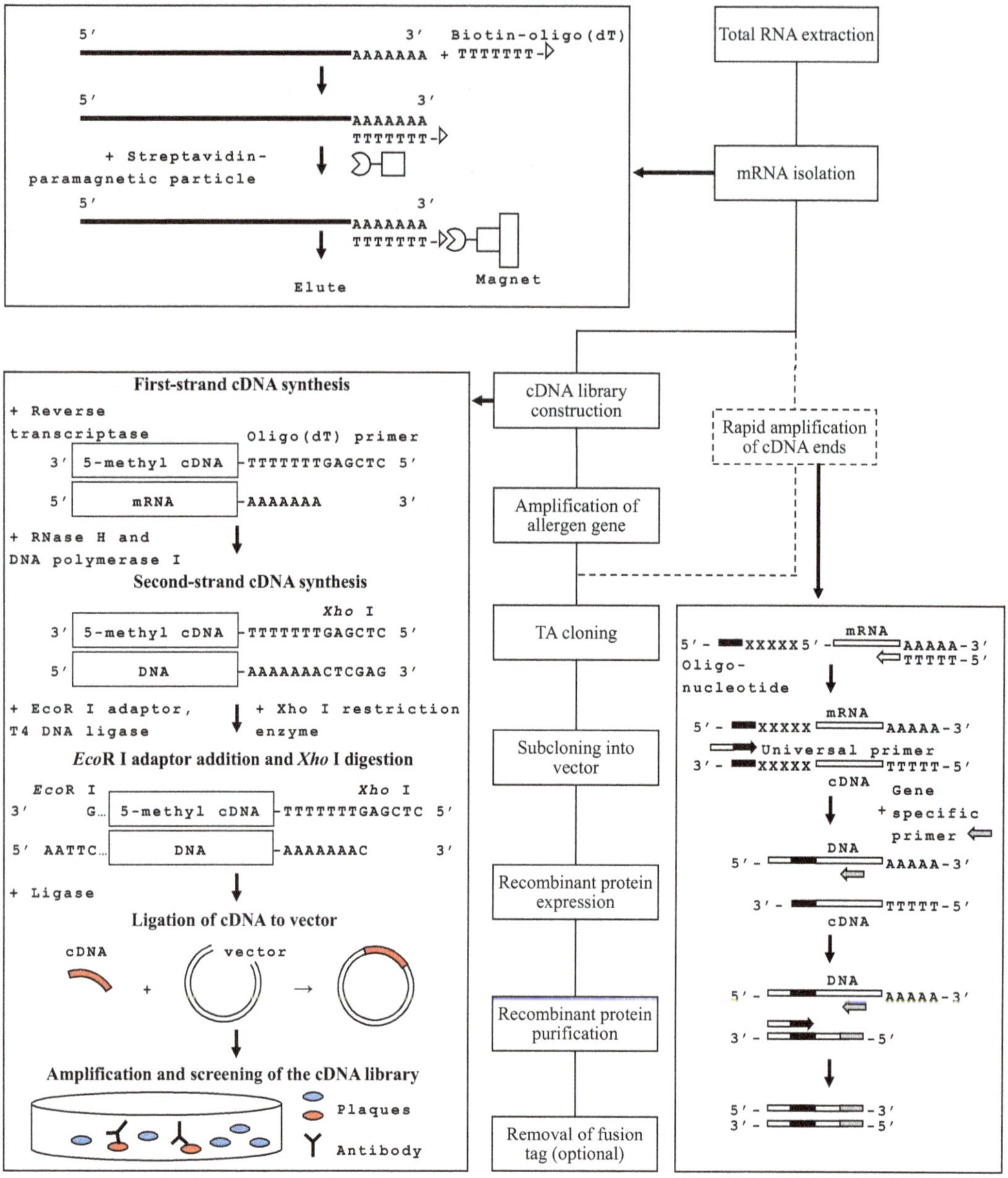

Fig. 2 Schematic diagram of the recombinant allergen production procedures

3.1 Tissue Collection

1. Collect tissues at various development stages to ensure the presence of the desired mRNA.
2. Proceed to Subheading 3.2 or freeze the tissues in liquid nitrogen immediately after harvest and store at −80 °C.

3.2 Total RNA Extraction

Extract total RNA as described by Chomczynski and Sacchi [15] or by using commercial total RNA extraction kit (e.g. Qiagen RNeasy kit).

1. Freeze the tissues in liquid nitrogen and grind to a fine powder with a mortar and pestle, add 1 mL solution D per 100 mg frozen tissue and mix well manually (*see* **Note 2**).
2. Transfer the tissue lysate to a polypropylene tube and add the following to 1 mL lysate in sequence: 0.1 mL 2 M sodium acetate, pH 4.0, mix thoroughly by inversion; 1 mL water-saturated phenol, mix thoroughly by inversion; 0.2 mL chloroform/isoamyl alcohol (49:1 v/v), shake vigorously by hand for 10 s.
3. Cool the samples on ice for 15 min followed by centrifugation at 10,000 × *g*, 4 °C for 20 min.
4. Transfer the upper aqueous phase containing RNA to a clean tube, add 1 mL isopropanol to precipitate RNA, and incubate the samples for at least 1 h at −20 °C.
5. Centrifuge at 10,000 × *g*, 4 °C for 20 min, and discard the supernatant.
6. Dissolve the RNA pellet in 0.3 mL solution D, transfer to a 1.5 mL microcentrifuge tube, add 0.3 mL isopropanol, and incubate at −20 °C for at least 30 min.
7. Centrifuge at 10,000 × *g*, 4 °C for 10 min, and discard the supernatant.
8. Resuspend the RNA pellet with 0.5–1 mL 75% ethanol and vortex for a few seconds.
9. Incubate samples at RT for 10–15 min, centrifuge at 10,000 × *g*, 4 °C for 5 min, and discard the supernatant.
10. Air-dry the RNA pellet at RT for 5–10 min (*see* **Note 3**), re-dissolve in 100–200 μL DEPC-treated water, and incubate at 60 °C for 10–15 min for complete solubilization.
11. The concentration of isolated RNA can be determined by measuring the absorbance at 260 nm (OD_{260}) in a spectrophotometer. An absorbance of 1 unit at 260 nm corresponds to 40 μg of RNA per mL ($OD_{260} = 1 = 40$ μg/mL). It is estimated that 1–5% of total RNA is mRNA [16].
12. Store the samples at −80 °C.

3.3 mRNA Isolation

mRNA is conventionally separated from total RNA using oligo(dT) cellulose gravity column that binds the poly(A) tail of the mRNA [17]. Faster and more convenient methods using oligo(dT) cellulose packed in spin columns or bound to magnetic particles are available (Thermo Fisher Scientific, New England BioLabs, ClonTech Laboratories, or Invitrogen). Detailed protocols for oligo(dT) cellulose packed gravity and spin column can be found in reference [18]. We describe here the recommended protocol for the PolyATtract mRNA isolation kit available from Promega (Fig. 2). This kit uses a biotinylated oligo (dT) primer to hybridize mRNA. The hybrids are captured and separated using streptavidin-coupled paramagnetic particles and a magnetic separation stand [19].

1. Transfer 1–5 mg total RNA to a sterile, RNase-free tube, add nuclease-free water to a final volume of 2.43 mL.
2. Heat at 65 °C for 10 min, add 10 μL biotinylated-oligo(dT) probe solution and 60 μL 20× SSC. Mix gently and cool to RT.
3. Resuspend the SA-PMPs by gently flicking the tube, then capture the particles by placing the tube in the magnetic stand until the particles are collected at the side of the tube.
4. Carefully remove the supernatant and wash the SA-PMPs three times with equal volume of 0.5× SSC (discard supernatant each time), then resuspend the washed SA-PMPs in 0.5 mL 0.5× SSC (*see* **Note 4**).
5. Add the entire contents of the **step 2** to the washed SA-PMPs, incubate for 10 min at RT, gently mix by inverting every 1–2 min.
6. Capture the SA-PMPs using the magnetic stand and carefully remove the supernatant.
7. Wash the SA-PMPs four times with 0.1× SSC by gently flicking the tube until all particles are resuspended. Remove as much supernatant as possible without disturbing the SA-PMPs.
8. Resuspend the final SA-PMP pellet in 1.0 mL nuclease-free water and gently flicking the tube to resuspend the particles.
9. Magnetically capture the SA-PMPs and transfer the eluted mRNA to a sterile, RNase-free tube (*see* **Note 5**).
10. The concentration and purity of eluted mRNA can be determined by spectrophotometry. Pure mRNA has an OD_{260}/OD_{280} absorbance ratio greater than or equal to 2.0.

3.4 cDNA Library Construction

Synthesis of cDNA can be accomplished by a number of different methods. For detailed information refer to protocols in [5]. cDNA production protocols for cDNA library construction (Subheading 3.4) and RACE (Subheading 3.5) are described below (Fig. 2). The protocol provided by ZAP Express cDNA Gigapack III Gold cloning kit (Agilent Technologies) is used to prepare cDNA library [20].

3.4.1 First-Strand cDNA Synthesis

1. Gently mix 5 μg mRNA isolated in Subheading 3.3 with 5 μL 10× first-strand buffer, 3 μL first-strand methyl nucleotide mixture, 2 μL linker-primer, and 1 μL RNase block ribonuclease inhibitor in a RNase-free microcentrifuge tube. Add DEPC-treated water to a final volume of 47 μL. Prepare a control mixture by replacing the isolated mRNA with the kit-provided mRNA.

2. Incubate at RT for 10 min then add 3 μL of AccuScript RT to synthesize the first-strand cDNA sample. Mix gently and spin down the contents.
3. Transfer 5 μL of the mixture to another tube containing 0.5 μL [α-^{32}P]dNTP as the first-strand synthesis control.
4. Incubate the first-strand cDNA sample and the first-strand control at 42 °C for 1 h.
5. Keep the first-strand cDNA sample on ice and freeze the first-strand control at −20 °C.

3.4.2 Second-Strand cDNA Synthesis

1. Add 20 μL 10× second-strand buffer, 6 μL second-strand dNTP mixture, 114 μL sterile deionized water, and 2 μL [α-^{32}P]dNTP to the first-strand cDNA sample.
2. Add 2 μL RNase H and 11 μL DNA polymerase I to start the second-strand cDNA synthesis.
3. Gently vortex and centrifuge (16,100 × *g*, RT) the mixture and incubate in a 16 °C water bath for 2.5 h (*see* **Note 6**), then immediately place the tube on ice.

3.4.3 Blunting the cDNA Termini

After synthesis, the frayed termini of the double-strand cDNA are repaired by the *Pfu* DNA polymerase.

1. Add 23 μL blunting dNTP mix and 2 μL *Pfu* DNA polymerase to the double-strand cDNA.
2. Quickly vortex and centrifuge (16,100 × *g*, RT) the mixture and incubate at 72 °C for exactly 30 min (do not exceed).
3. Add 200 μL phenol–chloroform, vortex and centrifuge at 16,100 × *g* for 2 min at RT. Transfer the upper aqueous layer containing the cDNA to a new tube.
4. Add equal volume of chloroform and repeat vortex mixing and centrifugation. Transfer the upper layer to a new tube.
5. Add 2 μL 3 M sodium acetate, 400 μL 100% (v/v) ethanol, vortex and precipitate the cDNA overnight at −20 °C.
6. Centrifuge at 16,100 × *g* for 60 min at 4 °C. Carefully remove the supernatant and discard in a radioactive waste container.
7. Gently wash the pellet with 500 μL 70% (v/v) ethanol. Do not mix or vortex.
8. Centrifuge at 16,100 × *g* for 2 min at RT, and dry the pellet by vacuum centrifugation.
9. Resuspend the pellet in 9 μL *Eco*R I adapters and incubate for 30 min at 4 °C. Transfer the cDNA to a new tube and ensure the cDNA is in solution.
10. Transfer 1 μL of the solution to a new tube as the second-strand control.

11. Run the first-strand and second-strand samples on an alkaline agarose gel to determine the cDNA size range and the secondary structures.

3.4.4 Addition of the EcoR I Adaptors

Addition of adaptors to the termini of the cDNAs is required to attach the generated cDNAs into the vector.

1. Add 1 μL 10× ligase buffer, 1 μL 10 mM rATP, and 1 μL T4 DNA ligase to the tube containing the blunted cDNA and the *Eco*R I adapters.
2. Centrifuge at 16,100 × *g* and incubate at 8 °C overnight.
3. Heat in a 70 °C water bath for 30 min to inactive the ligase.
4. Centrifuge at 16,100 × *g* for 2 s and cool at RT for 5 min.
5. Add 1 μL 10× ligase buffer, 2 μL 10 mM rATP, 5 μL sterile water, and 2 μL T4 polynucleotide kinase and incubate at 37 °C for 30 min to phosphorylate the adapter ends.
6. Inactivate the kinase by heating at 70 °C for 30 min.
7. Centrifuge at 16,100 × *g* for 2 s and cool to RT for 5 min.
8. Add 28 μL *Xho* I buffer and 3 μL *Xho* I to the reaction and incubate at 37 °C for 1.5 h.
9. Add 5 μL 10× STE buffer and 125 μL 100% (v/v) ethanol and precipitate the cDNA at −20 °C overnight.
10. Centrifuge at 16,100 × *g* for 60 min at 4 °C, discard the supernatant, dry the pellet and resuspend the pellet in 14 μL 1× STE buffer.
11. Add 3.5 μL column loading dye to each sample.

3.4.5 Fractionation of cDNA

Before insertion into the vector, cDNA is fractionated by gel filtration to remove excess adaptors and low molecular weight DNA.

1. Pack a sterile 1 mL pipette with a cotton plug at the narrow end with Sepharose CL-2B medium. Add the resin till the packed bed is 0.25 inch below the wide end of the pipette. Wash the column with at least 10 mL 1× STE buffer.
2. Gently load the cDNA sample using a pipettor and keep the column filled with 1× STE buffer.
3. Collect three drops per fraction in microcentrifuge tubes when the leading edge of the dye reaches the 0.4 mL gradation on the pipette. Stop fraction collection when the trailing edge of the dye reaches the 0.3 mL gradation or until all radioactive nucleotides are eluted.
4. Remove 8 μL sample from each fraction. Electrophorese the aliquots on a 5% non-denaturing acrylamide gel to assess the effectiveness of the fractionation and to determine which fractions to be used for ligation.

5. Adding an equal volume of phenol–chloroform (1:1, v/v) to the collected fractions. Vortex and centrifuge at 16,100 × *g* at RT for 2 min.
6. Collect the upper aqueous layer, add an equal volume of chloroform, vortex and centrifuge at 16,100 × *g* at RT for 2 min. Transfer the upper aqueous layer to a new microcentrifuge tube.
7. Add twice volume of 100% (v/v) ethanol and precipitate the cDNA at −20 °C overnight.
8. Centrifuge at 16,100 × *g* at 4 °C for 60 min. Discard the supernatant if the majority of radioactivity is present in the pellet. Otherwise repeat the centrifugation.
9. Carefully wash the pellet with 200 μL 80% (v/v) ethanol without vortex mixing. Centrifuge at 16,100 × *g* at RT for 2 min. Remove the ethanol and vacuum evaporate the pellet until dry (*see* **Note 7**).
10. Measure the counts per second (cps) of each fraction using a handheld Geiger counter. Resuspend each cDNA pellet in 3.5 μL (<30 cps) or 5 μL (>30 cps) sterile water and mix by pipetting up and down.
11. Quantify the cDNA using ethidium bromide plate assay.

3.4.6 Ligation of cDNA to the Vector

1. Prepare a control ligation by mixing 1 μL ZAP Express vector, 1.6 μL test insert, 0.5 μL 10× ligase buffer, 0.5 μL 10 mM rATP, and 0.9 μL deionized water.
2. Prepare the sample ligation by mixing 100 ng resuspended cDNA, 0.5 μL 10× ligase buffer, 0.5 μL 10 mM rATP, and 1 μL ZAP Express vector, then add deionized water to a final volume of 4.5 μL.
3. Add 0.5 μL T4 DNA ligase to the control and sample ligations, incubate at 12 °C overnight.
4. Remove Gigapack III Gold packaging extracts from −80 °C freezer and place on dry ice.
5. Add 1–4 μL experimental DNA (0.1–1 μg ligated DNA) to the packaging extract once it begins to thaw.
6. Gently mix with a pipette tip, centrifuge at 16,100 × *g* at RT for 3–5 s, and incubate at RT for 2 h (*see* **Note 8**).
7. Add 500 μL SM buffer, 20 μL chloroform and mix gently.
8. Centrifuge at 16,100 × *g* at RT for 3–5 s, collect the supernatant containing the phage, store at 4 °C.

3.4.7 cDNA Library Titration and Amplification

1. Streak the XL1-Blue MRF' and VCS257 cells onto LB agar plates containing appropriate antibiotic and incubate at 37 °C overnight.

2. Grow separate 50 mL cultures of XL1-Blue MRF' and VCS257 cells in LB broth with supplements at 37 °C for 4–6 h.
3. Centrifuge the cells at 1,000 × *g* for 10 min. Resuspend the cell pellet in 25 mL sterile 10 mM $MgSO_4$. Dilute the cell suspensions to an OD_{600} of 0.5 in 10 mM $MgSO_4$.
4. Add 1 μL lambda phage to 200 μL VCS257 cell suspension. Incubate at 37 °C for 15 min.
5. Add 2–3 mL melted NZY top agar cooled to ~48 °C, 15 μL 0.5 M IPTG, and 50 μL 250 mg/mL X-gal in dimethylformamide.
6. Plate immediately onto NZY agar plates, set for 10 min, invert, and incubate at 37 °C overnight.
7. Count the number of plaques and determine the titer using the following formula:

$$\frac{\text{Number of plaques} \times \text{dilution factor} \times \text{total packing volume}}{\text{Micrograms packed} \times \text{Microliters plated}}$$

8. Combine aliquots of the packaged mixture containing ~5 × 10^4 pfu bacteriophage with 600 μL XL1-Blue MRF' cells. Incubate at 37 °C for 15 min.
9. Mix each aliquot with 6.5 mL melted NZY top agar cooled to ~48 °C and spread evenly onto a freshly poured NZY agar plate, set for 10 min, invert the plates, and incubate at 37 °C for 6–8 h.
10. Add 8–10 mL SM buffer, store at 4 °C overnight.
11. Collect bacteriophage suspension from each plate, rinse the plates with 2 mL SM buffer and pool. Add chloroform to a 5% (v/v) final concentration. Mix and incubate at RT for 15 min.
12. Centrifuge at 500 × *g* for 10 min and collect the supernatant.
13. Repeat **steps 11** and **12** until the supernatant is clear. Add chloroform to a 0.3% (v/v) final concentration and store at 4 °C. Store aliquots of the amplified library in 7% (v/v) dimethyl sulfoxide (DMSO) at −80 °C.
14. Check the titer of the amplified library.

3.4.8 Screening of the cDNA Library

1. Combine 5 × 10^4 pfu/plate bacteriophage and 600 μL freshly prepared XL1-Blue MRF' cells at an OD_{600} of 0.5, incubate at 37 °C for 15 min.
2. Add 6.5 mL melted NZY top agar cooled to ~48 °C, quickly pour onto a NZY agar plate (at least 2 days old). Spread the cells evenly, allow set for 10 min, invert the plates, and incubate at 37 °C for 8 h.
3. Cool the plates at 4 °C for 2 h. Place a nitrocellulose membrane onto each NYZ agar plate for 2 min (*see* **Note 9**).

4. Submerge the membrane in a 1.5 M NaCl and 0.5 M NaOH solution for 2 min followed by submerging the membrane in a 1.5 M NaCl and 0.5 M Tris–HCl (pH 8.0) solution for 5 min.
5. Submerge the membrane in a 0.2 M Tris–HCl (pH 7.5) and 2× SSC buffer for <30 s and blot dry on a Whatman 3MM paper.
6. Oven-bake the membrane at 80 °C for 1.5–2 h. Store the stock agar plates at 4 °C.
7. Screen the membrane with antibodies of interest to identify the immunopositive plaques. Follow a basic Western blotting protocol.
8. Pick and purify the immunopositive clones, and store in SM buffer with 2% (v/v) chloroform at 4 °C.
9. Proceed to Subheading 3.6.

3.5 Generating RACE-Ready cDNA

When antisera and a cDNA library are not available and the specific sequence of the targeted gene is unknown, 5′ or 3′ RACE using degenerate primers can be performed to derive the genetic sequence of the target of interest. The SMARTer RACE cDNA amplification kit (Clontech Laboratories) protocol is used to synthesis the first-strand cDNA [21]. This first-strand cDNA can be directly used in 5′ and 3′ RACE without the need for second-strand synthesis and adaptor ligation.

1. Combine 1.0–2.75 μL mRNA and 1.0 μL 5′ CDS Primer A for 5′ RACE, add sterile water to a final volume of 3.75 μL. In a separate tube, combine 1.0–3.75 μL mRNA and 1.0 μL 3′ CDS Primer A for 3′ RACE, add sterile water to a final volume of 4.75 μL.
2. Mix and spin briefly in a microcentrifuge.
3. Incubate at 72 °C for 3 min, then cool to 42 °C for 2 min. Centrifuge at 14,000 × *g* for 10 s.
4. Add 1 μL SMARTer IIA oligo to the 5′ RACE.
5. Add 5.25 μL Master Mix to the 5′ RACE and 3′ RACE.
6. Mix by gentle pipetting and centrifuge briefly.
7. Incubate the tubes at 42 °C for 90 min followed by heating at 70 °C for 10 min.
8. Add 250 μL Tricine-EDTA buffer and store the synthesized first-strand cDNA at −20 °C.
9. Proceed to Subheading 3.7.

3.6 Amplification of the Immunopositive Phage Clones (cDNA Library)

1. Add the immunopositive phage clones containing 1–200 ng DNA, 200 nM each forward and reverse primers (primers designed based on the known target gene sequence or M13 primers), and 45 μL Platinum PCR SuperMix High Fidelity reagent (Invitrogen) to a microcentrifuge tube and mix.

2. Load the tube into a thermal cycler, incubate at 94 °C for 30 s to 2 min.
3. Perform 35 cycles of PCR amplification as follows: denature at 94 °C for 15–30 s, anneal at 55 °C for 15–30 s, extend at 68 °C for 1 min/kb [22].

3.7 Rapid Amplification of cDNA Ends (RACE)

3.7.1 Primer Design

Conserved DNA sequences in homologous proteins of related species are used to design the degenerate primers. For example, conserved homologous sequences in cashew, hazelnut, sesame, soybean, and fava bean 7S vicilins were used to design primers for pistachio vicilin gene amplification [14].

3.7.2 cDNA Amplification

1. Combine 2.5 μL 5′ RACE-ready cDNA, 5 μL universal primer A mix, 1 μL 5′ degenerate primer (10 μM), and 41.5 μL RACE Mix for 5′ RACE. Combine 2.5 μL 3′ RACE-ready cDNA, 5 μL universal primer A mix, 1 μL 3′ degenerate primer (10 μM), and 41.5 μL RACE Mix for 3′ RACE.
2. Start the following thermal cycling program:

   Five cycles: 94 °C 30 s, 72 °C 3 min.

   Five cycles: 94 °C 30 s, 70 °C 30 s, 72 °C 3 min.

   20 cycles: 94 °C 30 s, 68 °C 30 s, 72 °C 3 min.

3.8 Gel Purification of PCR Products

Check the purity of the PCR product by agarose gel electrophoresis. If a single, discrete band is not obtained, gel purify the fragment using the following protocol [23].

1. Electrophorese the PCR products on a low-melt TAE agarose gel (0.8–12%).
2. Visualize the DNA fragment under UV light and excise the band of interest.
3. Place the gel slice in a microcentrifuge tube and heat at 65 °C until the gel melts.
4. Keep the tube at 37 °C and use 4 μL of the melted agarose for TA cloning (Subheading 3.9).

3.9 TA Cloning of the Targeting Allergen cDNA

The PCR amplicon is TA cloned according to [23].

1. Mix 0.5–4 μL fresh PCR product with 1 μL salt solution, add deionized water to a total volume of 5 μL. Add 1 μL TOPO vector, mix gently, and incubate at RT for 5 min.
2. Add 4 μL of the mixture into a vial of One Shot chemically competent *E. coli*, mix gently, and incubate on ice for 5 min.
3. Spread 50 μL of the cells on a LB plate containing 50–100 μg/mL ampicillin and incubate at 37 °C overnight.

3.10 Sequencing of the Plasmid cDNA

The M13 forward and reverse primer sites are used for sequencing the PCR inserts on an ABI 3100 Genetic analyzer by using capillary electrophoresis and Version 2 Big Dye Terminators.

3.11 Subcloning and Expression of Recombinant Allergens

A wide variety of expression systems are available for the production of the recombinant allergen [4]. The selection of a suitable system depends on the desired yield, a need for post-translational modifications, ease of purification, the overall cost, and size of the allergen. The most common systems for recombinant allergen production are the pGEX (GE Healthcare Biosciences) which generates an allergen GST fusion protein, pET (Novagen) which generates a His tagged allergen protein, and pMAL (New England BioLabs) which generates an allergen MBP fusion protein [24, 25]. Schematic representation of common vectors used to generate recombinant allergens is illustrated in Fig. 3. The pMAL expression vector is demonstrated in this chapter [26].

3.11.1 Ligation of the cDNA into the Expression Vector

1. Digest 0.5 μg pMAL vector DNA in 20 μL 1× CutSmart buffer with 10 units each of *Xmn*I and *Sbf*I at 37 °C for 1 h. Inactivate the enzyme at 65 °C for 10 min.
2. Run 4 μL pMAL digest on an agarose gel to check for complete digestion.
3. Digest 0.5 μg cDNA insert in 20 μL 1× CutSmart Buffer with 10 units of *Sbf*I at 37 °C for 1 h.
4. Purify the pMAL vector backbone and the cut cDNA insert by gel extraction. A kit such as the QIAquick Gel Extraction Kit (QIAGEN) can be used.
5. Run the vector backbone and cDNA insert on a gel to check the concentrations.
6. Prepare the ligation reaction. Mix 20–40 ng vector backbone, 20 ng cDNA insert, 10 μL deionized water, and 10 μL 2× Quick Ligation reaction buffer. Add 1 μL Quick T4 DNA ligase, incubate at RT for 10 min.

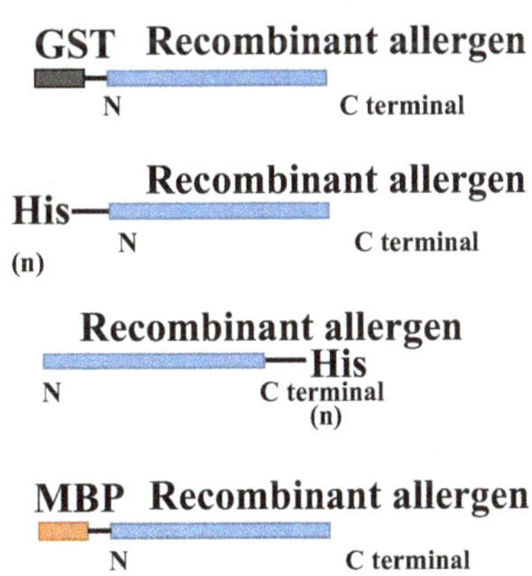

Fig. 3 Schematic representation of common vectors used to generate recombinant allergens. His tags can vary in length and location based upon the particular pET vector selected for expression. The molecular mass of GST and MBP is approximately 26 and 43 kDa, respectively

3.11.2 Transformation and Expression of the Recombinant Allergens

1. Mix 2 μL of the ligated vectors with 50 μL BL21 Competent *E. coli* cells (*see* **Note 10**). Incubate on ice for 5 min then heat to 42 °C for 30 s (*see* **Note 11**).
2. Add 0.2 mL LB and incubate at 37 °C for 20 min (*see* **Note 12**). Spread on an LB plate containing 100 μg/mL ampicillin. Incubate, inverted at 37 °C overnight.
3. Inoculate 10 mL overnight culture in 1 L rich broth containing glucose and ampicillin.
4. Grow to 0.5 OD_{600}, add IPTG to a 0.3 mM final concentration, incubate at 37 °C for 2 h (*see* **Note 13**).

3.12 Purification of Recombinant Allergens

3.12.1 Affinity Chromatography

1. Harvest the cells by centrifugation at 4,000 × *g* at 4 °C for 20 min and discard the supernatant. Resuspend the cells in 25 mL column buffer.
2. Freeze sample at −20 °C overnight. Thaw in cold water.
3. Keep sample in an ice-water bath and sonicate in 15 s short pulses until the released protein reaches a maximum concentration. Protein concentration can be monitored by mixing 5 μL sonicate with 1 mL Bradford reagent.
4. Centrifuge at 20,000 × *g* at 4 °C for 20 min to pellet cell debris and collect the supernatant. Dilute the supernatant 1:6 (v/v) in column buffer.
5. Pack amylose resin in a 2.5 × 10 cm column. The volume of resin is dependent upon the site of recombinant protein expression. Larger volumes of recombinant protein will be expressed in cytoplasm-directed expression as opposed to periplasm-directed expression (*see* **Note 14**).
6. Wash the column with five bed volumes of column buffer.
7. Load the diluted supernatant at a flow rate of 5 mL/min.
8. Wash with 12 bed volumes of column buffer at 10 mL/min.
9. Elute the fusion protein with 10 mM maltose in column buffer. Collect 10–20 fractions of 3 mL each to ensure all the recombinant allergen is eluted and collected from the column.
10. Pool the protein-containing fractions. Concentrate to ~1 mg/mL.
11. Amylose resin can be regenerated by washing with three column volumes of deionized water, three column volumes of 0.1% (w/v) SDS, one column volume of deionized water and five column volumes of column buffer (*see* **Note 15**). Store the regenerated resin at 4 °C.

3.12.2 Cleavage of the Fusion Protein

The fusion tag can be removed using the following protocol. However, removal of the tag may result in nonspecific degradation or protein insolubilization. In such cases, the recombinant allergens can be analyzed without cleavage of the fusion protein [8].

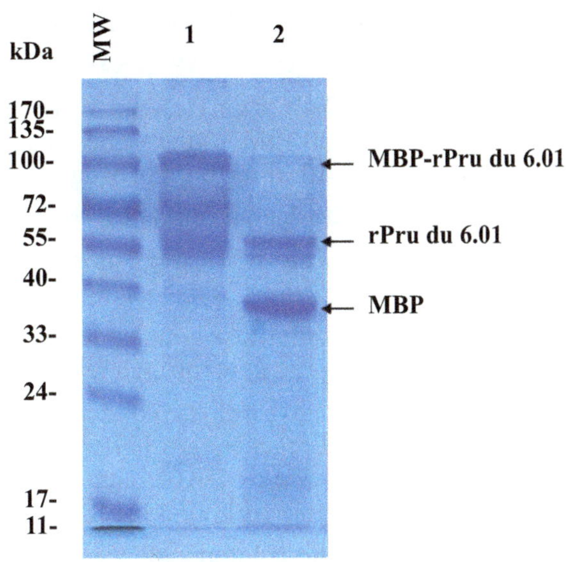

Fig. 4 Digestion of the recombinant almond allergen rPru du 6.01 expressed in the pMAL expression system by Factor Xa. *MW* Molecular weight marker, *1* undigested recombinant allergen, *2* recombinant allergen digested for 2 h at RT with Factor Xa. The liberated MBP must be removed from the sample by chromatography

SDS-PAGE of recombinant almond allergen rPru du 6.01 in presence and absence of fusion tag is illustrated in Fig. 4.

1. Mix 20 μL 1 mg/mL fusion protein with 1 μL 200 μg/mL Factor Xa. In a separate tube, add 5 μL fusion protein with no protease as control. At 2, 4, 8, and 24 h, remove 5 μL of the cleavage reaction.
2. Perform SDS-PAGE analysis of the cleavage samples to determine the success of the digestion. Add 5 μL SDS-PAGE sample buffer to the control and samples (*see* **Note 16**).
3. Boil for 5 min and run on an SDS-PAGE gel.
4. Scale up for the fusion proteins to be cleaved.
5. Stain gels using Colloidal Coomassie blue to visualize protein bands. MBP should be present at ~43 kDa. Recombinant allergen size will vary depending on the specific allergen expressed (*see* **Note 17**).

3.12.3 Separating the Recombinant Protein from MBP

Removal of MBP and Factor Xa can be performed using various column chromatography methods. If the recombinant allergen is <20 kDa or >100 kDa it can be separated from MBP using a sizing column. If the recombinant allergen and MBP are similar in size ion exchange chromatography is ideal for separation. Anion exchange chromatography is typically used as MBP and Factor Xa bind to a positively charged resin at pH 5.5, where most other proteins will flow through the column. Therefore, the recombinant allergen can be separated from the cleavage mixture by passage over an anion exchange column.

1. Dialyze the cleavage mixture in 100 volumes of running buffer (20 mM sodium phosphate buffer, 25 mM NaCl, pH 5.5) with three buffer changes, 2 h each.
2. Wash a HiTrap Q FF column with 15 mL running buffer.
3. Load the cleavage mixture onto the column. Collect 2.5 mL fractions of the column flow-through.
4. Wash the column with 3–5 mL running buffer until the OD_{280} of the flow through reaches baseline.
5. Regenerate the column by washing with five column volumes of regeneration buffer (running buffer with 1 M NaCl) followed by 5–10 columns volumes of running buffer. This will removed bound MBP and Factor Xa.
6. The column can now be stored at 4 °C to purify additional recombinant allergen.
7. Assess the purity of the recombinant allergen by SDS-PAGE (as described above) to ensure all contaminating MBP has been removed.
8. The purified recombinant allergen can be dialyzed into a desired phosphate containing buffer like phosphate buffered saline (PBS)-10 mM PO_4^{3-}, 137 mM NaCl, and 2.7 mM KCl, pH 7.4 for subsequent immunoassays.

3.13 Characterization and Applications of Recombinant Allergens

Recombinant allergens provide a source of molecularly defined homogenous protein preparations. This makes them ideal for both in vitro and ex vivo assays. Recombinant allergens are routinely used in a variety of immunoassays including: Western blots, dot blots, skin prick tests, basophil degranulation assays, ELISA, site directed mutagenesis, and epitope mapping studies. These assays aim to assess patient IgE reactivity, investigate cross-reactivity between various foods, assist in structural studies, identify IgE reactive epitopes, and analyze the effects of enzymatic digestion, and denaturation on allergenicity. The information gathered is important in diagnosis of allergies, furthering our understanding of the mechanism by which allergies are induced, and understanding the effect of the food matrices/digestions on the allergenicity of a protein. Commonly used physicochemical and immunological characterization methods for the recombinant allergens are listed in Table 1.

4 Notes

1. All agar plates and antibiotic containing media should be stored at 4 °C. This will prevent contaminating bacteria growth and antibiotic breakdown. Allow media to reach RT before use. Plates should be used within several weeks.

Table 1
Physicochemical and immunological characterization methods of recombinant food allergens

Parameter	Method	Example	Reference
Molecular mass	SDS-PAGE	rAna o 1, 2, 3; rAra h 8; rBer e 1; rCar i 1, 4; rCor a 1, 2, 8, 11, 12, 13, 14; rCyp c 1; rJug r 1, 2, 4; rMal d 4; rPis v 1, 2, 3, 4; rPru av 1, 4; rPru du 4, 5, 6	[7–14, 27–43]
	MALDI-TOF-MS	rBer e 1	[27]
	ESI-QTOF-MS	rMal d 4	[41]
Sequence verification	N-terminal sequence	rBer e 1; rCor a 1, 2, 8; rMal d 4	[27, 30, 41]
	MALDI-TOF-MS	rCor a 1, 2, 8; rCyp c 1	[30, 40]
Protein structure	Circular dichroism	rAra h 8; rBer e 1; rCor a 1, 2, 8, 11; rCyp c 1; rJug r 1; rMal d 4	[27, 28, 30, 31, 40, 41, 43, 44]
	NMR	rBer e 1; rCor a 1, 2, 8	[30, 45]
	Electron microscopy	rAna o 2	[46]
	Small angle X-ray scattering	rMal d 4	[41]
Disulfide mapping	HPLC-MS/MS	rBer e 1	[27]
Glycan analysis	Agglutinin binding	rBer e 1	[27]
	1D-NMR	rBer e 1	[27]
Digestibility	SGF digestion	rBer e 1; rMal d 4	[28, 41]
Epitope mapping	Solid-phase peptide synthesis	rAna o 1, 2, 3; rCar i 1, 4; rJug r 1; rPru du 6	[8–13, 44]
	LC-ESI FT-ICR MS (H/D exchange)	rAna o 1, 2; rPru du 6	[47–50]
	Chimeric molecule	rAna o 2; rPru du 6	[46, 48]
	Alanine mutation	rPru du 6	[48]
Immunoreactivity	Immunoblotting	rAna o 1, 2, 3; rAra h 8; rBer e 1; rCar i 1, 4; rCor a 1, 2, 8, 11, 12, 13, 14; rCyp c 1; rJug r 1, 2, 4; rMal d 4; rPis v 1, 2, 3, 4; rPru av 1, 4; rPru du 4, 5, 6	[7–14, 27–43]
	ELISA	rBer e 1; rCar i 1; rCyp c 1; rJug r 1; rMal d 4; rPru du 4, 6	[7, 8, 12, 28, 40, 41, 44]
	EAST	rAra h 8; rCor a 1; rPru av 1, 4	[29, 42, 43]
	RAST	rAra h 8; rMal d 4	[41, 43]
	Histamine/β-hexosaminidase release	rAra h 8; rCor a 1, 11; rCyp c 1; rJug r 1; rMal d 4	[29, 31, 40, 41, 43, 44]
	ImmunoCAP	rAra h 8; rCor a 1, 2, 8, 11, 14; rJug r 1	[29–31, 33, 34, 43]
	Skin prick test	rMal d 4	[41]

2. Samples should not be mixed with solution D for more than 30 min.
3. Never dry the RNA pellet completely, which greatly decreases RNA solubility.

4. The washing step is important as SA-PMPs are provided in a solution of phosphate buffered saline. 1 mg/mL bovine serum albumin, and 0.02% (w/v) sodium azide. Use the SA-PMPs within 30 min after washing for optimal performance.
5. If particles are transferred with the mRNA, remove by centrifugation at 12,000 × *g* for 1 min. The SA-PMPs cannot be washed and reused.
6. Temperatures above 16 °C may cause hairpin structure formation. It is therefore important to keep all reagents under 16 °C before adding the DNA polymerase I.
7. Do not over dry the pellet or the cDNA becomes difficult to solubilize.
8. Do not incubate for longer than 2 h as the packaging efficiency may drop.
9. It is essential to mark both the nitrocellulose membrane and plate with identifying symbols such as pencil annotations or indentions in the agar. This will ensure that the membrane can be correctly re-aligned with the plate to pick immunoreactive plaques identified in screening.
10. If desired, the ligation reaction can initially be transformed into DH5-α competent cells (Thermo Fisher Scientific). These cells increase insert stability and improve the quality of plasmid DNA. Plasmid can be isolated from these cells using a DNA plasmid miniprep kit. The obtained plasmid can be sequenced using an ABI 3100 Genetic analyzer to verify insertion of the allergen PCR product and to check for possible mutations, then transformed into BL21 Competent *E. coli* cells (New England BioLabs).
11. A short heat shock is essential for facilitating the uptake of plasmid DNA.
12. This short outgrowth is necessary for expression of the ampicillin resistance gene in newly transformed cells. This will allow the selective growth of transformed cells on ampicillin containing media.
13. Smaller culture volumes can be inoculated and expression induced with IPTG. If small scale, trail expression is desired 5 mL of culture is sufficient for induction and detection of the expressed allergen MBP fusion protein by SDS-PAGE.
14. Amylose resin can bind 7–10 mg/mL of MBP fusion protein. Typically 3–6 mL of resin is sufficient to bind recombinant proteins expressed in a 1 L culture of *E. coli*.
15. Resin may be regenerated up to five times.

16. For fusions resistant to cleavage, adding 0.005–0.05% (w/v) SDS in the reaction or denaturing the fusion by 6 M guanidine hydrochloride may improve the cleavage.
17. Alternative staining options are available such as silver stain or fluorescent dye stains.

Acknowledgement

Financial support from USDA-NIFA 2009-65503-05797; 2011-67017-20079; and Almond Board of California (ABC), Modesto, CA is gratefully acknowledged.

References

1. Sathe SK, Liu C, Zaffran VD (2016) Food allergy. Annu Rev Food Sci Technol 7:191–220
2. Boyce JA, Assa'ad A, Burks AW, Jones SM, Sampson HA, Wood RA, Plaut M, Cooper SF, Fenton MJ, Arshad SH (2010) Guidelines for the diagnosis and management of food allergy in the United States: report of the NIAID-sponsored expert panel. J Allergy Clin Immunol 126:S1–S58
3. FDA (2004) Food allergen labeling and consumer protection act of 2004 (Public Law 108-282, Title II). http://www.fda.gov/Food/GuidanceRegulation/GuidanceDocumentsRegulatoryInformation/Allergens/ucm106187.htm. Accessed 19 May 2016
4. Willison LN, Sathe SK, Roux KH (2014) Production and analysis of recombinant tree nut allergens. Methods 66:34–43
5. Ausubel FM, Brent R, Kingston RE, Moore DD, Seidman JG, Smith JA, Struhl K (eds) (2003) Current protocols in molecular biology. John Wiley & Sons, New York
6. White BA (ed) (1997) PCR cloning protocls: from molecular cloning to genetic engineering. Humanna Press, Totowa
7. Tawde P, Venkatesh YP, Wang F, Teuber SS, Sathe SK, Roux KH (2006) Cloning and characterization of profilin (Pru du 4), a cross-reactive almond (*Prunus dulcis*) allergen. J Allergy Clin Immunol 118:915–922
8. Willison LN, Tripathi P, Sharma G, Teuber SS, Sathe SK, Roux KH (2011) Cloning, expression and patient IgE reactivity of recombinant Pru du 6, an 11S globulin from almond. Int Arch Allergy Immunol 156:267–281
9. Wang F, Robotham JM, Teuber SS, Tawde P, Sathe SK, Roux KH (2002) Ana o 1, a cashew (*Anacardium occidentale*) allergen of the vicilin seed storage protein family. J Allergy Clin Immunol 110:160–166
10. Wang F, Robotham JM, Teuber SS, Sathe SK, Roux KH (2003) Ana o 2, a major cashew (*Anacardium occidentale* L.) nut allergen of the legumin family. Int Arch Allergy Immunol 132:27–39
11. Robotham JM, Wang F, Seamon V, Teuber SS, Sathe SK, Sampson HA, Beyer K, Seavy M, Roux KH (2005) Ana o 3, an important cashew nut (*Anacardium occidentale* L.) allergen of the 2S albumin family. J Allergy Clin Immunol 115:1284–1290
12. Sharma GM, Irsigler A, Dhanarajan P, Ayuso R, Bardina L, Sampson HA, Roux KH, Sathe SK (2011) Cloning and characterization of 2S albumin, Car i 1, a major allergen in pecan. J Agric Food Chem 59:4130–4139
13. Sharma GM, Irsigler A, Dhanarajan P, Ayuso R, Bardina L, Sampson HA, Roux KH, Sathe SK (2011) Cloning and characterization of an 11S legumin, Car i 4, a major allergen in pecan. J Agric Food Chem 59:9542–9552
14. Willison L, Tawde P, Robotham J, Penney R, Teuber S, Sathe S, Roux K (2008) Pistachio vicilin, Pis v 3, is immunoglobulin E-reactive and cross-reacts with the homologous cashew allergen, Ana o 1. Clin Exp Allergy 38:1229–1238
15. Chomczynski P, Sacchi N (2006) The single-step method of RNA isolation by acid guanidinium thiocyanate-phenol-chloroform extraction: twenty-something years on. Nat Protoc 1:581–585
16. Sambrook J, Russell D (2001) Molecular cloning: a laboratory manual. Cold Spring Harbor Laboratory, New York

17. Aviv H, Leder P (1972) Purification of biologically active globin messenger RNA by chromatography on oligothymidylic acid-cellulose. Proc Natl Acad Sci USA 69:1408–1412
18. Surzycki S (2000) Basic techniques in molecular biology. Springer, New York
19. PolyATtract mRNA Isolation Systems Technical Manual (2012) Promega. http://www.promega.com/resources/protocols/technical-manuals/0/polyattract-mrna-isolation-systems-protocol/. Accessed 3 Apr 2016
20. ZAP Express cDNA Gigapack III Gold Cloning Kit Instruction Manual (2010) Agilent Technologies. http://www.agilent.com/cs/library/usermanuals/public/200403-12_ZAPExpresscDNA_Manual.pdf. Accessed 5 Apr 2016
21. SMARTer RACE cDNA Amplification Kit User Manual (2012) Clontech Laboratories. http://www.clontech.com/xxclt_ibcGetAttachment.jsp?cItemId=17335. Accessed 19 May 2016
22. Platinum PCR SuperMix High Fidelity (2010) Invitrogen. https://tools.thermofisher.com/content/sfs/manuals/platinumsupermixhifi_man.pdf. Accessed 20 May 2016
23. TOPO TA Cloning Kit User Guide (2015) Invitrogen. https://tools.thermofisher.com/content/sfs/manuals/topota_man.pdf. Accessed 19 May 2016
24. Terpe K (2003) Overview of tag protein fusions: from molecular and biochemical fundamentals to commercial systems. Appl Microbiol Biotechnol 60:523–533
25. Bell MR, Engleka MJ, Malik A, Strickler JE (2013) To fuse or not to fuse: what is your purpose? Protein Sci 22:1466–1477
26. pMAL Protein Fusion and Purification System Instruction Manual (2015) New England BioLabs. https://www.neb.com/~/media/Catalog/All-Products/FF91B67397D945E0956F3483174CF7E3/Datacards%20or%20Manuals/manualE8200.pdf. Accessed 20 May 2016
27. Alcocer MJ, Murtagh GJ, Bailey K, Dumoulin M, Meseguer AS, Parker MJ, Archer DB (2002) The disulphide mapping, folding and characterisation of recombinant Ber e 1, an allergenic protein, and SFA8, two sulphur-rich 2S plant albumins. J Mol Biol 324:165–175
28. Murtagh G, Archer D, Dumoulin M, Ridout S, Matthews S, Arshad S, Alcocer M (2003) In vitro stability and immunoreactivity of the native and recombinant plant food 2S albumins Ber e 1 and SFA-8. Clin Exp Allergy 33:1147–1152
29. Lüttkopf D, Müller U, Skov PS, Ballmer-Weber B, Wüthrich B, Hansen KS, Poulsen LK, Kästner M, Haustein D, Vieths S (2002) Comparison of four variants of a major allergen in hazelnut (*Corylus avellana*) Cor a 1.04 with the major hazel pollen allergen Cor a 1.01. Mol Immunol 38:515–525
30. Lauer I, Alessandri S, Pokoj S, Reuter A, Conti A, Vieths S, Scheurer S (2008) Expression and characterization of three important panallergens from hazelnut. Mol Nutr Food Res 52:S262–S271
31. Lauer I, Foetisch K, Kolarich D, Ballmer-Weber BK, Conti A, Altmann F, Vieths S, Scheurer S (2004) Hazelnut (*Corylus avellana*) vicilin Cor a 11: molecular characterization of a glycoprotein and its allergenic activity. Biochem J 383:327–334
32. Akkerdaas JH, Schocker F, Vieths S, Versteeg S, Zuidmeer L, Hefle SL, Aalberse RC, Richter K, Ferreira F, van Ree R (2006) Cloning of oleosin, a putative new hazelnut allergen, using a hazelnut cDNA library. Mol Nutr Food Res 50:18–23
33. Garino C, Zuidmeer L, Marsh J, Lovegrove A, Morati M, Versteeg S, Schilte P, Shewry P, Arlorio M, van Ree R (2010) Isolation, cloning, and characterization of the 2S albumin: a new allergen from hazelnut. Mol Nutr Food Res 54:1257–1265
34. Teuber SS, Dandekar AM, Peterson WR, Sellers CL (1998) Cloning and sequencing of a gene encoding a 2S albumin seed storage protein precursor from English walnut (*Juglans regia*), a major food allergen. J Allergy Clin Immunol 101:807–814
35. Teuber SS, Jarvis KC, Dandekar AM, Peterson WR, Ansari AA (1999) Identification and cloning of a complementary DNA encoding a vicilin-like proprotein, Jug r 2, from English walnut kernel (*Juglans regia*), a major food allergen. J Allergy Clin Immunol 104:1311–1320
36. Wallowitz M, Peterson WR, Uratsu S, Comstock SS, Dandekar AM, Teuber SS (2006) Jug r 4, a legumin group food allergen from walnut (*Juglans regia* Cv. Chandler). J Agric Food Chem 54:8369–8375
37. Ahn K, Bardina L, Grishina G, Beyer K, Sampson H (2009) Identification of two pistachio allergens, Pis v 1 and Pis v 2, belonging to the 2S albumin and 11S globulin family. Clin Exp Allergy 39:926–934
38. Noorbakhsh R, Mortazavi SA, Sankian M, Shahidi F, Assarehzadegan MA, Varasteh A (2010) Cloning, expression, characterization, and computational approach for cross-reactivity prediction of manganese superoxide dismutase allergen from pistachio nut. Allergol Int 59:295–304

39. Mohsen A, Roux KH (2009) cDNA Cloning, expression and characterization of an allergenic 60s ribosomal protein of almond (*Prunus dulcis*). Iran J Allergy Asthma Immunol 8:77–84
40. Swoboda I, Bugajska-Schretter A, Verdino P, Keller W, Sperr WR, Valent P, Valenta R, Spitzauer S (2002) Recombinant carp parvalbumin, the major cross-reactive fish allergen: a tool for diagnosis and therapy of fish allergy. J Immunol 168:4576–4584
41. Ma Y, Zuidmeer L, Bohle B, Bolhaar S, Gadermaier G, Gonzalez-Mancebo E, Fernandez-Rivas M, Knulst A, Himly M, Asero R (2006) Characterization of recombinant Mal d 4 and its application for component-resolved diagnosis of apple allergy. Clin Exp Allergy 36:1087–1096
42. Scheurer S, Pastorello EA, Wangorsch A, Kästner M, Haustein D, Vieths S (2001) Recombinant allergens Pru av 1 and Pru av 4 and a newly identified lipid transfer protein in the in vitro diagnosis of cherry allergy. J Allergy Clin Immunol 107:724–731
43. Mittag D, Akkerdaas J, Ballmer-Weber BK, Vogel L, Wensing M, Becker W-M, Koppelman SJ, Knulst AC, Helbling A, Hefle SL (2004) Ara h 8, a Bet v 1-homologous allergen from peanut, is a major allergen in patients with combined birch pollen and peanut allergy. J Allergy Clin Immunol 114:1410–1417
44. Sordet C, Culerrier R, Granier C, Rancé F, Didier A, Barre A, Rougé P (2009) Expression of Jug r 1, the 2S albumin allergen from walnut (*Juglans regia*), as a correctly folded and functional recombinant protein. Peptides 30:1213–1221
45. Rundqvist L, Tengel T, Zdunek J, Björn E, Schleucher J, Alcocer MJ, Larsson G (2012) Solution structure, copper binding and backbone dynamics of recombinant Ber e 1-the major allergen from brazil nut. PLoS One 7:e46435
46. Xia L, Willison LN, Porter L, Robotham JM, Teuber SS, Sathe SK, Roux KH (2010) Mapping of a conformational epitope on the cashew allergen Ana o 2: a discontinuous large subunit epitope dependent upon homologous or heterologous small subunit association. Mol Immunol 47:1808–1816
47. Guan X, Noble KA, Tao Y, Roux KH, Sathe SK, Young NL, Marshall AG (2015) Epitope mapping of 7S cashew antigen in complex with antibody by solution-phase H/D exchange monitored by FT-ICR mass spectrometry. J Mass Spectrom 50:812–819
48. Willison LN, Zhang Q, Su M, Teuber SS, Sathe SK, Roux KH (2013) Conformational epitope mapping of Pru du 6, a major allergen from almond nut. Mol Immunol 55:253–263
49. Zhang Q, Noble KA, Mao Y, Young NL, Sathe SK, Roux KH, Marshall AG (2013) Rapid screening for potential epitopes reactive with a polycolonal antibody by solution-phase H/D exchange monitored by FT-ICR mass spectrometry. J Am Soc Mass Spectrom 24:1016–1025
50. Zhang Q, Willison LN, Tripathi P, Sathe SK, Roux KH, Emmett MR, Blakney GT, Zhang H-M, Marshall AG (2011) Epitope mapping of a 95 kDa antigen in complex with antibody by solution-phase amide backbone hydrogen/deuterium exchange monitored by Fourier transform ion cyclotron resonance mass spectrometry. Anal Chem 83:7129–7136

Chapter 4

Recombinant Allergens Production in Yeast

Maria Neophytou and Marcos Alcocer

Abstract

The methylotropic yeast *Pichia pastoris* has been extensively used in large-scale production of properly folded recombinant proteins. As an eukaryotic organism *P. pastoris* presents a series of advantages at expression and processing of heterologous proteins such as post-translational modifications, protein processing, and a reasonably sophisticated quality control of protein folding when compared against *Escherichia coli*. In this chapter, we describe the modified lab procedure for cloning and expression in *Pichia pastoris* of common food allergens sequences from the raw fruit to the fully folded biotinylated protein product.

Key words Food allergens, In vivo biotinylation, *Pichia pastoris*, Protein expression, Protein tagging, Yeast expression

1 Introduction

Pichia pastoris has become an interesting alternative to *E. coli* in recombinant antibody production. It presents the advantages of single-celled organisms, such as ease of handling and cost-effectiveness, combined with the benefits of eukaryotic systems that include post-translational modifications, protein processing, and a reasonably sophisticated quality control of protein folding. Additionally, it is a more manageable and sturdy system than higher eukaryotes, such as insects and mammalian tissue culture cells systems, that besides been auxotrophic they can employ cheap methanol as the sole source of carbon and energy [1, 2].

In this work, we describe the modified lab procedure for cloning and expression in *Pichia pastoris* of common food allergens. As an example of this application, the following steps describe the amplification of Pru p 3 gene from the raw fruit (*Prunus persica*), sequencing, and the target DNA sequence cloning into yeast expression vector driven by methanol. In this system, the AOX promoter drives the alpha-mating type pre-prosequence that directs the fusion product to the ER and subsequent GOLGI and cell secretion. The fusion protein is then cleaved from the

Jing Lin and Marcos Alcocer (eds.), *Food Allergens: Methods and Protocols*, Methods in Molecular Biology, vol. 1592, DOI 10.1007/978-1-4939-6925-8_4, © Springer Science+Business Media LLC 2017

pre-prosequence by an internal protease system (Kex II) [3–6]. Most of the general steps of this procedure are described in details in the Pichia expression system brochures produced by INVITROGEN using the vector pPICZ that is easily accessible on line.

In addition to the procedure described by the manufacturer we added few essential selection steps (dot blots) that make an effective contribution toward a successful expression. Further, we describe our latest generic tagging system where a biotinylation C-terminal target sequence was engineered [7, 8] for in vivo biotinylation of the target protein [9–12]. The procedure described here has been successfully used in the production of biotinylated scFv [13, 14] and others not yet published, and is now routine in our lab.

2 Materials

2.1 Gene Amplification

1. RNA Extraction: RNeasy mini Kit (QIAGEN, UK).
2. Complementary DNA: M-MLV reverse transcriptase and Random Primers.
3. End-point PCR: ZymoTaq DNA Polymerase Set including enzyme, buffer and dNTPs (Zymoresearch Cambridge Biosciences, UK or similar). Synthetic DNA oligonucleotides (5 μM each).

2.2 Agarose Gel Electrophoresis

1. 1% Agarose gel: Weigh 1 g agarose and dissolve in 100 mL of 1× TAE Buffer.
2. Tris-acetate EDTA running buffer (TAE Buffer; 1×): 40 mM Tris (pH 7.6), 20 mM acetic acid, 1 mM EDTA.
3. Gel electrophoresis apparatus.
4. Power pack (Bio-Rad, UK).
5. DNA Stain: Midori Green Direct DNA Stain.

2.3 PCR Product Purification and Cloning

1. QIAquick PCR Purification Kit (QIAGEN, UK).
2. TOPO TA Cloning Kit with pCR 2.1vector (Life Technologies, UK).
3. Purified PCR product.
4. TOP 10 Chemically Competent *E. coli*.
5. DNA midi kit Plasmid purification (QIAGEN, UK).

2.4 General Media

1. Luria-Bertani medium (LB): 1% Tryptone, 0.5% Yeast Extract, 0.5% NaCl. Autoclave at 121 °C for 15 min cycle. Store at 4 °C.
2. Luria-Bertani agar plates (LBA): 1% Tryptone, 0.5% Yeast Extract, 0.5% NaCl, 1.5% agar pH 7.5. Autoclave at 121 °C for 15 min cycle. Cool down before adding the selective antibiotic.

3. Yeast Extract Peptone Dextrose (YPD) medium: 1% yeast extract, 2% peptone, 2% dextrose. Store at 4 °C. Autoclave at 121 °C for 15 min cycle. Cool down before adding the selective antibiotic.
4. Yeast Extract Peptone Dextrose Sorbitol (YPDS) agar plates: 1% Yeast Extract, 2% peptone, 2% dextrose, 1 M sorbitol, 2% agar with 100 μg/mL of Zeocin.
5. Buffered Glycerol-complex Medium (BMGY): 1% yeast extract, 2% peptone, 100 mM potassium phosphate pH 6.0, 1.34% Yeast Nitrogen Base (YNB), 1% glycerol, 4.10^{-5}% biotin.
6. Buffered Methanol-complex Medium (BMMY): 1% yeast extract, 2% peptone, 100 mM potassium phosphate pH 6.0, 1.34% YNB, 1% methanol, 4.10^{-5}% biotin.
7. Glycerol stocks: Luria-Bertani medium with 25% final concentration of glycerol.

2.5 Pichia Protein Production

1. Plasmid DNA linearization: SacI restriction enzyme.
2. Pichia Electrocompetent cells: pMJA180-GS115 Pichia, cold (4 °C) sterile 1 M sorbitol.
3. Electroporator: BioRad MicroPulser electroporation apparatus and 0.2 cm cuvettes (Bio-Rad, UK).
4. Selection antibiotics: 100 μg/mL Zeocin, 500 μg/mL Blasticidin.

2.6 Dot Blot Analysis

1. Acrylic Dot blot microfiltration unit.
2. PVDF membrane.
3. Phosphate-buffered saline (PBS): One tablet dissolved in 200 mL of deionized water yields 0.01 M phosphate buffer, 0.0027 M potassium chloride and 0.137 M sodium chloride, pH 7.4, at 25 °C.
4. Tris Buffered Saline (TBS; 10×): 1.5 M NaCl, 0.1 M Tris–HCl, pH 7.4.
5. Blocking solution: 3% BSA (w/v) TBS (50 mM Tris–HCl, 150 mM NaCl, pH 7.5).
6. Washing buffer: TBST (0.05% v/v Tween-20).
7. Streptavidin Alkaline Phosphatase dilution: (1:5000 v/v) in 1% BSA (w/v) TBST.
8. Develop agent: a ready-to-use solution of 5-bromo-4-chloro-3-indolyl-1-phosphate and nitroblue tetrazolium.

2.7 SDS-PAGE

1. NuPAGE XCell SureLock System Mini-cell electrophoresis system.
2. Mini Gel: NuPAGE Bis-Tris, Novex Pre-Cast Gel 12%.

3. NuPAGE LDS Sample Buffer 4×.
4. Reducing agent: 1 M DTT.
5. Running Buffer; 1×: 50 mL of 20× NuPAGE MES Running buffer diluted in 950 mL of distilled water.
6. NuPAGE Antioxidant: contains Dimethylformamide and Sodium bisulfite.
7. Protein Molecular marker: Precision Plus All Blue Pre-stained Protein Marker.
8. Staining solution: 0.1% Coomassie Brilliant Blue R250 in 50% Methanol (v/v), 10% Glacial acetic acid (v/v), and 40% water.
9. Destaining solution: 40% Methanol (v/v), 10% Glacial acetic acid (v/v).

2.8 Western Blotting

1. Xcell II Blot Module.
2. Transfer Buffer: 1× NuPAGE Transfer Buffer with 10% Methanol and 0.1% Antioxidant.
3. Blotting pads.
4. PVDF membrane (Immuno-Blot, Bio-Rad).
5. Filter paper.

3 Methods

The following procedure describes the cloning and expression of peach allergens from the native fruit to the final protein expression in Pichia. All procedures should be carried out at room temperature and under sterile conditions unless otherwise specified.

3.1 RNA Extraction and Amplification

1. The peach (*Prunus persica*) RNA is isolated from 30 mg of frozen raw fruit using RNA extraction kit essentially as described by the manufacturer (QIAGEN, UK).
2. Complementary DNA: Each reverse transcription (RT) reaction is carried out in duplicate, one containing the Reverse Transcriptase enzyme (+RT) and one where RT is substituted with water (−RT) (*see* **Note 1**). Complementary DNA (cDNA) is synthesized from 0.5 μg of total RNA incubated with 200 units of the M-MLV reverse transcriptase enzyme, primers in 5× reaction buffer in a final volume of 25 μL, for 1 h at 42 °C.
3. End-point Polymerase Chain Reaction (PCR): The peach-specific genes are amplified by PCR using specific primers containing the PstI site in frame with the alpha-mating restriction site at 5′ end and a NotI site at 3′ end. All primers are designed based on the mature protein and with a Tm of ca. 58 °C (*see* **Note 2**). The amplification is carried out at 30 cycles of

94 °C 30 s, 58 °C 30 s, 72 °C 30 s using the cDNA produced in **step 2** (2 μL), ZymoTaq DNA Polymerase (2 units/50 μL), enzyme buffer and dNTPs according to the manufacturer's instructions (Zymoresearch Cambridge Biosciences, UK or similar).

4. The PCR product size is confirmed by gel sizing in a 1% agarose gel electrophoresis (*see* **Note 3**). Running conditions are 90 V for 45 min.

3.2 TA Cloning TOPO and Screening

1. The correct size amplified product is excised from the gel or if single intense band, purified directly essentially as described in QIAquick PCR Purification Kit.
2. The purified product (2 μL) is then ligated to the TOPO pCR 2.1vector (0.5 μL) in a 30 min room temperature reaction essentially as described by the manufacturer (*see* **Note 4**).
3. The ligated mixture is then transformed into either electro or chemically competent *E. coli* cells and spread on pre-warmed low salt Luria-Bertani agar plates containing 50 μg/mL Ampicillin.
4. Plates are incubated overnight at 37 °C.

3.3 Plasmid Purification

1. PCR colony screening: In a sterile flow cabinet, 5–10 growing colonies are picked and inoculated into 100 μL of LB medium containing 50 μg/mL Ampicillin and grown for 1 h at 37 °C with 200 rpm shaking. The positive clones are confirmed by PCR using the LB culture (2 μL) as template, M13 oligonucleotides specific for TOPO-pCR 2.1vector at 30 cycles of 94 °C 30 s, 58 °C 30 s, 72 °C 30 s using DyNazyme II DNA Polymerase (0.5 units/25 μL), enzyme buffer and dNTPs according to the manufacturer's instructions (*see* **Note 5**).
2. Positive *E. coli* clones are then inoculated into either 10 mL or 100 mL LB containing 50 μL/mL Ampicillin accordingly to the amount of plasmid required by the plasmid purification Kits following the manufacturer's instructions (*see* **Note 6**).
3. Purified plasmids are then sent for sequencing.

3.4 pPICZ Cloning

1. Once the sequence is confirmed the TOPO vector (5 μg) produced in **step 3** is digested for 2 h at 37 °C with PstI and NotI (10 U/each) in 100 μL reaction (*see* **Note 7**).
2. The digested product size is confirmed by 1% agarose gel to electrophoresis.
3. The correct size fragment is then excised from the gel and purified using the QIAquick PCR Purification Kit according to the manufacturer's instructions.

4. The purified fragment (10–20 ng) is then ligated to the PstI/NotI digested plasmid pMJA167 (90 ng) for 2–4 h at 15 °C using T4 Ligase (5 U) in a 20 μL reaction mixture containing enzyme buffer and ATP.
5. The ligated mixture is then transformed into *E. coli* competent cells and spread on pre-warmed low salt LB agar plates containing 50 μg/mL of Zeocin and incubated O/N at 37 °C.
6. The positive clones are again selected by PCR essentially as described in Subheading 3.3 **step 1** but using the primer-specific oligonucleotides.
7. The positive clones are then inoculated in 100 mL LB medium containing 50 μg/mL Zeocin and grow O/N at 37 °C with 200 rpm shaking for Midi or Maxi purification according to the Kit's manufacturer.

3.5 *Pichia* Transformation [15]

1. Inoculate pMJA180-GS115 into 100 mL of YPD containing 500 μL/mL of Blasticidin and grow O/N at 30 °C with 200 rpm shaking.
2. Measure the OD_{600} density of the overnight culture until reaching 1.3–1.5. Then centrifuge cells (3000 g, 10 min), wash pellet in 30 mL of cold (4 °C) sterile water. Vortex the cell pellet to dissolve and centrifuge again (3000 g, 5 min).
3. Repeat once the wash step then resuspend cell pellet in 2 mL of cold (4 °C) sterile 1 M sorbitol and centrifuge (3000 g, 5 min). Finally, resuspend cell pellet in about 200 μL cold (4 °C) sterile 1 M sorbitol (*see* **Note 8**).
4. The pPICZ plasmid DNA (10 μg) from each protein of interest is linearized by SacI digestion followed by ethanol precipitated [15].
5. The plasmids are then transformed into *P. pastoris* BirA-GS115 competent cells (**step 3** above) by electroporation, following the electroporator manufacturer's instructions.
6. Transformed cells are spread on Yeast Extract Peptone Dextrose Sorbitol Medium (YPDS) agar plates containing 100 μg/mL Zeocin and 500 μg/mL Blasticidin and incubate for 72 h at 30 °C.
7. 24 isolated colonies from each construct plate are selected and grown again on an YPDS 96-well plate containing100 μg/mL Zeocin and 500 μg/mL Blasticidin and incubate for 48 h at 30 °C (*see* **Note 9**).
8. 24 colonies from the backup plate are inoculated in 2 mL of Buffered Glycerol-complex Medium (BMGY) in 24-well plates containing 100 μg/mL Zeocin and 500 μg/mL Blasticidin and incubate for 72 h at 30 °C with 200 rpm shaking.
9. Plates are then centrifuged (1800 g, 10 min, 4 °C), the supernatant removed and cells resuspended in Buffered Methanol-

complex Medium (BMMY) to induce the production of protein of interest incubated for 72 h at 30 °C with 200 rpm shaking.

10. Methanol (1% v/v) is replenished every 12 h for 72 h.
11. Finally, plates are centrifuged (1800 g, 10 min, 4 °C) and the supernatant is analyzed by dot blot analysis in search for the expression of each protein.

3.6 Dot Blot Analysis

1. 400 μL of supernatant from 24 selected *P. pastoris* clones are filtered through a dot blot microfiltration unit containing a PVDF membrane (*see* **Note 10**).
2. Membrane is then blocked with 3% BSA (w/v) TBS at 37 °C for 1 h (*see* **Note 11**).
3. After washing the membrane three times for 5 min with TBST, incubate with Streptavidin Alkaline Phosphatase (1:5000 v/v) at 37 °C for 2 h (*see* **Note 12**).
4. Membrane is then washed three times with TBST and once with distilled water.
5. Finally, add a ready-to-use solution of 5-bromo-4-chloro-3--indolyl-1-phosphate and nitro blue tetrazolium to detect the alkaline phosphatase enzyme activity.
6. Reaction is stopped by rinsing the membrane with water.
7. Figure 1 shows a typical dot blot analyses.

3.7 SDS-PAGE

1. Sample preparation: samples from Subheading 3.5 **step 11** are dialyzed (3.5 K cutoff) against water overnight followed by freeze-drying.
2. Dried samples are then resuspended in LDS Sample buffer (*see* **Note 13**).
3. Samples are separated by SDS electrophoresis using a NuPAGE Bis-Tris, Novex Pre-Cast Gel 12% essentially according to the manufacturer's protocol (*see* **Note 14**).
4. The gel is fixed and stained in Coomassie blue into a staining container overnight on a shaking platform. Next morning the gel is destained completely until the bands easily visualized.

3.8 Western Blotting

1. The blotting procedure is performed essentially according to the manufacturer's protocol (Novex). Briefly, the SDS-PAGE gel was blotted onto a PVDF membrane at 30 V/1 h using the dedicated Transfer buffer.
2. The membrane is washed three times in TBST and water and the biotinylated proteins detected essentially as described in Subheading 3.6 for dot blot analysis or through the use of specific antibody.
3. Figure 2 shows a typical Western blotting for the biotinylated protein Pru p 3.

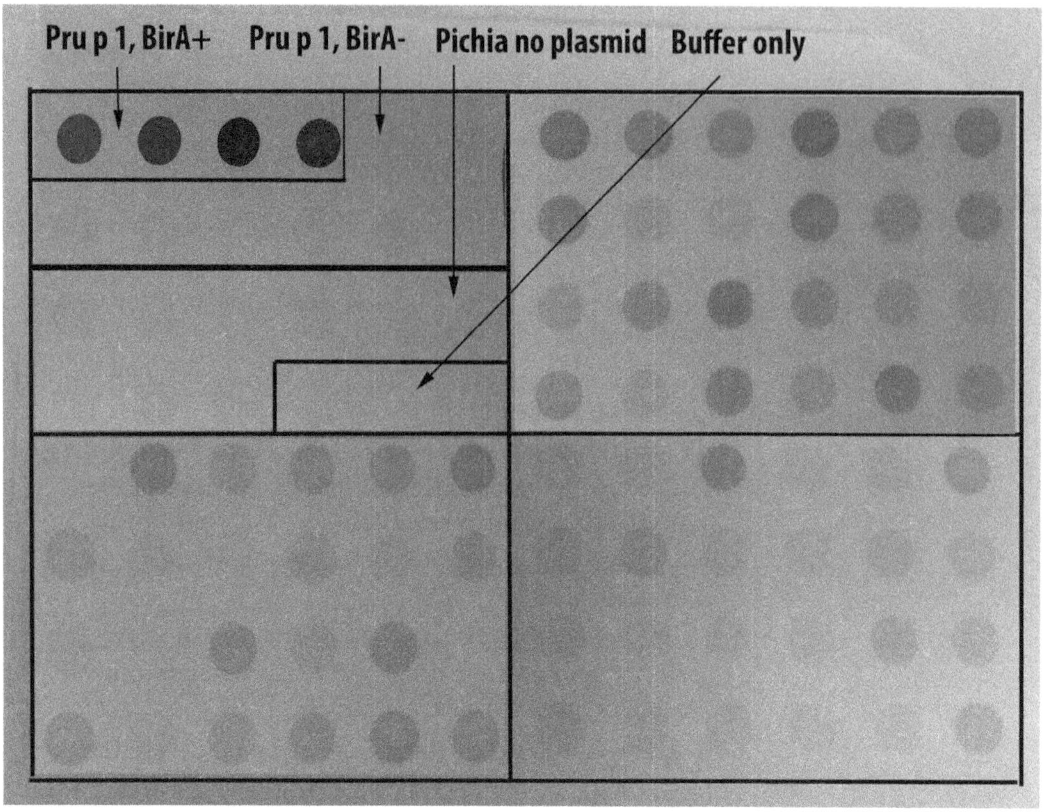

Fig. 1 Representative screening of 24-well expression plates after methanol induction. After induction for 72 h the supernatants were dot blotted into PVDF membrane and probed with avidin-Alkaline Phosphatase. Pru p 1, a peach allergen was used as positive control. No to very low expression of Pru p 1 was detected in the absence of BirA. The other three panels are representative expression of different scFv clones under the BirA+ background. The selection of the higher expressers is carried out visually

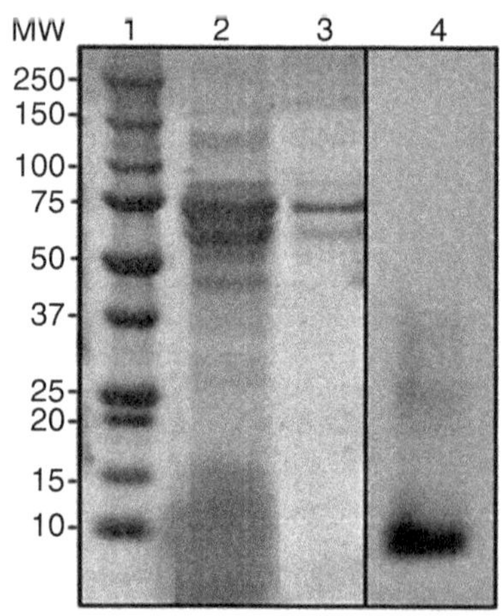

Fig. 2 SDS-PAGE and Western Blot of the biotinylated protein Pru p 3. *Lane 1* shows pre-stained SDS-PAGE molecular weight standards; *Lane 2* shows Pru p 3 supernatant extract; *Lane 3* shows Pru p 3 supernatant diluted 1:10; *Lane 4* shows Western Blot of Pru p 3 supernatant diluted 1:10 using Streptavidin-AP as detection in a 1:1000 dilution

4 Notes

1. The Reverse Transcriptase enzyme is substituted with water (−RT) to control for any genomic contamination in our RNA samples as well as other reaction components. RNA denaturation is carried out at 70 °C for 5 min and then on ice for 1 min. Random primers or specific gene primers can be used at this stage.
2. More information and tips for the primer design can be found in the INVITROGEN pPICZ manual.
3. Midori Green Dye is a safer replacement for the ethidium bromide. Mix samples and DNA markers with Midori Green Direct stain at 1:10 (dye:samples) dilution rate. If you expect only one or few DNA bands in a lane do not use more than 0.5 μL Midori Green Direct per sample even if you use more than 5 μL sample volume. If you apply DNA ladders or samples with a lot of bands use 1 μL of Midori Green Direct. After the electrophoresis, view the results on the FastGene Blue LED Illuminator.
4. For the ligation reaction use half of the recommended amount, i.e. 0.5 μL of TOPO vector, 0.5 μL of Salt solution, and 2 μL of purified PCR product. Incubate the maximum recommended time.
5. DyNazyme II DNA Polymerase diluted and added separately after the second cycle in a conventional hot-start procedure. We find that way give us better results. By using M13 external primers, the absence of ligated band will result in a 100–120 bp product so the successful amplification can be easily monitored.
6. On the step where applying the supernatant that contains the plasmid DNA into the QIAGEN-tip filter, pass it through a Whatman paper first. This is to make sure that the tip will not be blocked from any precipitation that might be leftover in supernatant.
7. We use PCR machine for all the incubation reactions.
8. BirA Pichia cells contain the *E. coli* biotinylation enzyme that will recognize the C-terminal Tag sequence in the construct. Dissolve cell pellet in a suitable volume of cold (4 °C) sterile 1 M sorbitol, depending on the size of cell pellet.
9. We use that 96-well plate as a backup plate by adding Glycerol at final concentration of 20%. The plates are then stored at −80 °C.
10. The dot blots are carried out in duplicates, with one dot from neat supernatant and another diluted 100× in PBS [16]. The dot blot step is essential to this procedure as it ensures that the highest expresser clones are selected.

11. We find that it is best to prepare this fresh each time.
12. Streptavidin Alkaline Phosphatase is used for the detection of biotinylated molecules.
13. LDS sample buffer is used to prepare protein samples for denaturing gel electrophoresis. Heat the samples at 70 °C for 10 min and make sure there is a hole on the top of the lid to avoid any lid explosion from the high temperature.
14. NuPAGE® Antioxidant is added to the running buffer in the upper (cathode) buffer chamber when performing protein gel electrophoresis under reducing conditions.

References

1. Cai H, Chen L, Wan L et al (2009) High-level expression of a functional humanized anti-CTLA4 single-chain variable fragment antibody in Pichia pastoris. Appl Microbiol Biotechnol 82(1):41–48
2. Cregg JM, Cereghino JL, Shi JY et al (2000) Recombinant protein expression in Pichia pastoris. Mol Biotechnol 16(1):23–52
3. Ellis SB, Brust PF, Koutz PJ et al (1985) Isolation of alcohol oxidase and 2 other methanol regulatable genes from the yeast pichia-pastoris. Mol Cell Biol 5(5): 1111–1121
4. Koutz P, Davis GR, Stillman C et al (1989) Structural comparison of the pichia-pastoris alcohol oxidase genes. Yeast 5(3):167–177
5. Tschopp JF, Brust PF, Cregg JM et al (1987) Expression of the lacz gene from 2 methanol-regulated promoters in pichia-pastoris. Nucleic Acids Res 15(9):3859–3876
6. Tschopp JF, Sverlow G, Kosson R et al (1987) High-level secretion of glycosylated invertase in the methylotrophic yeast, pichia-pastoris. Bio-Technol 5(12):1305–1308
7. Beckett D, Kovaleva E, Schatz PJ (1999) A minimal peptide substrate in biotin holoenzyme synthetase-catalyzed biotinylation. Protein Sci 8(4):921–929
8. Cull MG, Schatz PJ (2000) Biotinylation of proteins in vivo and in vitro using small peptide tags. Methods Enzymol 326:430–440. doi:10.1016/S0076-6879(00)26068-0
9. Chapman-Smith A, Mulhern TD, Whelan F et al (2001) The C-terminal domain of biotin protein ligase from E-coli is required for catalytic activity. Protein Sci 10(12):2608–2617
10. Predonzani A, Arnoldi F, Lopez-Requena A et al (2008) In vivo site-specific biotinylation of proteins within the secretory pathway using a single vector system. BMC Biotechnol 8:41. doi:10.1186/1472-6750-8-41
11. Scholle MD, Kriplani U, Pabon A et al (2006) Mapping protease substrates by using a biotinylated phage substrate library. Chembiochem 7(5):834–838
12. Thie H, Binius S, Schirrmann T et al (2009) Multimerization domains for antibody phage display and antibody production. N Biotechnol 26(6):314–321
13. de la Cruz S, Cubillos-Zapata C, Lopez-Calleja IM et al (2015) Isolation of recombinant antibody fragments (scFv) by phage display technology for detection of almond allergens in food products. Food Control 54:322–330
14. de la Cruz S, Alcocer M, Madrid R et al (2016) Production of in vivo biotinylated scFv specific to almond (*Prunus dulcis*) proteins by recombinant Pichia pastoris. J Biotechnol 227:112–119
15. Cregg JM and Russell KA (1998) Transformation, in Methods in Molecular Biology™; Pichia protocols. In: D.R. Higgins and J.M. Cregg (eds). pp. 27–39
16. Arbulu S, Jimenez JJ, Gutiez L et al (2015) Cloning and expression of synthetic genes encoding the broad antimicrobial spectrum bacteriocins SRCAM 602, OR-7, E-760, and L-1077, by Recombinant Pichia pastoris. Biomed Res Int 015:767183

Part II

Food Allergen Discovery, Detection, and Quantification

Chapter 5

2D-Electrophoresis and Immunoblotting in Food Allergy

Galina Grishina, Luda Bardina, and Alexander Grishin

Abstract

Two-dimensional polyacrylamide gel electrophoresis (2DE) and Western immunoblotting have proven to be invaluable and fundamental techniques for comprehensive characterization of food allergens. Here, we describe and discuss detailed protocols used in our studies on identification of allergenic proteins in shrimp, sesame, hazelnut, and pistachio.

Key words Food allergen, Proteomics, 2D electrophoresis, Immunoblotting, Hazelnut, Pistachio

1 Introduction

In the last two decades, food allergies have been increasingly important health concern worldwide [1, 2]. Identification and characterization of food allergens are essential for understanding mechanisms, improving diagnostic and prognosis of the disease and for assessing food safety. A remarkable effort made by many research teams including ours has yielded in identification at molecular level of more than 600 food allergens with over 200 officially registered by the allergen nomenclature subcommittee at International Union of Immunological Societies (IUIS) (http://www.allergen.org).

Owing to complexity of food products, investigation of food allergens has always required implementation of a multistep procedure involving a variety of separation and analytical methods including immuno-assays (enzyme-linked immunosorbent assay (ELISA) and immunoblotting), gel electrophoresis and isoelectric focusing, liquid chromatography, molecular cloning, protein and nucleic acid sequencing, and introduced later on mass spectroscopy. While most of these techniques have been extensively used since pioneering studies, overall approach and methodology for identification and characterization of food allergens have remarkably changed over the last decades [3–12]. Introduction of advanced high-resolution mass spectrometry, improved bioinformatics tools and highly efficient separation techniques has widened experimental horizons and

Jing Lin and Marcos Alcocer (eds.), *Food Allergens: Methods and Protocols*, Methods in Molecular Biology, vol. 1592,
DOI 10.1007/978-1-4939-6925-8_5, © Springer Science+Business Media LLC 2017

provided a platform for large-scale proteomics-based research of food allergens. For more discussion on application of proteomics methodology in food allergen studies and on basics of individual techniques, we would like to refer you to a wealth of recent excellent reviews, tutorials, and books [8–12]. In this chapter, we are focusing on detailed procedure of two-dimensional polyacrylamide gel electrophoresis under denaturing conditions and Western blot analysis which have been extensively used for identification and characterization of food allergens in many laboratories including ours ([7], and references in [13–21]).

High-resolution modification of 2D-PAGE using denaturing conditions in both dimensions has been a powerful tool for analysis of complex protein mixture from biological samples since it was introduced by Patric O'Farell in 1975 [22]. This technique allows separation of hundreds to thousands of proteins in gel and has been recognized over the years as robust and fundamental method in protein studies. However, there are well-understood built-in limitations of 2-DE including low reproducibility, difficulties in separation of hydrophobic proteins and resolving basic proteins with pI above 7, low dynamic range and protein losses in different steps of the workflow [11, 12, 23]. Early days low reproducibility caused by instabilities of the pH gradients was overcome later on with introduction of immobilized pH gradients (IPG) which also allow using narrow range pH gradients for more accurate analysis of closely arrayed protein spots [11, 12, 23]. Furthermore, non-equilibrium pH gel electrophoresis (NEPHGE) techniques have been developed to resolve proteins with high pI (≥7) which cannot be separated by conventional isoelectrofocusing [11, 12, 23]. At the same time, while there are approaches to address difficulties in separation of hydrophobic proteins by IEF and low dynamic range, these two remain unsolved built in limitations of the method [11, 12, 23]. Despite of these technical drawbacks, 2-DE continues to be one of the best methods suitable for discovery phase of research on proteome. Furthermore, 2-DE coupled with downstream Western immunoblotting and mass spectroscopy remains powerful and essential approach in proteomics.

In the next sections, detailed protocols for 2-DE and immunoblotting are described. Combination of these methods was instrumental in our work on identification and characterization of novel allergenic proteins from shrimp, sesame, hazelnut, and pistachio nuts [16, 17, 19, 20]. We made use of commercially available ready-to-use immobilized pH gradient (IPG) strips and pre-cast polyacrylamide mini-gels followed by immunoblotting with sera from subjects with confirmed sensitization to hazelnut and pistachio. Final identification of each protein spot was done by mass spectroscopy and by internal Edman sequencing.

Recently, detailed outline of 2-DE and Western blotting procedures have been described ([7, 23], for example). While the already published protocols and the one discussed below are similar in many aspects, there are differences as well. We hope that all this information should be helpful to researchers in designing procedure most suitable for their goals.

2 Materials

Prepare all solutions using ultrapure water (preferably MilliQ quality or similar) and analytical grade reagents. All reagents should be prepared and stored at room temperature unless indicated otherwise.

2.1 IEF

1. Reagent 2, lyophilized (Bio-Rad). Add 6 mL of water to lyophilized Reagent 2, dissolve by gentle mixing. Make 1 mL aliquots in 1.5 mL polypropylene tubes. Store aliquots at −80 °C.
2. 200 mM of Tributylphosphine (TBP) stock solution, stored at −20 °C (*see* **Note 1**).
3. 7 cm IPG gel strips with immobilized linear pH gradient: broad range, 3–10 and narrow range, 4–7 and 5–8 (Bio-Rad). Strips are stored at −20 °C. Take appropriate number of strips from the freezer and bring them to room temperature.
4. Rehydration Buffer: Reagent 2 containing 2 mM TBP (*see* **Notes 1** and **2**).
5. Protein extract prepared in 1× phosphate buffered saline (PBS) with protease inhibitor cocktail.
6. 0.5 M of Dithiothreitol (DTT) stock solution (*see* **Note 2**).
7. Electrode wicks (Bio-Rad).
8. Tweezers to handle IPG strips.
9. Mineral oil (any PCR quality oil).
10. The focusing tray (Bio-Rad).
11. Protean IEF cell (Bio-Rad).

2.2 SDS PAGE and Transfer

1. SDS PAGE running buffer: Make 1 L of 1× running buffer from 20× stock MES NuPAGE buffer. Add 50 mL of 20× running buffer to 1 L cylinder and bring up to 1 L with water.
2. Precast NuPAGE gradient (4–12%) Bis-Tris ZOOM gels (Invitrogen).
3. 1 M Tris–HCl (pH 8.8): Add about 400 mL water to a glass beaker. Weigh 157.6 g of Tris–HCl and transfer to a beaker with water. Mix and adjust pH with NaOH. Top up to 500 mL with water; filter the solution by using any 500 mL Filter System; use in the next step.

4. 2D Equilibration buffer stock: 6 M Urea, 2% SDS, 0.375 M Tris–HCl, pH 8.8, 20% Glycerol. Weigh 80 g of urea and dissolve it in about 200 mL of water in a glass beaker by mixing. Add to Urea solution 10 g of SDS, 182.5 mL of 1 M Tris–HCl stock solution, 100 mL of glycerol and mix. Transfer the buffer into 500 mL cylinder and adjust the volume to 500 mL. Filter Equilibration buffer by using any 500 mL sterile unit.
5. 2D Equilibration buffer I: 6 M Urea, 2% SDS, 0.375 M Tris–HCl, pH 8.8, 20% Glycerol, 5 mM TBP; usually prepared immediately prior to use (*see* **Notes 2** and **4**).
6. Iodoacetamide (optional, *see* **Note 3**).
7. NuPAGE LDC Sample buffer (4×) (Invitrogen).
8. 2D Equilibration buffer II: 1× NuPAGE Sample buffer.
9. SeeBlue Plus2 Prestained Standard (Invitrogen or equivalent).
10. Disposable rehydration/equilibration tray (Bio-Rad).
11. SimplyBlue Protein Stain.
12. Heat Block (water bath) at 70 °C.
13. XCell *SureLock*™ Mini-Cell system with Blot Module and Blotting Pads.
14. Methanol.
15. NuPAGE® MES 20× Transfer buffer. Make 1 L of transfer buffer by adding 50 mL of 20× stock solution and 200 mL methanol (20% methanol for 2 gels) to 750 mL deionized water.
16. Immobilon-P transfer membrane, PVDF, 0.45 μm (Millipore) or similar quality.
17. Whatman No. 3 Filter paper.
18. Plastic container.
19. Power Supply.

2.3 Immunoblotting

1. Phosphate buffered saline (PBS; 10× and 1×).
2. 1× PBS containing 0.05% Tween-20 (PBST).
3. Bovine serum albumin (BSA) grade V.
4. Antibody dilution buffer: 10% normal goat serum (NGS), 1% BSA in PBST. Prepare 500 mL of antibody dilution buffer: Dissolve 5 g BSA in 400 mL of PBST, add 50 mL NGS and adjust the volume to 500 mL with PBST. Filter the buffer by using sterile filter unit. Make 45 mL aliquots in 50 mL conical tubes and store at −20 °C (*see* **Note 4**).
5. 0.05 M Tris (pH 9.6): Dissolve 6.05 g of Tris-base in 400 mL of water in a glass beaker. Mix and adjust pH with ~10 M HCl. Transfer the solution into the cylinder and adjust the volume to 500 mL.

6. Phosphatase substrate BCIP/NBT.
7. Kodak X-OMAT Imagine Film.
8. Cassette with mounted intensifying screen on both sides (*see* **Note 5**).

2.4 Antigens and Conjugates

1. Subject' serum is diluted five to twenty times depending on the level of antigen-specific IgE in diluent solution. Choice of secondary antibody (*see* **Note 6**).
2. Iodine-125-labeled goat anti-human IgE antibody.
3. Phosphatase-conjugated goat anti-human IgE antibody.

3 Methods

All procedures are performed at room temperature unless otherwise specified. The following protocol was optimized for our specific research projects.

To identify all potential allergenic proteins, protein extracts should be first separated on IPG gel strips with broad range of pH. Then resolve proteins by molecular weights on SDS PAGE and transfer to ImmobilonP membranes (Figs. 1 and 2). Identify the allergens by immunolabeling of the separated proteins with

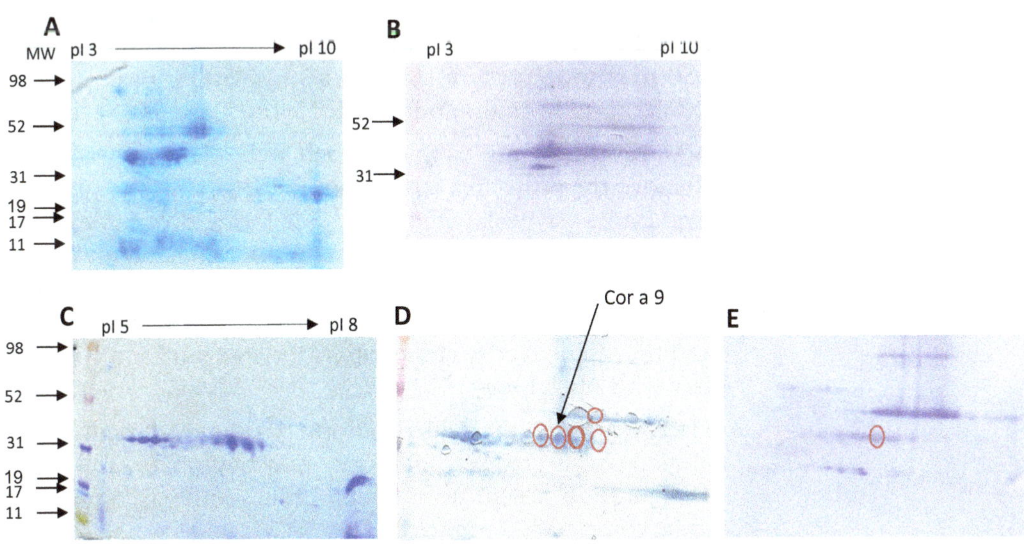

Fig. 1 2D Proteomics map of hazelnut proteins. 50 μg of the extract was first separated at broad pH range (3–10) and stained with Colloidal Blue stain for total protein analysis (**a**). The transferred proteins were immunolabeled with serum pool of five subjects to identify the clusters of allergenic proteins (**b**). For identification of the individual allergens, the extract was separated at narrow pH (5–8) range. The gel was stained with Coomassie Blue stain (**c**). The membrane with transferred protein was stained with Amido Black stain to confirm the efficiency of the transfer (**d**). Immunolabeling with individual patient serum is shown (**e**). Alkaline Phosphatase-conjugated secondary antibody diluted five thousand times was used for immunolabeling

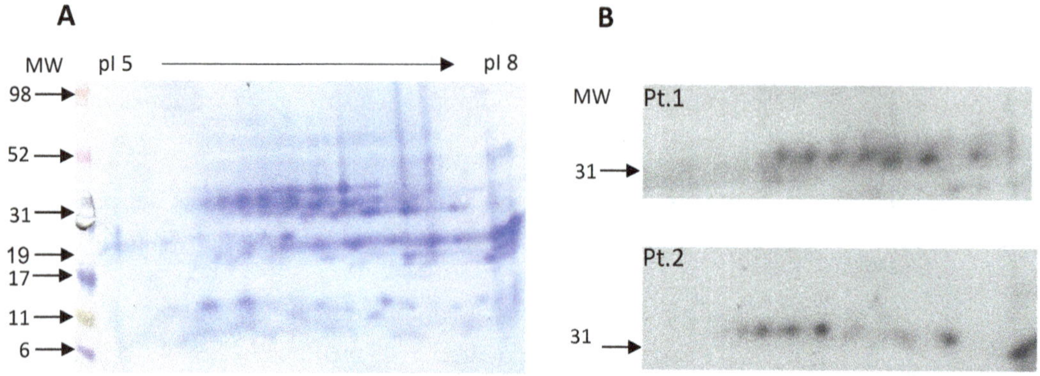

Fig. 2 Two-dimensional proteomic map of pistachio proteins separated at narrow pH range. The membrane was stained with Coomassie Blue stain (**a**) and immunolabeled with two representative patients (**b**). For identification of pistachio allergens, iodinated secondary antibody was used at dilution factor of 5

the pool of diluted sera from five to ten allergic subjects. For identification of the individual proteins use IPG gel strips with immobilized narrow pH range. Two strips needs to be tested for validation of replicability.

3.1 Isoelectric Focusing

In our isoelectrofocusing procedure, we always use the rehydration method with sample.

1. Prepare the sample in Rehydration buffer enough for two to four IPG strips. Sample loading volume per strip should be at 150 μL. Add no more than 10–15 μL (50 μg of protein) of extract to Rehydration buffer (*see* **Notes 7** and **10**).
2. Add 150 μL of the sample to each well of the focusing tray. Remove the protective cover from the IPG strip and place the strip into a tray well with the gel side facing down. Make sure that the strips are positioned in the focusing tray in correct polarity. Wet the strip by sliding it through the rehydration solution. Slide the damp electrode wicks between electrodes and the strip. Overlay each strip with mineral oil and cover the tray with the lid.
3. Place the tray on the Peltier platform. Use a preset method with linear voltage gradient and active rehydration. It takes about 18 h for the isoelectric focusing procedure with rehydration step to be completed (*see* **Note 8**).
4. Upon completion of the isoelectrofocusing step transfer the IPG strips into equilibration tray or plastic container with the gel side facing up and keep at 4 °C for a short time (1–2 days). For longer storage, transfer the strips to −20 °C freezer.

3.2 SDS PAGE and Transfer

Always wear gloves and use tweezers when working with ImmobilonP transfer membrane.

1. Take needed number of IPG strips (add two more strips for replicability test, which will not be used for immunoblotting) from the freezer, place into equilibration tray and warm up to room temperature.
2. Prepare 2D equilibration buffer I for both strips (enough to use twice). Mix 25 μL of TBP stock with 975 μL of stock of 2D equilibration buffer and add about 450 μL to each strip. The buffer should cover the strip. Place the tray on the rocking table for 10 min, then replace equilibration buffer I in the tray with a fresh aliquot of the same solution and equilibrate for another 10 min.
3. Transfer the strips into the same volume of equilibration buffer II and continue the incubation for 10 min. While the strips are being incubated in equilibration buffers I and II, prepare NuPAGE Bis-Tris ZOOM gels, 1× NuPAGE running buffer and 1× transfer buffer (*see* **Note 9**).
4. Take the strip from the sample buffer, cut plastic ends of the strip and load the strip on the gel. Load 5 μL of Plus2 standard in the single well and electrophorese at 200 V until the dye front has reached the bottom of the gel (Fig. 1a, c, *see* **Note 10**).
5. Start preparing membrane, filter paper, and sponges for transfer when the dye front is about 1 inch from the bottom of the gel. Place sponges in the container, add transfer buffer, enough to cover, and use roller to remove any trapped air bubbles. Wet ImmobilonP membrane in methanol for 15 s, then rinse in water for 2 min and leave membrane in transfer buffer until the gel is ready (5–10 min).
6. Following SDS PAGE, immediately remove the gels from the running buffer. Open the plates with the help of a spatula. Rinse the gel in transfer buffer and assemble the gel membrane sandwich. Transfer two gels in one Blot Module at 30 V for 1 h.
7. After transfer is completed, rinse ImmobilonP blots in 100% methanol for 5 min.
8. Transfer all blots onto filter paper to remove the excess of the liquid.
9. Leave the blots between filter paper to dry overnight or over the weekend (*see* **Note 11**).

3.3 Immonublotting

For identification of allergenic proteins, modified rapid immunodetection procedure suggested by Millipore were followed. To avoid any unspecific binding, the membranes have to be completely dry before starting immunolabeling with subjects' sera.

1. Bring the antibody dilution buffer to room temperature. Keep subject's and control sera on wet ice (*see* **Note 10**).

2. Dilute serum pool in antibody dilution buffer according to the specific IgE (sIgE) levels as follows: sera with sIgE levels at <5 kU/L were diluted four times, with sIgE at 5–10 kU/L-five times, with sIgE at 10–20 kU/L-ten times, and with above 20 kU/L of sIgE-twenty times. As a control for unspecific binding, negative control serum diluted four times should be used (*see* **Note 12**).

3. Place each blot in a dish and add diluted pool or individual serum enough to cover the blots.

4. Incubate the blots with agitation for 1 h. The solution should move freely across the surface on the membrane. At the end of the incubation with sera, prepare a dilution of the secondary antibody.

5. Remove antibody and add PBS to the blots.

6. Wash blots with PBS four times for 10–15 s each.

7. Add phosphatase-conjugated secondary antibody at 5000 times dilution and incubate with agitation for 45 min. [^{125}I]-labeled secondary antibody is to be used at five times dilution.

8. Repeat the washes as in **steps 5** and **6**. For phosphatase-conjugated secondary antibody, follow **steps 9a–12a**. For [^{125}I]-labeled secondary antibody, skip **steps 9a–12a** and follow **steps 9b–13b**.

9a. Aspirate PBS and rinse the blots in 50 mM (pH 9.6) Tris buffer for 1 min.

10a. Add Phosphatase substrate (BCIP/NBT) enough to cover the membrane and leave blots in the substrate for 5–10 min.

11a. As soon as the protein bands are visible on the blot with negative control serum, rinse the membranes in water and dry the blots with filter paper.

12a. Analyze images of the blots on any available Imaging System (Fig. 1b, e).

9b. If using [125I]-labeled secondary antibody, after **step 8** from above: Remove the blots from PBS; dry the excess of the liquid with filter paper; mount the membranes on the new sheet of filter paper; wrap in clear plastic film.

10b. Place the wrapped blots in the cassette. In the dark room place Kodak X-OMAT Imagine Film on the blots.

11b. Insert the cassette in the light protective bag and leave the cassette at −80 °C for 2–3 h or overnight (*see* **Note 13**).

12b. Before developing the film, bring the cassette to room temperature. Usually it takes about 2 h.

13b. Develop the film (Fig. 2b, *see* **Notes 6** and **13**).

4 Notes

1. TBP is a toxic reagent and should be always opened under the fume hood. The reagent is not stable at lower concentrations. Any buffer containing TBP has to be prepared immediately before use.
2. TBP could be replaced with DTT in Rehydration and Equilibration buffers. Prepare 0.5 M stock solution: Dissolve 0.78 g of DTT in 10 mL of water, filter through 0.22 μm syringe filter, make 0.5 mL aliquots and store the tubes at −20 °C.
3. We have tested Rehydration buffer prepared with DTT at concentrations 0.05, 0.075, and 0.1 M. With 0.05 M DTT in the solution, the proteins were well separated. However, protein extracts separation showed better resolution in TBP containing buffer.
4. Leave one or two aliquots of the diluent in the refrigerator if using it next day.
5. The [^{125}I]-labeled antibody has very low specific radioactivity. Therefore, intensifying screens have to be placed on both sides of the cassette.
6. Advantages of using [^{125}I]-secondary antibody are clean Negative Controls and generation of multiple X-Ray images with various intensity of exposure. Disadvantages are the cost, requirement of Lab License for Isotope use and limited shelf life (about 2 months).
7. Salt concentration in the sample is most critical during electrofocusing procedure. The volume of the extract mixed with Rehydration buffer should be less than 10% of the total sample volume. The protein concentration in the extract loaded on IPG strips has to be at 5 mg/mL or higher. Use any desalting/concentrating columns with cut off ≥ 3 kDa to concentrate the extract. It is convenient to precipitate the proteins and then dissolve the pellet in Rehydration buffer. In our experiment we used “Perfect Focus” kit from Geno Technology Inc. for protein precipitation.
8. We found that it is practical to start the separation of the proteins in first dimension early afternoon. Then on next day morning, IPG strips are ready for equilibration and proteins separated in 1D would be loaded on SDS PAGE gels. First of all it is a must to validate IEF for replicability. Use two strips

for the second dimension and stain the gels with protein stain. Then the proteins from the rest of the strips could be transferred onto the membranes.

9. If DTT is used instead of TBP in Equilibration buffer, two buffers have to be prepared and used -I-1 and I-2. Equilibrate the IPG strips for 10 min in each. To make up I-1 buffer add 25 μL of 0.5 M DTT to 975 μL of 2D stock equilibration buffer (enough for two strips). Buffer I-2 contains 0.135 M of Iodoacetamide (25 μg per 1 mL of buffer). It is important to equilibrate IPG strips in the buffer with DTT first followed by incubation in the Iodoacetamide containing buffer.
10. It is important at the beginning to separate the extract at broad pH range to see the map of all proteins and stain 2 gels for replicability of isoelectrofocusing. Coomassie Blue protein stain is less sensitive than Colloidal Blue stain but it is easy to use. In our experiments, we used Colloidal Blue stain for staining the extract separated at 3–10 pH range. Then the proteins were transferred onto the membrane and tested with serum pool from five patients to identify the clusters of allergens (Fig. 1a, b). For identification of individual allergenic proteins, extract was isoelectrofocused at narrow pH range. Membrane with transferred proteins could be stained with Amido Black or Coomassie Blue stain (Figs. 1d and 2a). Sensitivity of both stains are similar.
11. This is an important step before starting the immunolabeling, which helps to avoid unspecific binding to separated proteins. In addition, put a heavy weight (book or catalog usually works well) on the filter paper/membrane sandwich to keep the blots flat. The membranes with transferred proteins could be stored between filter paper up to 1 month at room temperature.
12. In our immunolabeling experiments, we used sera from non-food allergic subjects as a control for unspecific binding.
13. In case specific IgE of tested sera are very high, keep the cassette at room temperature for 2–3 h, develop the film, then put a new film and leave it overnight in the freezer. Always include negative control serum in each immunolabeling experiment.

References

1. Elizur A, Katz Y (2016) Timing of allergen exposure and the development of food allergy: treating before the horse is out of the barn. Curr Opin Allergy Clin Immunol. doi:10.1097/ACI.0000000000000243
2. Sicherer SH, Sampson HA (2014) Food allergy: epidemiology, pathogenesis, diagnosis, and treatment. J Allergy Clin Immunol 133 (2):291–307; quiz 308. doi:10.1016/j.jaci.2013.11.020. [pii]:S0091–6749(13)01836–8
3. Burks AW, Williams LW, Connaughton C, Cockrell G, O'Brien TJ, Helm RM (1992) Identification and characterization of a second major peanut allergen, Ara h II, with use of the sera of patients with atopic dermatitis and positive peanut challenge. J Allergy Clin Immunol 90(6 Pt 1):962–9694
4. Vallier P, DeChamp C, Valenta R, Vial O, Deviller P (1992) Purification and characterization of an allergen from celery immuno-

chemically related to an allergen present in several other plant species. Identification as a profilin. Clin Exp Allergy 22(8):774–782

5. Eigenmann PA, Burks AW, Bannon GA, Sampson HA (1996) Identification of unique peanut and soy allergens in sera adsorbed with cross-reacting antibodies. J Allergy Clin Immunol 98(5 Pt 1):969–978 [pii]:S0091674996003156
6. Sanchez-Monge R, Blanco C, Diaz-Perales A, Collada C, Carrillo T, Aragoncillo C, Salcedo G (1999) Isolation and characterization of major banana allergens: identification as fruit class I chitinases. Clin Exp Allergy 29(5):673–680
7. Nakamura R, Teshima R (2014) Immunoproteomics analysis of food allergens. Methods Mol Biol 1072:725–735. doi:10.1007/978-1-62703-631-3_50
8. Di Girolamo F, Muraca M, Mazzina O, Lante I, Dahdah L (2015) Proteomic applications in food allergy: food allergenomics. Curr Opin Allergy Clin Immunol 15(3):259–266. doi:10.1097/ACI.0000000000000160
9. Cunsolo V, Muccilli V, Saletti R, Foti S (2014) Mass spectrometry in food proteomics: a tutorial. J Mass Spectrom 49(9):768–784. doi:10.1002/jms.3374
10. Kurien BT, Scofield RH (eds) (2015) Western blotting. Methods in molecular biology, vol 1312. Humana Press. doi:10.1007/978-1-4939-2694-7
11. Westermeier R (2014) Looking at proteins from two dimensions: a review on five decades of 2D electrophoresis. Arch Physiol Biochem 120(5):168–172. doi:10.3109/13813455.2014.945188
12. Magdeldin S, Enany S, Yoshida Y, Xu B, Zhang Y, Zureena Z, Lokamani I, Yaoita E, Yamamoto T (2014) Basics and recent advances of two dimensional-polyacrylamide gel electrophoresis. Clin Proteomics 11(1):16. doi:10.1186/1559-0275-11-161559-0275-11-16
13. Hird H, Pumphrey R, Wilson P, Sunderland J, Reece P (2000) Identification of peanut and hazelnut allergens by native two-dimensional gel electrophoresis. Electrophoresis 21(13):2678–2683. doi:10.1002/1522-2683(20000701)21:13<2678::AID-ELPS2678>3.0.CO;2-V
14. Park JW, Kang DB, Kim CW, koh SH, Yum HY, Kim KE, Hong CS, Lee KY (2000) Identification and characterization of the major allergens of buckwheat. Allergy 55(11):1035–1041
15. Sander I, Flagge A, Merget R, Halder TM, Meyer HE, Baur X (2001) Identification of wheat flour allergens by means of 2-dimensional immunoblotting. J Allergy Clin Immunol 107(5):907–913. doi:10.1067/mai.2001.113761. [pii]:S0091–6749(01)34567–0
16. Beyer K, Bardina L, Grishina G, Sampson HA (2002) Identification of sesame seed allergens by 2-dimensional proteomics and Edman sequencing: seed storage proteins as common food allergens. J Allergy Clin Immunol 110(1):154–159 [pii]:S0091674902000556
17. Beyer K, Grishina G, Bardina L, Grishin A, Sampson HA (2002) Identification of an 11S globulin as a major hazelnut food allergen in hazelnut-induced systemic reactions. J Allergy Clin Immunol 110(3):517–523 [pii]:S009167490200146X
18. Yu CJ, Lin YF, Chiang BL, Chow LP (2003) Proteomics and immunological analysis of a novel shrimp allergen, Pen m 2. J Immunol 170(1):445–453
19. Ayuso R, Grishina G, Bardina L, Carrillo T, Blanco C, Ibanez MD, Sampson HA, Beyer K (2008) Myosin light chain is a novel shrimp allergen, Lit v 3. J Allergy Clin Immunol 122(4):795–802. doi:10.1016/j.jaci.2008.07.023 [pii]:S0091-6749(08)01352-3
20. Ahn K, Bardina L, Grishina G, Beyer K, Sampson HA (2009) Identification of two pistachio allergens, Pis v 1 and Pis v 2, belonging to the 2S albumin and 11S globulin family. Clin Exp Allergy 39(6):926–934. doi:10.1111/j.1365-2222.2009.03259.x [pii]:CEA3259
21. Krishnan HB, Kim WS, Jang S, Kerley MS (2009) All three subunits of soybean beta-conglycinin are potential food allergens. J Agric Food Chem 57(3):938–943. doi:10.1021/jf802451g10.1021/jf802451g
22. O'Farrell PH (1975) High resolution two-dimensional electrophoresis of proteins. J Biol Chem 250(10):4007–4021
23. Magdeldin S (ed) (2012) Gel electrophoresis–principles and basics. InTech, Rijeka, Croatia

Chapter 6

Two-Dimensional Electrophoresis and Identification by Mass Spectrometry

Fernando de la Cuesta, Gloria Alvarez-Llamas, and Maria G. Barderas

Abstract

Two-dimensional electrophoresis (2-DE) is a classical separation technique for complex protein mixtures based on a first-separation step by isoelectric point (pI) followed by SDS-PAGE. Due to its high resolving power (including protein isoforms) and the capability to display post-translational modifications, 2-DE has been the technique of choice in many studies focused in characterizing allergens. In this chapter, we describe a standard protocol which enables efficient protein separation and subsequent protein identification by tandem mass spectrometry (MALDI-MS/MS).

Key words 2-DE, Two-dimensional electrophoresis, MALDI-TOF, Mass spectrometry, Allergens

1 Introduction

Two-dimensional electrophoresis (2-DE) is a classical technique able to provide an extended picture of the proteins present in the sample of interest. It is based on a first-separation step by protein isoelectric point, followed by a second separation by molecular weight (SDS-PAGE) [1]. The result is a protein map highly resolved where one spot usually contains a unique protein. Despite of the most recent appearance of mass spectrometry-based approaches for protein separations (LC-MS/MS) [2], 2-DE is still the technique of choice in many studies aimed at the characterization of allergens, particularly when SDS-PAGE protein separation does not provide sufficient resolution to guarantee a unique protein per gel band [3–5]. 2-DE has high resolution power to separate complex mixtures and proved capacity to identify up- or down-regulation in a biological context when combined with quantitative assays based on fluorescence labeling as DIGE [6]. Additionally, 2-DE allows displaying post-translational modifications (PTMs) as glycosylation, phosphorylation, oxidation, and nitrosylation. Main limitation of

Jing Lin and Marcos Alcocer (eds.), *Food Allergens: Methods and Protocols*, Methods in Molecular Biology, vol. 1592, DOI 10.1007/978-1-4939-6925-8_6, © Springer Science+Business Media LLC 2017

2-DE is the difficulty to study certain subsets of proteins which show impaired separation affecting subsequent MS identification, such as membrane proteins, proteins with isoelectric point higher than 11 or lower than 3, and proteins with molecular weight higher than 120 kDa or lower than 7 kDa.

The successful implementation of 2-DE in the laboratory demands a previous careful optimization of the experimental protocol. Sample preparation should guarantee an efficient protein extraction and subsequent removal of potential matrix interferents to ensure compatibility with the isoelectric focusing (IEF) step, otherwise resulting in a defective protein separation. Instrumental parameters (IEF program) should be set-up and optimum conditions should be adjusted for every sample type. Once proteins have been separated, bidimensional immunoblot may follow or direct protein identification from spots of interest by MALDI-MS/MS. In this case, the method of choice for protein spots visualization should be compatible with mass spectrometric analysis, and proteins have to be extracted from the gel spot and efficiently enzymatically digested. Resulting peptides are extracted from the gel and analyzed by mass spectrometry.

In this chapter, we describe a general procedure to carry out 2-DE analysis and protein identification by MALDI-MS/MS which can be applied to allergens characterization.

2 Materials

2.1 Equipment

2.1.1 Two-Dimensional Gel Electrophoresis

1. Electrophoresis apparatus (Protean isoelectric focusing (IEF) cell, PROTEAN II, Bio-Rad, Hercules, CA).
2. ReadyStrip immobilized pH gradient (IPG) 17 cm 4.0–7.0, 3.0–10.0, 6.0–9.0 (Bio-Rad).
3. Protean IEF cell (Bio-Rad).
4. Mili Q® System (Millipore, Bedford, MA).
5. Shaker.
6. Thermomixer compact.
7. Ultrasonic bath.
8. Glass plates 16 × 20 cm (Bio-Rad).
9. Reswelling cassette (Bio-Rad).
10. Clamps (Bio-Rad).
11. Scanner (DUO Scan Hid, Agfa-Geavaert, Marstel, Belgium).

2.1.2 Identification of Allergens by MS/ MS

1. ExQuest Spot Cutter.
2. 5424 Microcentrifuge.
3. Ettan Digester (GE Healthcare).
4. Speedvac vacuum concentrator.

5. MALDI plate (AB Sciex).
6. 4800 MALDI TOF/TOF Analyzer (AB Sciex).
7. 4000 Series Explorer Software (AB Sciex).
8. GPS Explorer Software (AB Sciex).

2.2 Reagents

2.2.1 Two-Dimensional Gel Electrophoresis

1. Bradford protein assay (Bio-Rad).
2. Sample solubilization buffer: 7 M Urea, 2 M Thiourea, 4% CHAPS, 1% dithiothreitol (DTT). To prepare 50 mL of solubilization buffer, dissolve 7.02 g of thiourea, 21.02 g of urea, and 2 g of CHAPS in deionized water and make up to 50 mL, stir, and filter. Sample solubilization buffer can be stored at −80 °C in small aliquots of 0.5 mL. Never refreeze.
3. Rehydration solution: 8 M urea, 0.5–4% CHAPS, 20–100 mM DTT, 0.5–2% Pharmalyte. It is important not to heat urea solutions above 37 °C in order to reduce the risk of protein carbamylation.
4. Equilibration buffer: 8 M urea, 1.5 M Tris–HCl, 87% glycerol (99% purity), 2% sodium dodecyl sulfate (SDS) (97% purity), bromophenol blue. During the first equilibration step, 100 mg of DTT is added to 10 mL equilibration buffer. In the second step, 250 mg of iodoacetamide is added to 10 mL equilibration buffer.
5. Acrylamide/*bis*-acrylamide solution: Acrylamide/*bis*-acrylamide 30%. Stir for 10 min, filter, and fill up to 100 mL with deionized water.
6. Ammonium persulfate solution: 10% Ammonium persulfate (98% purity).
7. Phosphated-buffered saline (PBS) buffer pH 7.2: NaCl (99.5% purity), KCl (99% purity), Na_2HPO_4 (99.5% purity), KH_2PO_4 (99% purity).
8. Fixation solution: 30% Ethanol (99.8% purity), 5% acetic acid.

2.2.2 Identification of Allergens by MS/MS

1. 100 mM ammonium bicarbonate (99% purity; Scharlau) in water. Make daily and discard after use.
2. DTT solution: 10 mM dithiothreitol (DTT) (Sigma-Aldrich) in 100 mM ammonium bicarbonate. Prepare shortly before use.
3. Iodoacetamide solution: 55 mM iodoacetamide (Sigma-Aldrich) in 100 mM ammonium bicarbonate. Prepare shortly before use.
4. Methanol (gradient, HPLC grade, Scharlau).
5. Acetonitrile (gradient, HPLC grade, Scharlau).
6. Trypsin buffer: Modified porcine trypsin (sequencing grade; Promega) 20 ng/μL in 20 mM ammonium bicarbonate. Prepare shortly before use.
7. Trifluoroacetic acid (99.5% purity; Sigma Aldrich).

3 Methods

3.1 Two-Dimensional Gel Electrophoresis

3.1.1 Sample Preparation

1. Solubilize 300 μg of protein in 200 μL of solubilization buffer and freeze at −80 °C until use (*see* **Note 1**).
2. Sonicate the protein mixture for 1 min at room temperature.
3. Heat the protein sample at 80 °C for 5 min.
4. Cool the sample at room temperature.
5. Incubate the protein mixture with 200 μL of Benzonase to eliminate nucleic acids.
6. Incubate again for 50 min at room temperature.
7. Quantify the protein content using the Bradford method [7].
8. Dilute 200–250 μL in rehydration solution (350 μL final volume).

3.1.2 Sample Application

1. 250 μg of proteins are mixed with 350 μL of rehydration solution.
2. Pipet the entire sample containing rehydration solution into the groove of a swelling tray.
3. Peel off the protective cover sheets from the IPG Gel Strips (17 cm, pH 3.0–10.0, 4.0–7.0, 6.0–9.0, 6.0–11.0) and position them such that the gel of the strip is in contact with the sample (*see* **Note 2**).
4. Cover the IPG Gel Strips and the sample with mineral oil.

3.1.3 First Dimension: IEF Separation

IEF is performed in a Protean IEF Cell (Bio-Rad). The strips are actively rehydrated for 12 h at 30 V to enhance protein uptake and then the voltage is increased according to the following program:

1. 1 min at 50 V (ramping) for a total of 300 V.
2. 30 min at 300 V (ramping) for a total of 1000 V.
3. 1 h and 30 min at 1000 V (ramping) for a total of 5000 V.
4. 1 h. and 30 min at 5000 V (ramping) for a total of 29,000 V.

For strips in the 6.0–9.0, 6.0–11.0 pH range a different protocol is used:

1. 16 h of rehydration at 30 V.
2. 30 min at 500 V.
3. 1 h at 1000 V.
4. 30 min at 5000 V.
5. 8000 V for a total of 60,000 V.

3.1.4 Second Dimension: SDS-Polyacrylamide Gel Electrophoresis

A number of gel concentrations and gradients as well as different buffering systems can be used in the second dimension [8]. We perform SDS-polyacrylamide gel electrophoresis according to the

Laemmli system [9], as previously described [10], using a Protean II system (Bio-Rad). Prepare a 12.5% acrylamide gel. Perform the equilibration as follows:

1. Place the IPG Gel Strips in a clean cassette for equilibration. Add 5 mL of equilibration buffer with DTT and rock for 15–20 min on a shaker. After that, discard the equilibration buffer and rinse with deionized water.
2. Add 5 mL of equilibration buffer with iodoacetamide and equilibrate for another 15–20 min on a shaker. Finally rinse again with deionized water and put on a piece of filter paper to remove excess of equilibration buffer (*see* **Note 3**).

Transfer the equilibrated IPG gel strips onto the top of the SDS gel and run it at 25 mA/gel at 4°C.

3.1.5 Fixing Gels

Remove the gels from the apparatus and separate the glass plates and place them fixation solution overnight.

3.1.6 Staining

When gels are fixed, stain with Silver staining kit (GE-Healthcare) or with different reagents (Coomassie Blue (Bio-Rad), Sypro Ruby Protein Gel Staining (Thermo Fisher Scientific, etc.)).

3.2 Identification of Allergens by MS/MS

From Shevchenko et al. with modifications [11] (*see* **Note 4**).

1. Excise the positive band/s from the 1-DE gel or spot/s from the 2 DE gel (*see* **Note 5**).
2. Cut bands into 1 × 1 mm cubes to facilitate in-gel digestion.
3. Transfer gel pieces into a microcentrifuge tube or 96-well plate, spin them down in a bench-top microcentrifuge (*see* **Note 6**).

3.2.1 Destaining of Coomassie Blue Stained Bands and Spots

1. Cover gel pieces with 100 μL (*see* **Note 7**) of 50 mM ammonium bicarbonate, 50% acetonitrile (mix 1:1 100 mM ammonium bicarbonate and acetonitrile). Incubate under constant agitation for 30 min at room temperature. Remove supernatant. Repeat until gel pieces have been mostly destained of Coomassie blue (*see* **Note 8**).
2. Shrink gel pieces by adding 100 μL acetonitrile for 5 min. Gel pieces should look whitish.

3.2.2 Reduction and Alkylation

1. Incubate with 50 μL of DTT solution for 30 min at 37 °C in a thermomixer under constant agitation.
2. Remove DTT solution (*see* **Note 9**).
3. Add 100 μL of 100 mM ammonium bicarbonate to let DTT come out of the gel pieces, incubate for 5 min at room temperature under constant agitation.

4. Shrink gel pieces by adding 100 μL of acetonitrile for 5 min.
5. Incubate with 50 μL of iodoacetamide solution for 20 min at room temperature in the dark.
6. Remove iodoacetamide solution.
7. Add 100 μL of 100 mM ammonium bicarbonate to let iodoacetamide come out of the gel pieces, incubate for 5 min at room temperature under constant agitation.
8. Wash with 50 mM ammonium bicarbonate in 50% methanol for 5 min at room temperature under constant agitation.
9. Repeat gel shrinking by adding acetonitrile and dry in a Speedvac.

3.2.3 Trypsin Digestion

1. Add 50 μL of trypsin buffer, or as much as needed to cover all gel pieces.
2. Incubate at 37 °C overnight (*see* **Note 10**).

3.2.4 Elution of Peptides and MALDI-TOF/TOF

1. Extract peptides from gel pieces with 60% acetonitrile and 0.1% formic acid for 15 min at 37 °C under constant agitation.
2. Mix an aliquot of the trypsin digestion solution with an aliquot of α-cyano-4-hydroxycinnamic acid in 30% aqueous acetonitrile, 15% 2-propanol and 0.1% trifluoroacetic acid.
3. Deposit onto the MALDI plate and allow drying at room temperature.
4. Obtain MALDI-MS and MS/MS data in a MALDI TOF/TOF Analyzer (*see* **Note 11**).

4 Notes

1. Sample preparation and solubilization are crucial factors for the performance of the 2-DE technique. Protein complexes and aggregates should be completely disrupted in order to allow the appearance of all possible spots.
2. For the correct development of the first dimension, it is very important that when the strip is placed over the sample no bubbles are present.
3. DTT is used to facilitate the conversion of disulfide bonds to free sulfhydryl groups. Sulfhydryl groups are then alkylated with iodoacetamide (carboxiamidomethylation), since the reducing reaction is reversible and the re-formation of the disulfide bridges must be prevented.
4. Special care has to be taken in order to avoid contamination with dust and particularly hair and skin keratins. Wear gloves at all times, rinse or dispose gloves if in contact with uncleaned surfaces. Perform all manual procedures in a laminar flow hood.

5. For excising positive band/s from a 1-DE gel or spot/s from a 2-DE gel, an automated picker can be used or can be done manually if not available. For the latter, excise positive band/s from the 1-DE gel using a sterile scalpel. For excising spot/s from the 2-DE gel, a 100–1000 μL pipette tip can be used. Keep gels humid with double-distilled water during whole process. Carefully excise gel areas avoiding contamination with other bands or spots, which may result in misleading identification of potential allergen(s).
6. If in-gel digestion protocol is going to be performed in an automatic digester, gel pieces should not be smaller than 1 × 1 mm as they might be absorbed by the digester's suction tubes and get trapped, or clog pipette tips if doing manually.
7. The volumes specified during the whole protocol may be increased in order to cover all gel pieces.
8. Normally two washes of 30 min are enough to destain gel bands and spots. The majority of Coomassie blue has to be destained, but there is no problem if a bit is remaining.
9. Notice that most of the volume would have been absorbed by the dehydrated gel pieces.
10. After 30 min, check volume and add more trypsin buffer to cover entire gel pieces, if needed.
11. Analysis of mass data may be performed using the 4000 Series Explorer Software. MALDI-MS and MS/MS data are combined through the GPS Explorer Software to search a non-redundant protein database, such as Swiss-Prot or nrNCBI. Identification of allergens by MS/MS coming from positive bands excised after overlapping immunoblot and Coomassie blue-stained gels can result in identification of one or more top abundant proteins in the band. Bands from 1-DE gels (and sometimes 2-DE gel spots too if the extract is very complex) would normally contain more than one protein and special care has to be taken before affirming the identification of a novel allergen. Confirmation by additional experiments, such as inhibitory assays, is needed to prove these findings.

Acknowledgments

This work was supported by grants from the Instituto de Salud Carlos III (FIS PI070537, IF08/3667-1, PI11-02239, PI14/01917, PI11/01401, PI11/02432, PI13/01873, PI13/01746, PI13/01581, PI14/01650, PI14/01841) by PT13/0001/0013, IDCSalud (3371/002) and Redes Temáticas de Investigación Cooperativa (FONDOS FEDER, RD06/0014/1015, RD12/0042/0071).

References

1. Bruno B (2012) Two-dimensional gel electrophoresis (2-DE), gel electrophoresis—principles and basics. In: Sameh M (ed) InTech. doi: 10.5772/38312
2. Monaci L, Visconti A (2009) Mass spectrometry-based proteomics methods for analysis of food allergens. Trends Analyt Chem 28(5):581–591
3. Castro L, Crespo JF, Rodríguez J et al (2015) Immunoproteomic tools are used to identify masked allergens: Ole e 12, an allergenic isoflavone reductase from olive (*Olea europaea*) pollen. Biochim Biophys Acta 1854(12): 1871–1880
4. Abou Chakra OR, Sutra JP, Demey Thomas E et al (2012) Proteomic analysis of major and minor allergens from isolated pollen cytoplasmic granules. J Proteome Res 11(2):1208–1216
5. Perez-Gordo M, Cuesta-Herranz J, Maroto AS et al (2011) Identification of sole parvalbumin as a major allergen: study of cross-reactivity between parvalbumins in a Spanish fish-allergic population. Clin Exp Allergy 41(5):750–758
6. Unlü M, Morgan ME, Minden JS (1997) Difference gel electrophoresis: a single gel method for detecting changes in protein extracts. Electrophoresis 18(11):2071–2077
7. Ausubel FM, Brent R, Kingston RE et al (2005) Current Protocols in Molecular Biology, vol 10. John Wiley & Sons, New York, NY, pp 97–106
8. Gorg A, Weiss W, Dunn MJ (2004) Current two-dimensional electrophoresis technology for proteomics. Proteomics 4(12):3665–3685
9. Laemmli UK (1970) Cleavage of structural proteins during the assembly of the head of bacteriophage T4. Nature 227(5259): 680–685
10. Barrio E, Antón L, Marques G, Sánchez A, Vivanco F (1991) Formation of covalently linked C3-C3 dimers on IgG immune aggregates. Eur J Immunol 21(2):343–349
11. Shevchenko A, Tomas H, Havlis J, Olsen JV, Mann M (2006) In-gel digestion for mass spectrometric characterization of proteins and proteomes. Nat Protoc 1(6):2856–2860

Chapter 7

Enzyme-Linked Immunosorbent Assay (ELISA)

George N. Konstantinou

Abstract

Food allergy is a public health concern especially after recognizing its constantly increased prevalence and severity. Despite careful reading of food ingredient statements, food allergic individuals may experience reactions caused by "hidden", "masked", or "contaminated" proteins that are known major allergens. Many techniques have been developed to detect even small traces of food allergens, for clinical or laboratory purposes. Enzyme-linked immunosorbent assay (ELISA) is one of the best validated and most routinely used immunoassay in allergy research, in allergy diagnosis in allergy-related quality control in various industries. Although as a technique it has been implemented for the last 45 years, the evolution in biochemistry allowed the development of ultrasensitive ELISA variations that are capable of measuring quantities in the scale of picograms, rendering ELISA attractive, robust, and very famous.

Key words Enzyme-linked immunosorbent assays (ELISA), Protocol, Method, Food allergy, Allergen

1 Introduction

1.1 Background

Food allergy is one of the major public health issues with prevalence between 5 and 10% that is constantly increasing [1]. It is not known what is causing this increase, but seems to be multifactorial with significant components being the genetic susceptibility, the interacting environment, cultural, behavioral, and dietary particularities [2–6].

The food allergens are proteins capable of stimulating a type-I hypersensitivity reaction in sensitized individuals through immunoglobulin E (IgE)-mediated reactions even at very small amounts [7, 8]. Till now there is no known etiological treatment for food allergy, therefore all efforts rely on prevention [9]. It can be relatively easy for an allergic individual to recognize food products made by ingredients they are allergic to, but it might be tricky to identify hidden, masked, or contaminated small amounts of allergens.

Prevention is based upon: (a) appropriate food labeling practices by food manufacturers to make it easy for food allergic

Jing Lin and Marcos Alcocer (eds.), *Food Allergens: Methods and Protocols*, Methods in Molecular Biology, vol. 1592, DOI 10.1007/978-1-4939-6925-8_7, © Springer Science+Business Media LLC 2017

individuals to identify the presence of clinically important food allergens in their packed products [10], and (b) patients training to follow correct label reading practices to recognize and avoid everything they are allergic to. Teleologically, the identification of the traces that may exist in processed food is of major importance and for that reason the detection techniques that will be applied should be highly sensitive. The most commonly used analytical method for food allergen detection is based on the enzyme-linked immunosorbent assay (ELISA) technique.

1.2 ELISA Principles

The ELISA is a sensitive and specific analytic biochemistry assay utilized for detection and quantitative or qualitative analysis of an analyte without the requirement of sophisticated or expensive equipment [11–13]. The analyte could be any specific substance, either a specific protein or a more complex mixture of more than one protein (e.g. a biomolecular complex).

As a methodology, ELISA is based on a few important scientific advances the most important of which is the production of antigen-specific antibodies either monoclonal or polyclonal. Secondly, the development of radioimmunoassay techniques has been a milestone. With this technique the detection antibodies can be labeled with radioisotopes providing an indirect way of quantifying a protein by measuring the radioactivity. Alternatively, the indirect quantification can be performed by measuring the signal that is produced when utilizing the appropriate substrate, with antibodies that are chemically linked to biological enzymes. Similarly, fluorescence tag technology (a form of luminescence also known as a label or probe) allows the indirect quantification of protein chemically attached with a fluorescent dye by measuring fluorescence quantum yields and compare it with a standard. Generally, ELISA has good sensitivity with a limit of detection/limit of quantification (LOD/LOQ) down to lower nanogram scale [14, 15].

In ELISA, a liquid sample, that has specific binding properties, is added onto a stationary solid phase inside a reaction chamber or a microplate well. Then, different liquid reagents are sequentially incubated resulting in some optical change (e.g. color development by the product of an enzymatic reaction) in the final liquid. This change is integrated as a dynamic variable into mathematical formulas which compare the optical density with a known standard parameter, and are able to indirectly quantify the analyte of interest.

The detection of an antigen by ELISA relies on the recognition and specific binding of that antigen (potential allergen), which is known as ligand, to a specific antibody. Allergen-antibody binding depends on the solubility and integrity of the protein. These antigen-specific antibodies may recognize a particular epitope on an allergen (monoclonal antibodies), a mixture of allergens in the same source (e.g. Ara h 1, Ara h 2, Ara h 3, Ara h 6, etc. allergens in peanut) (polyclonal antibodies) or allergens with homolog epitopes (cross reactive allergens). [16]. Cross-reactivity is the ability of an antibody to react with similar antigenic structures/epitopes on different proteins. This may occur on unrelated proteins from the same (e.g. Ara h 2 and Ara h 6 allergens in peanut) or different species (e.g. hevein-like protein in banana and latex, or LTP allergens in different foods of plant origin) and can be a result of lack of protein purification or measuring a protein in a mixture of unknown proteins with cross-reacting epitopes. Both cases may lead to false-positive results [17] rendering cross-reactivity the main shortcoming in protein quantification.

Some food products contain several major allergens (e.g. peanut contains Ara h 1, Ara h 2, Ara h 3, etc.) that may all cause an immunological response, although they may have dissimilar chemical and structural properties. This does not preclude the possibility of someone being allergic to only one protein (e.g. only Ara h 2, in peanut) [16].

1.3 Variations Between ELISA Protocols

There are two principle methods that vary in the way the antigen of interest is immobilized. In the *direct coating* approach the antigen is diluted usually in a carbonate/bicarbonate buffer with pH > 9 and directly attached to the inner surface of the wells of a microtiter plate by passive adsorption (Fig. 1a, b). In the capture, or *indirect coating*, also known as Sandwich ELISA approach, an antigen-specific antibody that is adsorbed onto the wells, immobilizes the antigen

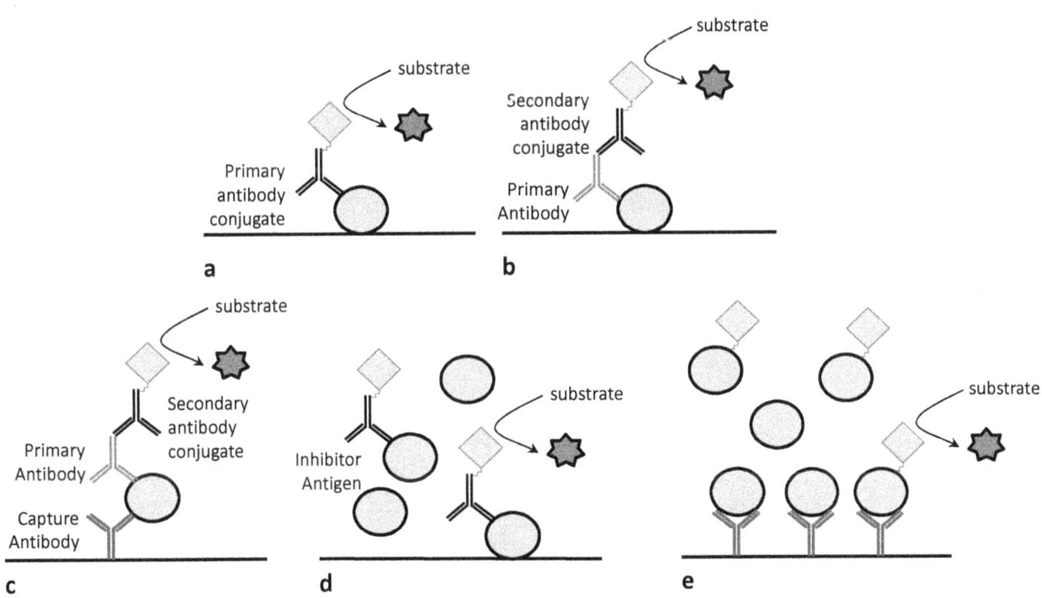

Fig. 1 Popular ELISA formats. (**a**) Direct ELISA, (**b**) Indirect ELISA, (**c**) Sandwich ELISA, (**d**) Competitive ELISA with labeled antibody, (**e**) Competitive ELISA with labeled antigen

of interest after incubation with the antigen sample (Fig. 1c). This approach is more sensitive and commonly used when the antigen to be detected is in small amounts, or its physicochemical properties do not allow sufficient adherence to the wells, or when the samples include more than one protein. With this approach only the antigen of interest is bound to that antigen-specific antibody.

There is a more complicated ELISA format that is called competition or competitive ELISA. The distinguishing feature of competitive ELISA is that the combination of the reference/standard analyte with an unknown amount of the same analyte (introduced from the unknown sample) competes for binding to a limited number of antibody binding sites. The competitive ELISA assay can be performed with either the analyte or the antibody absorbed to the solid phase. In the first variation of this format (Fig. 1d), the added sample analyte is competing with solid phase absorbed reference/standard analyte for binding to a limited amount of labeled antibody. In the second variation of this format (Fig. 1e), the labeled reference/standard analyte in solution is combined with the unknown sample analyte and they both compete for binding to a limited amount of solid phase absorbed antibody.

For the first variation, after the incubation period of the competitive mixture, any unbound antibody is washed off. The more antigen the sample has, the more conjugated antibody will be bound to the sample antigen and, consequently, the smaller the amount of the unbound antibody that will be available to bind to the coated antigen. In the second variation, the same approach applies for the conjugated antigen. Absence of color indicates the presence of antigen in the sample [18].

The selection of the format used depends mainly on the size of the target molecules. For instance, the sandwich format can be used to measure intact allergenic proteins or big fragments. On the other hand, the competitive format has to be used in certain circumstances like, for instance, in the case of small peptides which contain only one binding epitope that an antibody can recognize [19].

In all aforementioned approaches, the antigen of interest can be detected with two ways: in the *direct detection*, the primary antibody is labeled with an enzyme or a fluorescent chemical compound known as fluorophore (Fig. 1). The *indirect detection* method involves an additional step using another antibody (a secondary antibody that specifically binds to the primary antigen-specific antibody) conjugated with a detectable tag [e.g. horseradish peroxidase (HRP) or alkaline phosphatase (AP) enzymes], or biotin. In the case of a biotinylated antibody the detectable tag is bound to avidin or streptavidin, two molecules that bind very strongly with biotin molecule. The direct detection approach is faster and eliminates the potential extra background signal due to cross-reactivity between the secondary antibody and the coating antibody, however is less sensitive than the indirect detection method which can provide signal amplification. This amplification can be explained either from the fact that biotinylated antibodies have multiple biotin tags per antibody molecule, thus allowing more than one avidin/streptavidin molecules to bind to each antibody molecule, or from the fact that avidin/streptavidin conjugation process with enzymes result in conjugates with more than one enzyme. Therefore, the indirect detection method is preferable when the target antigen is expected to be in low amounts.

Last but not least, a final chemical reaction is needed in order to generate a measurable signal from an enzyme. The catalysis of a specific substrate produces a fluorescent compound, chemiluminescence or, the most commonly used, colored compound. These signals can be measured with an appropriately filtered fluorometer, a luminometer or a spectrophotometric plate reader, respectively. Although chemiluminescent detection is considered more sensitive, the colorimetric approach is the most commonly used. Colorimetric substrates like 2-2′-azino-di-(3-ethylbenzthiazoline sulfonic acid (ABTS), 3,3′,5,5′-Tetramethylbenzidine (TMB) and o-Phenyl-diamine-dihydrochloride for peroxidase (OPD) for HRP, and p-Nitrophenyl Phosphate for Alkaline Phosphatase (pNPP) for AP, form a soluble colored product that can be measured directly or halted using a stop solution for direct measurements.

All these different ELISA types may be implemented in different settings (laboratory-research or clinical-diagnostic) but they are all based on similar technical procedures [16]:

1. **Coating or Capture**: Direct or indirect (by the coated captured antibody) immobilization of the standards (e.g. allergens/ antigens) to the inner surface of the wells of a polystyrene microtiter plate by adsorption.
2. **Blocking**: Addition of an irrelevant protein/molecule to cover all unsaturated surface-binding sites of the microtiter plate wells.
3. **Detection (or Probing)**: Incubation with antigen-specific antibodies that are bound to the immobilized antigens.
4. **Signal Measurement**: Detection of the signal generated via the direct or secondary tag bound on a specific antibody.

1.4 Producing the Standards—Food Allergen Isolation

Regardless of the format that will be followed, there is always a need to obtain standardized extracts and pure allergens. Ideally, a purified recombinant standard can be used, but there might be a need to extract the standard protein directly from the examined food. Food allergens are denatured mixtures of proteins in complex matrices with different physicochemical properties, and therefore there is not a single, standard extraction method suitable for all foods [20].

Almost always the extraction starts with a tissue and cell disruption which is most of the times accomplished with homogenization (the process of reducing a substance to extremely small particles and distributing it uniformly throughout a fluid). Homogenization is followed by different procedures aiming at solubilization and precipitation, fractionation and purification and allergen enrichment techniques (Fig. 2).

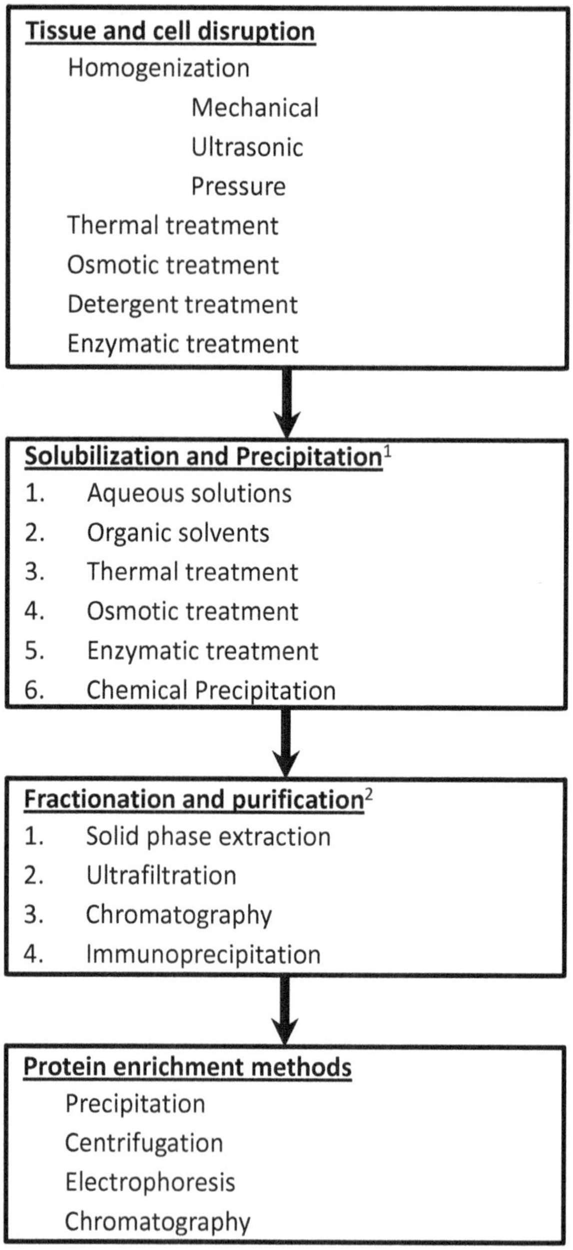

Fig. 2 Extraction and fractionation techniques for proteins from foods of plant or animal origin.
Superscript 1 protein separation from lipids, carbohydrates, nucleic acids, and mineral.
Superscript 2 sample cleanup and protein isolation

Protein extraction from foods of plant origin is generally more problematic because plant tissues are rich in proteases and other interfering compounds [21]. The method of choice of plant protein extraction (e.g. cereals, legumes, and fruits) is based on trichloroacetic acid (TCA)/acetone precipitation [22]. The combination of acetone with the negative charge of TCA and the extreme pH causes immediate denaturation and precipitation of the proteins, while it deactivates the proteolytic and, in general, modifying activity of the enzymes included in the treated mixture. One disadvantage of TCA-precipitated proteins is that they are difficult to redissolve [23].

Sample solubility can be improved by using an appropriate mixture of agents that exert chaotropic activity (agents that can disrupt the hydrogen bonding network between water molecules) like urea or thiourea, detergents like sodium dodecyl sulfate (SDS) or the phenol extraction procedure. Phenol exerts strong solvent action on proteins but only has a little predisposition to dissolve polysaccharides and nucleic acids, although as a procedure is time-consuming and toxic [24]. For storage proteins extraction (e.g. soybean proteins glycinin and b-conglycinin) ammonium sulfate may be a good precipitant [25, 26].

Aqueous alcohols (ethanol, isopropyl alcohol, butanol) are also used in the extraction process to remove oligosaccharides, phenolics, or inhibitors from defatted meals and seeds [24]. However, they may change the structure of the proteins, induce coagulation, reduce the number of available epitopes and, as a consequence, reduce the functional properties of the protein. To minimize this consequence, mechanical and thermal treatments can be applied, which might also interfere with protein functionality but to a much less degree [27, 28].

An example of proteins difficult to dissolve and isolate is gliadin. Gliadin is one of the main components of the gluten fraction in wheat, rye and barley seed and a member of the prolamins (a group of plant storage proteins). Gliadins are slightly soluble in ethanol but there are a few extraction solutions that are able to extract prolamins in a quantitative manner without interfering with the ELISA results [e.g. "cocktail solution" by Garcia et al. [29]. and the "RIDA® extraction solution" R 7099 (R-Biopharm AG)].

Another type of protein isolation and enrichment that is widely used in food allergy is immunoprecipitation. With this technique, an antibody is used to precipitate the protein of interest by forming a precipitating antigen–antibody complex [30].

1.5 Must Knows Before Using ELISA

1. *Homemade vs commercial ELISA kits*

   Homemade ELISA kits may be sensitive and specific enough [31] but they require specialized, sometimes time-consuming extraction or isolation techniques and labor measurements of allergen concentration that can be affected by several variables like food matrix and thermal processing [32, 33]. Thus the involvement of an expert is recommended at least at the initial steps of the development of such an ELISA kit, in order to be confident that the technique is accurate and applicable. This is not the case for commercially available ELISA kits that offer advantages such as good sensitivity, need for only limited technical equipment, simultaneous sample analysis and ease in execution without need for specialized personnel. This is the reason these kits are widely used by the food industry [34].

2. *Information about antibody specificities*

   It is of crucial importance to know the clonality (monoclonal or polyclonal antibody), the host, the antibody isotype, the purification process and if possible which protein was used to generate the antibody (a fractionated and isolated protein from a natural source, a modified protein, a synthesized protein or a few specific peptides from that protein) [35].

3. *Information about cross-reactivity*

   Knowing the exact protein utilized to produce an antibody could be enough to hypothesize which might be the cross-reactive epitopes recognized by the produced antibody, and where these epitopes can be found. Since epitope-specific antibody production cannot be customized when whole protein extracts are used, any potential cross-reactivity must be tested against a variety of food commodities or purified proteins that might be cross-reactive candidates.

4. *Information on matrices*

   Epitope recognition is matrix-dependent as it has been shown for several foods with the most well examined paradigm being egg in which at least fat and gluten affect its allergenicity [36, 37]. Therefore, ELISA results are expected to be susceptible to matrix effects or perform differently in different matrices. Ideally, the antibody developer should have performed tests with different matrices and identify those that the antibody may have difficulties or may not be applicable for.

2 Materials

2.1 Disposables and Equipments

1. Clear ELISA microtiter 96-well plates (*see* **Note 1**).
2. Disposable plate sealers.
3. Assorted graduated cylinders.
4. Assorted volume, 8- or 12-channel multichannel precision pipettes.
5. Disposable plastic pipette tips.

6. Wash bottle and/or automatic plate washer.
7. ELISA plate reader or luminometer with appropriate software to detect the substrate (usually 405–650 nm).
8. ELISA plate shaker.
9. Incubator.
10. Vortex.
11. pH meter.
12. Adhesive plastic (Parafilm).
13. Small-volume bottles.
14. Timer.

2.2 Reagents

1. Coating buffer: 0.05 M sodium carbonate/bicarbonate buffer, pH 9.6.
2. Capture antibody: Diluted in Coating Buffer.
3. Wash buffer: phosphate-buffered saline containing 0.05% Tween-20 (PBST).
4. Blocking buffer: usually 2% (w/v) Bovine Serum Albumin (BSA) in Wash buffer. Alternatively, the following may be used: 1% human serum albumin (HSA) in PBS + 5% goat serum albumin (NGS), 1% human serum albumin (HSA) in PBS + 10% goat serum albumin (NGS), 1% HSA in PBST, 1% BSA in PBS + 10% NGS, 2% NGS in PBST, 1% normal sheep serum (NSS) in PBST, 2% NSS in PBST, 1% BSA in PBST, 2% BSA in PBST, etc. (*see* **Note 2**).
5. Standard: Purified antigen of interest. A standard curve span concentrations is dependent upon the predicted amount of antigen in the sample and the amount of standard protein available (usually from 0 to 3000 pg/mL). Dilution of the standard is performed with the blocking buffer.
6. Sample: The sample is diluted using the blocking buffer as many times needed to fit the standard curve concentrations span.
7. Conjugated detection antibody: dilute to the appropriate concentration in blocking buffer.
8. Enzyme conjugate: Streptavidin-HRP diluted to the appropriate concentration in blocking buffer.
9. Substrate: ABTS or TMB substrate.
10. Stop solution: 2 M sulfuric acid.
11. Control: As negative control use three wells coated with coating buffer and incubated in all following steps with blocking buffer.

3 Methods

3.1 ELISA Optimization

The following steps are needed for optimization. In all steps check for strong signal versus low background:

1. Use appropriate controls to account for any background signal/noise generated that cannot be attributed to the presence of the analyte under investigation. The best controls that can be used are wells coated according to the protocol but incubated in all other steps with the blocking buffer. In these wells, the conjugated detection antibody is added followed by the substrate, and in some others the conjugated antibody is omitted and only the substrate is added (*see* **Notes 3–5**).
2. In capture assay format, use two antibodies with different specificities. Titrate the primary antibody concentration between 500 ng/mL and 15 μg/mL. The latter concentration will be sufficient to demonstrate saturation.

   Optimize capture and detection antibody testing in at least three different concentrations. Check at the same plate different combination of capture versus detection antibody tested concentrations (*see* **Note 6**).
3. In direct assay format, titrate antigen concentration in the range of 1–20 μg/mL. Optimize detection antibody testing in at least three different concentrations. Check at the same plate different combination of antigen versus detection antibody tested concentrations (*see* **Note 6**).
4. Optimizing blocking time. Optimal blocking requires 1–2 h, but 15 min may be sufficient in some arrays.
5. Optimizing Signal Detection. Select substrate according to the expected amount of antigen in unknown sample and ELISA reader sensitivity. If the antigen is below the threshold for detection then consider selecting a more sensitive substrate.
6. The ELISA titration data that are generated when increasing the concentrations of labeled analyte (or antibody) are typically plotted either linear-linear, log-linear, log-log, or log-logit. The most useful plot of the data is usually the log-log plot. It provides the most precise estimate of true values in the unsaturated region of the curve and it is easy to fit the data to a curve by linear regression (*see* **Note 7**).

3.2 ELISA Representative Protocols

3.2.1 Direct ELISA (Fig. 1a)

1. To coat the plate with antigen, add 50–100 μL/well of different concentration of the antigen, seal the plate and incubate overnight at 4 °C.
2. Wash three times with wash buffer in an ELISA washer or for 3 × 5 min in a shaking platform. Wells should be filled and emptied to remove the solution by either aspiration or plate inversion (*see* also **Notes 8–10**).

3. Block (100–200 μL/well) the plate using blocking buffer, seal the plate and incubate for 60 min at 31 °C (*see* also **Note 11**).
4. Wash as **step 2**.
5. Add antibody conjugate solution (50–100 μL/well, same volume as used in **step 1** of the standard or sample), diluted in blocking buffer in a series of twofold dilutions (at least three). Apply in triplicates. Seal the plate and incubate for 1 h at 31 °C (*see* also **Note 12**).
6. Remove the solution and wash six times with wash buffer in an ELISA washer or for 6 × 5 min in a shaking platform.
7. Add substrate solution (same volume as used in **step 1** of the substrate), incubate for 30 min at 31 °C or until the desired color intensity is reached (expect a clear gradient for the standards) (*see* also **Notes 13–15**).
8. Stop the reaction, if necessary, by adding the same volume used in **step 1** of stop solution.
9. Measure the absorbance using an ELISA plate reader with the appropriate hardware (*see* also **Note 16**).
10. Analyze data and plot signal versus concentration of antigen.

3.2.2 Indirect ELISA (Fig. 1b)

Steps 1–4, same as **steps 1–4** in Subheading 3.2.1 direct ELISA.

5. Add primary antibody (same volume as used in **step 1** of the standard or sample), diluted in blocking buffer in a series of twofold dilutions (at least three). Apply in triplicates. Seal the plate and incubate for 1 h at 31 °C.

Then follow **steps 4–10** in Subheading 3.2.1 "Direct ELISA" for substrate addition, absorbance measurement, and data analysis.

3.2.3 Sandwich ELISA (Fig. 1c)

Sandwich ELISA (Fig. 1c) requires two different antibodies specific for the antigen to be detected. Each has to recognize different epitopes for this antigen. The first antibody (adsorbed to the plate) is called the capture or coating antibody, while the second antibody is called detection antibody. These antibodies must not compete for binding to the antigen. Not all combination of antibodies work properly and they have to be validated before used. Generally, monoclonal antibodies are used for coating and polyclonal for detection.

The recommended protocol steps are the following.

1. To coat the plate with capture antibody add 50–100 μL/well of a prespecified concentration, seal the plate and incubate overnight at 4 °C or for 2 h at room temperature.

   Steps 2–4, same as **steps 2–4** in Subheading 3.2.1 "Direct ELISA".

5. Add standards and samples (50–100 μL/well, same volume as used in **step 1** of the standard or sample), diluted in blocking buffer in a series of twofold dilutions (at least three). Apply in triplicates. Seal the plate and incubate for 2 h at 31 °C.

Then follow **steps 4–10** in Subheading 3.2.1 "Direct ELISA" for substrate addition, absorbance measurement, and data analysis.

3.2.4 Competitive ELISA with Labeled Antibody (Fig. 1d)

Steps 1–4, same as **steps 1–4** in Subheading 3.2.1 "Direct ELISA".

5. Competitive incubation:
   Dilute the standard/samples in blocking buffer. Dilute the conjugated ***antibody*** in blocking buffer. Mix the standards/sample and the conjugated antibody together.
6. Add competitive mixture:
   Add the mixture (50–100 μL/well, same volume as used in **step 1**), diluted in blocking buffer in a series of twofold dilutions (at least three). Apply in triplicates. Seal the plate and incubate for 1 h at 31 °C.

Then follow **steps 6–10** in Subheading 3.2.1 "Direct ELISA" for substrate addition, absorbance measurement, and data analysis.

3.2.5 Competitive ELISA with Labeled Antigen (Fig. 1e)

Steps 1–4, same as **steps 1–4** in Subheading 3.2.3 "Sandwich ELISA".

5. Competitive Incubation:
   Dilute the standard/samples in blocking buffer. Dilute the conjugated ***antigen*** in blocking buffer. Mix the standards/sample and the conjugated antigen together.
6. **Step 6** same as **step 6** in Subheading 3.2.4 "Competitive ELISA with Labeled Antibody".

Then follow **steps 6–10** in Subheading 3.2.1 "Direct ELISA" for substrate addition, absorbance measurement, and data analysis.

3.3 Signal Amplification Using Biotin-Streptavidin System

In all previous protocols if the detection antibody is conjugated with biotin, stop before the step of adding antibody conjugate solution and continue with the following steps:

1. Add biotinylated detection antibody (50–100 μL/well, same volume as used in the detection antibody), diluted to the appropriate concentration in blocking buffer. Seal the plate and incubate for 2 h at 31 °C.
2. Remove the solution and wash three times with wash buffer in an ELISA washer or for 3 × 5 min in a shaking platform.

3. Add enzyme conjugates with streptavidin/avidin (the same volume used for the biotinylated detection antibody) diluted to the appropriate concentration in blocking buffer. Seal the plate and incubate for 2 h at 31 °C.
4. Remove the solution and wash six times with wash buffer in an ELISA washer or for 6 × 5 min in a shaking platform.

Then follow **steps 7–10** in Subheading 3.2.1 "Direct ELISA" for substrate addition, absorbance measurement, and data analysis.

4 Notes

1. The type of plate used is of major importance. Gamma-irradiated plates are preferable since this treatment enhances coating via increasing positive charge of the material they are made of. It is essential to use a flat bottomed plate with clear, transparent base since the absorbances of the colorimetric substrates are measured by shining a laser through the base of each well. For fluorescence, black plates with clear bottom are preferable to minimize background signal, and for chemiluminescence white plates with clear bottom for signal amplification.
2. The blocking buffer is usually based on mammalian protein solution and is used to cover all unsaturated surface-binding sites of the microtiter plate wells. The blocking buffer should be tested for cross-reactivity, too. In cases of cross-reactivity attributed to blocking buffer, a non-mammalian protein should be considered as an alternative (e.g. salmon serum or a protein-free blocking solution). It is advised to consider the addition of a surfactant like Tweet®-20 in a final concentration of 0.05% (v/v) to the blocking buffer. Surfactants are capable of minimizing hydrophobic interactions between the antibody/antigens and the blocking protein preventing final weaker signals.
3. Background signal can be attributed to:
   (a) nonspecific binding of analyte to the plate,
   (b) insufficient blocking,
   (c) presence of unexpected antibody reactivity in the sample,
   (d) cross-reactivity of antibody to irrelevant antigens,
   (e) nonspecific binding of detection reagent to the plate, and
   (f) unstable substrate.
4. Use affinity purified antibodies (versus non-purified) for optimal signal:noise ratio.

5. Check for strong versus low background signal using the appropriate negative control wells. Check blank wells, too, to exclude unspecific signal from the type of plate used.
6. Once an optimal signal/noise ratio has been obtained, test several blocking and washing conditions to see if these will affect this ratio.
7. In homemade ELISAs it is advisable to first generate and optimize (sensitivity, range, and linearity) a standard curve for the analyte to be measured using a standard, the amount of which is known in advance, and afterward proceed to unknown samples testing.
8. Do not allow the plate to dry at any point.
9. Check washer alignment daily, ensure that the plate is leveled and examine the fill volume while wash (a slight dome should be observed at the top of the well) not allowing wells to overflow.
10. Examine the wells for complete aspiration of contents. Upon completion of wash cycle, blot to remove residual fluid.
11. To reassure constant condition, prefer incubation at constant known temperatures.
12. Prepare working dilution of conjugate just before you need it and do not leave it on the bench for excessive time. Excessively diluted conjugate should not be stored for future use.
13. Place plates in dark immediately after addition of light sensitive substrate solutions.
14. The commonly used substrates and their appropriate plate reader setting are
    (a) 2-2′-azino-di-(3-ethylbenzthiazoline sulfonic acid (ABTS: 405–410 nm),
    (b) 3,3′,5,5′-Tetramethylbenzidine (TMB: non-stopped 620–650 nm, stopped 450 nm),
    (c) o-Phenyl-diamine-dihydrochloride for peroxidase (OPD: non-stopped 450 nm, stopped 490 n) and
    (d) p-Nitrophenyl Phosphate for Alkaline Phosphatase (pNPP: 405–410 nm).
15. Do not hold substrate solution longer than 1 h. The temperature of solution is important because it affects rate of color reaction. Do not add fresh substrate to reagent bottle containing old substrate.
16. To remove fingerprints, clean bottom surface of plates with wash buffer. Wipe the bottom of the plate with a lint-free cloth/towel before reading.

References

1. Savage J, Johns CB (2015) Food allergy: epidemiology and natural history. Immunol Allergy Clin North Am 35(1):45–59. doi:10.1016/j.iac.2014.09.004
2. Gray CL, Levin ME, Zar HJ, Potter PC, Khumalo NP, Volkwyn L, Fenemore B, du Toit G (2014) Food allergy in South African children with atopic dermatitis. Pediatr Allergy Immunol 25(6):572–579. doi:10.1111/pai.12270
3. Baumann S, Lorentz A (2013) Obesity—a promoter of allergy? Int Arch Allergy Immunol 162(3):205–213. doi:10.1159/000353972
4. Lack G (2012) Update on risk factors for food allergy. J Allergy Clin Immunol 129(5):1187–1197. doi:10.1016/j.jaci.2012.02.036
5. Marrs T, Bruce KD, Logan K, Rivett DW, Perkin MR, Lack G, Flohr C (2013) Is there an association between microbial exposure and food allergy? A systematic review. Pediatr Allergy Immunol 24(4):311–320.e318. doi:10.1111/pai.12064
6. Prescott S, Allen KJ (2011) Food allergy: riding the second wave of the allergy epidemic. Pediatr Allergy Immunol 22(2):155–160. doi:10.1111/j.1399-3038.2011.01145.x
7. Wensing M, Penninks AH, Hefle SL, Akkerdaas JH, van Ree R, Koppelman SJ, Bruijnzeel-Koomen CA, Knulst AC (2002) The range of minimum provoking doses in hazelnut-allergic patients as determined by double-blind, placebo-controlled food challenges. Clin Exp Allergy 32(12):1757–1762
8. Hourihane JB, Kilburn SA, Nordlee JA, Hefle SL, Taylor SL, Warner JO (1997) An evaluation of the sensitivity of subjects with peanut allergy to very low doses of peanut protein: a randomized, double-blind, placebo-controlled food challenge study. J Allergy Clin Immunol 100(5):596–600
9. Ewan PW, Clark AT (2001) Long-term prospective observational study of patients with peanut and nut allergy after participation in a management plan. Lancet 357(9250):111–115
10. Joshi P, Mofidi S, Sicherer SH (2002) Interpretation of commercial food ingredient labels by parents of food-allergic children. J Allergy Clin Immunol 109(6):1019–1021
11. Fuller HR, Goodwin PR, Morris GE (2006) An enzyme-linked immunosorbent assay (ELISA) for the major crustacean allergen, tropomyosin, in food. Food Agric Immunol 17(1):43–52. doi:10.1080/09540100600572651
12. Mariager B, SØlve M, Eriksen H, Brogren CH (1994) Bovine β-lactoglobulin in hypoallergenic and ordinary infant formulas measured by an indirect competitive ELISA using monoclonal and polyclonal antibodies. Food Agric Immunol 6(1):73–83. doi:10.1080/09540109409354815
13. Sletten GB, Løvberg KE, Moen LH, Skarpeid HJ, Egaas E (2005) A comparison of time-resolved fluoroimmunoassay and ELISA in the detection of casein in foodstuffs. Food Agric Immunol 16(3):235–243. doi:10.1080/09540100500206020
14. Teuber SS, Sathe SK, Peterson WR, Roux KH (2002) Characterization of the soluble allergenic proteins of cashew nut (Anacardium occidentale L.). J Agric Food Chem 50(22):6543–6549
15. Sakai S, Adachi R, Akiyama H, Teshima R (2013) Validation of quantitative and qualitative methods for detecting allergenic ingredients in processed foods in Japan. J Agric Food Chem 61(24):5675–5680. doi:10.1021/jf3033396
16. Abbott M, Hayward S, Ross W, Godefroy SB, Ulberth F, Van Hengel AJ, Roberts J, Akiyama H, Popping B, Yeung JM, Wehling P, Taylor SL, Poms RE, Delahaut P (2010) Validation procedures for quantitative food allergen ELISA methods: community guidance and best practices. J AOAC Int 93(2):442–450
17. van Hengel AJ (2007) Food allergen detection methods and the challenge to protect food-allergic consumers. Anal Bioanal Chem 389(1):111–118. doi:10.1007/s00216-007-1353-5
18. Dobrovolskaia E, Gam A, Slater JE (2006) Competition enzyme-linked immunosorbant assay (ELISA) can be a sensitive method for the specific detection of small quantities of allergen in a complex mixture. Clin Exp Allergy 36(4):525–530. doi:10.1111/j.1365-2222.2006.02466.x
19. EFSA NDA Panel (EFSA Panel on Dietetic Products NaA) (2014) Scientific opinion on the evaluation of allergenic foods and food ingredients for labelling purposes. EFSA J 12(11):286. doi:10.2903/j.efsa.2014.3894
20. Pedreschi R, Hertog M, Lilley KS, Nicolaï B (2010) Proteomics for the food industry: opportunities and challenges. Crit Rev Food Sci Nutr 50(7):680–692. doi:10.1080/10408390903044214
21. Wang W, Tai F, Chen S (2008) Optimizing protein extraction from plant tissues for enhanced proteomics analysis. J Sep Sci 31(11):2032–2039. doi:10.1002/jssc.200800087

22. Damerval C, De Vienne D, Zivy M, Thiellement H (1986) Technical improvements in two-dimensional electrophoresis increase the level of genetic variation detected in wheat-seedling proteins. Electrophoresis 7(1):52–54. doi:10.1002/elps.1150070108
23. Nandakumar MP, Shen J, Raman B, Marten MR (2003) Solubilization of trichloroacetic acid (TCA) precipitated microbial proteins via NaOH for two-dimensional electrophoresis. J Proteome Res 2(1):89–93. doi:10.1021/pr025541x
24. Moure A, Sineiro J, Domínguez H, Parajó JC (2006) Functionality of oilseed protein products: a review. Food Res Int 39(9):945–963. doi:10.1016/j.foodres.2006.07.002
25. Bodzon-Kulakowska A, Bierczynska-Krzysik A, Dylag T, Drabik A, Suder P, Noga M, Jarzebinska J, Silberring J (2007) Methods for samples preparation in proteomic research. J Chromatogr B Analyt Technol Biomed Life Sci 849(1–2):1–31. doi:10.1016/j.jchromb.2006.10.040
26. Deak NA, Murphy PA, Johnson LA (2006) Effects of NaCl concentration on salting-in and dilution during salting-out on soy protein fractionation. J Food Sci 71(4):C247–C254. doi:10.1111/j.1750-3841.2006.00028.x
27. Barbin DF, Natsch A, MÜLler K (2011) Improvement of functional properties of rapeseed protein concentrates produced via alcoholic processes by thermal and mechanical treatments. J Food Process Preserv 35(3):369–375. doi:10.1111/j.1745-4549.2009.00476.x
28. Bader S, Oviedo JP, Pickardt C, Eisner P (2011) Influence of different organic solvents on the functional and sensory properties of lupin (Lupinus angustifolius L.) proteins. LWT–Food Sci Tech 44(6):1396–1404. doi:10.1016/j.lwt.2011.01.007
29. Garcia E, Llorente M, Hernando A, Kieffer R, Wieser H, Mendez E (2005) Development of a general procedure for complete extraction of gliadins for heat processed and unheated foods. Eur J Gastroenterol Hepatol 17(5):529–539
30. Pastorello EA, Trambaioli C (2001) Isolation of food allergens. J Chromatogr B Biomed Sci Appl 756(1–2):71–84. doi:10.1016/S0378-4347(01)00072-X
31. Konstantinou GN, Nowak-Wegrzyn A, Bencharitiwong R, Bardina L, Sicherer SH, Sampson HA (2014) Egg-white-specific IgA and IgA2 antibodies in egg-allergic children: is there a role in tolerance induction? Pediatr Allergy Immunol 25(1):64–70. doi:10.1111/pai.12143
32. Konstantinou GN, Kim JS (2012) Paradigm shift in the management of milk and egg allergy: baked milk and egg diet. Immunol Allergy Clin North Am 32(1):151–164. doi:10.1016/j.iac.2011.11.003
33. Taylor SL, Nordlee JA, Niemann LM, Lambrecht DM (2009) Allergen immunoassays–considerations for use of naturally incurred standards. Anal Bioanal Chem 395(1):83–92. doi:10.1007/s00216-009-2944-0
34. Schubert-Ullrich P, Rudolf J, Ansari P, Galler B, Fuhrer M, Molinelli A, Baumgartner S (2009) Commercialized rapid immunoanalytical tests for determination of allergenic food proteins: an overview. Anal Bioanal Chem 395(1):69–81. doi:10.1007/s00216-009-2715-y
35. Fremy JM, Usleber E (2003) Policy on characterization of antibodies used in immunochemical methods of analysis for mycotoxins and phycotoxins. J AOAC Int 86(4):868–871
36. Kato Y, Oozawa E, Matsuda T (2001) Decrease in antigenic and allergenic potentials of ovomucoid by heating in the presence of wheat flour: dependence on wheat variety and intermolecular disulfide bridges. J Agric Food Chem 49(8):3661–3665
37. Kato Y, Watanabe H, Matsuda T (2000) Ovomucoid rendered insoluble by heating with wheat gluten but not with milk casein. Biosci Biotechnol Biochem 64(1):198–201. doi:10.1271/bbb.64.198

Chapter 8

Detection of Food Allergens by Taqman Real-Time PCR Methodology

Aina García, Raquel Madrid, Teresa García, Rosario Martín, and Isabel González

Abstract

Real-time PCR (polymerase chain reaction) has shown to be a very effective technology for the detection of food allergens. The protocol described herein consists on a real-time PCR assay targeting the plant ITS (Internal Transcribed Spacer) region, using species-specific primers and hydrolysis probes (Taqman) dual labeled with a reporter fluorophore at the 5′ end (6-carboxyfluorescein, FAM) and a quencher fluorophore at the 3′ end (Blackberry, BBQ). The species-specific real-time PCR systems (primers/probe) described in this work allowed the detection of different nuts (peanut, hazelnut, pistachio, almond, cashew, macadamia, walnut and pecan), common allergens present in commercial food products, with a detection limit of 0.1 mg/kg.

Key words Real-time polymerase chain reaction, Taqman probe, Nuts, Food allergy

1 Introduction

Within the food industry and official food control agencies, the currently most commonly used methods to assess the presence of allergens in food products are based in protein detection [1]. Particularly, the enzyme-linked immunosorbent assay (ELISA), based on the interaction of species-specific proteins with specific antibodies either raised in animals [2, 3] or produced by recombinant technologies [4, 5], is the most widespread and commonly used protein-based test for allergen detection. Immunochemical methods can be highly sensitive and specific; however, depending on the epitopes recognized by the antibodies, they may be biased by cross-reactivity with other species. Moreover, the detection of the target proteins can be compromised by the variety of food

Jing Lin and Marcos Alcocer (eds.), *Food Allergens: Methods and Protocols*, Methods in Molecular Biology, vol. 1592, DOI 10.1007/978-1-4939-6925-8_8, © Springer Science+Business Media LLC 2017

processing methodologies, like heat treatment or roasting, which can strongly affect their integrity and quality [2]. An alternative to the direct detection of proteins is provided by DNA-based methods, where the target molecules are specific DNA sequences which are amplified by the polymerase chain reaction (PCR), either by qualitative end-point PCR (distinguished by their differential migration through agarose gel electrophoresis) or by real-time PCR using fluorescent-labeled probes or dyes. In real-time PCR, the crossing point value (*Cp*), which refers to the cycle number where the sample's fluorescence increases above the background level, is related to the amount of amplicon generated, so it provides quantitative information about the presence of the target species.

Real-time PCR has several advantages compared to conventional end-point PCR, for example: (1) the ability to detect very small size products, since it eliminates the need for gel visualization, (2) the reduced risks for crossover contamination, as reactions are kept confined during amplification and analysis, (3) the capability for large-scale processing and high automated throughput, and (4) the improvement in precision, sensitivity, dynamic range and resolution, since data are analyzed at the exponential phase of the PCR reaction.

Initially, intercalating dyes were used to measure real-time PCR products, but they have the disadvantage that both, specific and nonspecific PCR products, are detected. Besides, TaqMan® probes consisting on single-stranded oligonucleotides containing a fluorescent reporter (donor) dye on the 5′ end and a quencher (acceptor) dye on the 3′ end, are designed to hybridize within the amplification primers resulting in specific system detection. The proximity of the quencher dye greatly reduces the fluorescence emitted by the reporter dye by fluorescence resonance energy transfer (FRET) mechanism. However, the hydrolysis of the probe during the amplification due to the 5′–3′ double-strand–specific exonuclease activity of the *Taq* polymerase separates the donor fluorophore from the quencher resulting in a fluorescence increase. Fluorescence intensity registered will be proportional to the amount of target DNA present in the sample [6].

Here, we describe the development of a high-resolution species-specific Taqman® real-time PCR protocol to detect peanut [7], hazelnut [8], pistachio [9], almond [10], cashew, macadamia [11], walnut and pecan [12]; nuts that are included within the 14 major food allergens that should be declared in food labeling according to EU Regulation 1169/2011 [13].

2 Materials

Prepare all solutions using ultrapure water (PCR water if indicated) and analytical grade reagents (*see* **Note 1**).

2.1 Components and Reagents for DNA Extraction

1. DNA extraction buffer: 10 mM Trizma® base, 150 mM NaCl, 2 mM EDTA, 1% SDS, pH 8.0. Add about 200 mL water to a beaker provided with a magnetic stirring bar. Weight and transfer to the beaker: 0.6 g Trizma® base, 4.38 g NaCl, 0.37 g EDTA and 5 g SDS. Mix until complete dissolution of solids and adjust pH to 8.0 with 1 N HCl. Make up in a graduated flask to 500 mL with water and transfer the solution to a 1 L glass bottle. Autoclave for 20 min at 121 °C. Make 15–20 mL aliquots and store at room temperature for a period no longer than 3 months.
2. Guanidine hydrochloride (5 M): add about 80 mL water to a beaker provided with a magnetic stirring bar. Weight 47.76 g of guanidine hydrochloride and transfer into the beaker. Mix until complete dissolution and make up in a graduated flask to 100 mL with water. Autoclave for 20 min at 121 °C and make 500 μL aliquots in 1.5 mL microcentrifuge tubes. Store at room temperature for a period no longer than 3 months (*see* **Note 2**).
3. Proteinase K (20 mg/mL): weight in precision balance 20 mg of proteinase K and transfer to a microcentrifuge tube with 1 mL of PCR water. Vortex until complete dissolution. Make 200 μL aliquots into 500 μL microcentrifuge tubes and store at 4 °C.
4. Isopropanol (80%): prepare 50 mL by mixing 40 mL of isopropanol with 10 mL of PCR water in a conical tube. Make 2 mL aliquots in 2 mL microcentrifuge tubes and store at room temperature.
5. Chloroform. The volume required will be aliquoted in a conical tube and discarded after use.
6. DNA elution solution: water (DNase, RNase-safe certified, 0.1 μm filtered) or Tris-EDTA buffer solution (10 mM Tris–HCl, 1 mM EDTA, pH 8.0). Make 1 mL disposable aliquots in 1.5 mL microcentrifuge tubes and store at −20 °C.
7. Kit Wizard® DNA Clean-Up System (Promega, Madison, WI, USA): each Kit contains sufficient reagents for 100 samples (100 mL Wizard® DNA Clean-Up Resin, 100 Wizard® minicolumns and 100 syringe barrels). Aliquot the whole content of the resin into 1.5 mL microcentrifuge tubes at a volume of 1 mL. Store at room temperature and protected from direct sunlight exposure (*see* **Note 3**).

8. Vac-Man® Laboratory Vacuum Manifold (Promega): vacuum manifold capable of processing 20 samples simultaneously and provided with 20 one-way luer locks stopcock, so each port is controlled individually.
9. Vacuum pump "Fisher Scientific" mod. EYELA A-3S.
10. Incubator at 55 °C provided with a shaker.
11. Thermoblock at 65 °C.

2.2 Components and Reagents for Real-Time PCR

1. Water (DNase, RNase-safe certified, 0.1 μm filtered).
2. LightCycler® TaqMan® Master Mix (Roche Diagnostics GmbH, Mannheim, Germany): briefly spin one vial of enzyme (1a) and one vial of "reaction mix" (1b), pipet 10 μL from vial 1a into vial 1b and mix gently by pipetting up and down (do not vortex enzyme solutions). Re-label this master mix vial with number 1 (*see* **Note 4**). Vial number 2 contains water, PCR grade (*see* **Note 5**). Kit components must be stored at −20 °C.
3. Primers (forward and reverse) (*see* **Note 6**): resuspend the lyophilized oligonucleotides in 1 mL water to get the stock solution. Vortex and spin the stock solution before making two 200 μL aliquots into 1.5 mL microcentrifuge tubes to obtain two work solutions (label these solutions as A and B). Always vortex and gently spin the primer work solution before preparing the dilutions for real-time PCR assay. Into 500 μL microcentrifuge tubes, add the necessary volume of work solution A and PCR water to obtain the final primer concentration used in the PCR reaction (forward primers at 300 nM/μL and reverse primers at 900 nM/μL). Make 50 μL disposable aliquots and store at −20 °C.
4. *Taqman® probes*: resuspend the lyophilized oligonucleotides in the necessary volume (see manufacturer indications) of water to obtain a final concentration of 20 pmol/μL (stock solution). Once it is completely resuspended by pipetting up and down (do not vortex labeled oligonucleotides), prepare two 100 μL aliquots into 1.5 mL microcentrifuge tubes to obtain two work solutions (label solutions as A and B). Using 200 μL microcentrifuge tubes, prepare disposable 1/10 dilutions (2 pmol/μL) by mixing 3 μL of the work solution and 27 μL of PCR water. Store these aliquots at −20 °C.

   The primers and probes used for real-time PCR detection of each food allergen are listed and described in Table 1.
5. LightCycler® 2.0 (Roche Applied Science, Germany) equipped with LightCycler® 2.0 Sample Carousel.
6. LightCycler® Capillaries (*see* **Note 7**).
7. LightCycler® Capping Tools.

Table 1
DNA sequences and description of the primers and probes listed alphabetically

Primers	Length (bp)	Sequence (5′/3′)	Description	Target gene	Fragment length (bp)	Reference
AlmondITSfw AlmondITSrev	19 19	CTAGCCGAACGACCCGAGA CCGAGATAAAGGGGACGAG	Almond-specific forward primer Almond-specific reverse primer	ITS	76	[10]
CashewITSfw CashewITSrev	19 19	GAACGAACCCGATGATCC CCATCGAGGGTCAAGGAG	Cashew-specific forward primer Cashew-specific reverse primer	ITS	69	[11]
HazelnutITSfw HazelnutITSrev	20 17	GAGACACTCGTGCCTTCTTG GGAGCACTCTTTAGTTGAAGTTCC	Hazelnut-specific forward primer Hazelnut-specific reverse primer	ITS	70	[8]
MacITSfw MacITSrev	19 20	AGTCAAGGGCTCCTCGTGT ATGTCCGAACAATGGCAAAG	Macadamia-specific forward primer Macadamia-specific reverse primer	ITS	72	[11]
PeanutITSfw PeanutITSrev	20 17	AAGCCAAACGTTTCTGCTCT CGTTGCCGAGAGTCGTT	Peanut-specific forward primer Peanut-specific reverse primer	ITS	90	[7]
PecITSfw PecITSrev	18 18	ATGAAAGCTGCCCACCGC CATTGTTCGACCGGGAAG	Pecan-specific forward primer Pecan-specific reverse primer	ITS	69	[12]
PistITSfw PistITSrev	20 20	GGCGTTCGAAACAGAACCTA CGAGGGTCAAAGAGTCCGTA	Pistachio-specific forward primer Pistachio-specific reverse primer	ITS	72	[9]
WalITSfw WalITSrev	20 20	GACAATCGGTGGTTGAGAAA GTCGAGGAGCACCTTCACAG	Walnut-specific forward primer Walnut-specific reverse primer	ITS	70	[12]
18Sfw 18Srev	16 25	TGGTGCCAGCAGCCGC TCCAACTACGAGCTTTTTAACTGCA	Positive control forward primer Positive control reverse primer	18S rRNA	77	[7–12]
AlmondITSP	22	6FAM-ACTAGTTTCAAAGCGGGGG-BBQ	Almond probe	ITS		[10]
CashewITSP	22	6FAM-ACGCGCTCTCTCTGTGCC-BBQ	Cashew probe	ITS		[11]
HazelnutITSP	18	6FAM-GCGCCGGGGTTCGTTGTT-BBQ	Hazelnut probe	ITS		[8]
MacITSP	19	6FAM-TCACGATGAGTGGTGCGTC-BBQ	Mac probe	ITS		[11]
PeanutITSP	24	6FAM-TAACTCTTGTGGTCACTCGTCGCC-BBQ	Peanut probe	ITS		[7]
PecITSP	19	6FAM-CGGGTCAGTCTCCTCGTTC-BBQ	Pecan probe	ITS		[12]
PistITSP	22	6FAM-TCGTGCGGTTGCGTTCTACTGT-BBQ	Pistachio probe	ITS		[9]
WalITSP	18	6FAM-TGACCCGTCGTGTGTTGCCC-BBQ	Walnut probe	ITS		[12]
18SP	22	6FAM-CGCTATTGGAGCTGGAATTACC-BBQ	Universal probe	18S rRNA		[7–12]

8. LightCycler® Centrifuge Adapters in a dedicated aluminum cooling block. Store at 4 °C (*see* **Note 8**).
9. Centrifuge provided with a microcentrifuge tubes rotor.

3 Methods

3.1 Sample Digestion

1. Prepare working areas (*see* **Note 9**).
2. Grind sample in order to facilitate the DNA extraction. A pestle and mortar or a kitchen robot can either be used.
3. With a disposable spatula weigh 200 mg of the sample (in case of liquid sample, pipette 200 μL) into a 2 mL microcentrifuge tube and add 860 μL of extraction buffer, 100 μL of guanidine hydrochloride (5 M) and 40 μL of proteinase K (20 mg/mL) (*see* **Note 10**).
4. Homogenize samples with a vortex mixer and incubate overnight at 55 °C with shaking at 60 rpm.

3.2 DNA Purification

1. Remove the samples from the incubator and leave them to cool at room temperature for 10 min before adding 500 μL of chloroform to the lysate (*see* **Note 11**).
2. Homogenize with a vortex mixer and centrifuge at 20,000 × *g* for 10 min (*see* **Note 12**).
3. Carefully pipet 500 μL of the lysate (the clear aqueous supernatant containing the DNA) into 1 mL aliquot of the resin and gently mix by pipetting up and down.
4. Pipet the resin/supernatant mix into the syringe, open the stopcocks and apply vacuum to draw the whole solution through the minicolumn. Close the stopcocks and break vacuum.
5. Add 2 mL aliquot of 80% isopropanol to the syringe to wash the column and re-apply vacuum following the same procedure. Apply vacuum for 30 s after the solution has been pulled through the column in order to encourage column drying.
6. Remove the syringe and transfer the minicolumn to a clean 1.5 mL microcentrifuge tube with the cap previously cut away.
7. Centrifuge the minicolumn at 20,000 × *g* for 2 min to remove any residual isopropanol.
8. Transfer the minicolumn to a new microtube with the cap previously cut away. To elute the DNA, add 50–100 μL of prewarmed (65 °C) water or TE buffer to the minicolumn and wait for 1 min.
9. Centrifuge the minicolumn for 1 min at 20,000 × *g* to elute the bound DNA.

10. Discard the minicolumn and distribute the eluted DNA (referred to as "DNA extract") into two aliquots of 25–50 μL in 500 μL microcentrifuge tubes. DNA extracts may be stored at −20 °C.
11. Make a disposable aliquot of 3 μL in a 200 μL microcentrifuge tube to measure the DNA concentration with a NanoDrop ND-1000 spectrophotometer (NanoDrop Technologies Inc., Delaware, United States) (*see* **Note 13**).
12. After each extraction, wash with 70% ethanol the stopcock one-way luer locks connected to the vacuum manifold and change vacuum pump water.

3.3 Real-Time Polymerase Chain Reaction Protocol

1. Prepare working areas (*see* **Note 14**).
2. Program the LightCycler® instrument before preparing the reaction mixes (*see* **Note 15**). In this work, program shown in (Table 2) was suitable for all the real-time PCR primers/probe systems.

   The hydrolysis probes used in this assay are FAM-labeled at the 5′ end so the fluorescence default channel employed was 530 λ (emission maximum of the fluorescence reporter dye) with a gain value "1".
3. Prepare LightCycler® TaqMan® Master Mix and primers and probe solutions as previously indicated (forward primers at 300 nM/μL, reverse primers at 900 nM/μL, and probes at 2 pmol/μL).
4. Dilute DNA extracts to obtain the required concentration for PCR (2 μL of sample will be added to each reaction) (*see* **Note 16**).

Table 2
PCR program used in all real-time systems

Analysis mode	Cycles	Segment	Target temperature (°C)	Hold time	Acquisition mode
Pre-incubation					
None	1		95	10 min	None
Amplification					
Quantification	55	Denaturation	95	5 s	None
		Annealing	60	30 s	None
		Extension	72	1 s	Single
Cooling					
None	1		40	30 s	None
Temperature transition rate 20 °C/s					

Table 3
PCR primer mixtures

Component	Concentration (pmol)	Volume per sample (μL)
Forward primer	3	1
Reverse primer	9	1
Probe	2	1
LightCycler® TaqMan® Master (vial 1)		2
PCR water (vial 2)		3
Final volume PCR Mix		8

5. In the reagents cabinet, prepare a rack with empty labeled 200 μL microcentrifuge tubes, one per test sample, including the negative controls: (a) PCR negative control (NC) and (b) the DNA negative extraction control (NEC) (*see* **Note 17**).
6. Prepare PCR Mix as described in (Table 3) for a volume of 10 μL per reaction (*see* **Note 18**).
7. Add 8 μL of PCR Mix to each tube.
8. In the tubes corresponding to the negative controls, NC and NEC, add 2 μL of PCR water (vial 2) and 2 μL of the negative extraction control, respectively.
9. Transfer the rack to the DNA cabinet and in the tubes corresponding to the test DNA samples, add 2 μL of DNA template at the required concentration.
10. Mix and briefly spin all the microcentrifuge tubes.
11. Bring the cooling block with the LightCycler® Centrifuge Adapters out of the fridge and clean it with 70% ethanol.
12. Fill the capillaries as follows: with clean forceps, carefully place a capillary into the adapter, pipet the complete PCR reaction volume (10 μL) into the capillary head and seal it with a stopper with the help of the LightCycler® Capping Tool (*see* **Note 19**).
13. Centrifuge the adapters at 500 ×*g* for 1 min (if a higher speed is used, the risk of capillaries breakage increases).
14. Transfer the capillaries to the LightCycler® 2.0 Sample Carousel.
15. Introduce Carousel in the instrument and run the real-time PCR program.
16. Obtain and interpret results: the crossing point value (*Cp*) is calculated automatically by the LightCycler® software as the first maximum of the second derivative of the curve (*see* **Note 20**).

3.4 Selection of Genetic Marker and Design of Primers and Probes

The next steps are followed to develop and assess the applicability of the real-time PCR assay to detect allergenic nut species in food products. In this work, the plant ITS-DNA region has been used as suitable genetic marker for the design of species-specific primers and Taqman® probes. NCBI (National Center of Biotechnology Information) database was used to search for the ITS sequences available for various plant species. EMMA program (EMBOSS software) allowed the alignment and computer analysis of the sequences. Primer Express 2.0 software helped in primer design. Taqman® probes were located within the gene fragment delimited by each species-specific primer pair and were designed and synthesized by TibMolBiol (Berlin, Germany). A positive amplification control (PAC) system (primers/probe) was designed in a conserved region of the nuclear 18S rRNA of eukaryotes (Table 1).

3.5 Assay Specificity and Efficiency (See Note 21)

1. Perform the DNA extraction from the target nuts: peanut, hazelnut, pistachio, almond, cashew, macadamia, walnut, and pecan (stored at room temperature in the dark). Whenever possible, try to test different available commercial varieties of each target species.
2. Perform the DNA extraction of different plant and animal species typically used in the manufacture of commercial food products (test at least 50 species for representative results).
3. Analyze all the samples with each species-specific PCR system, as well as with the PAC system.
4. When the species-specific system is employed, a *Cp* value should be obtained for the corresponding target DNA, whereas no amplification signal should be obtained for heterologous species DNA. For all the eukaryotic species, a *Cp* value should be obtained with the 18S rRNA system (PAC).
5. Prepare two binary mixtures of every allergenic target species (raw and heat-treated) in wheat flour at different concentrations ranging between 100,000 mg/kg and 0.1 mg/kg by (1) roasting 100 g of every sample at 160 °C for 13 min, (2) finely grinding the different varieties of nuts (both raw and roasted) with the aid of a pestle and mortar or a kitchen robot, (3) in order to obtain the first target concentration (100,000 mg/kg), mix thoroughly 50 g of ground sample with 450 g of wheat flour at maximum speed for 5 min in a kitchen robot (Thermomix, Vorwerk).
6. Repeat the process described in **item 5** with tenfold dilutions (50 g of previous mixture and 450 g of wheat flour) to obtain the rest of mixture concentrations: 10,000 mg/kg, 1,000 mg/kg, 100 mg/kg, 10 mg/kg, 1 mg/kg, and 0.1 mg/kg.
7. Perform DNA extraction for each binary mixture in triplicate.

8. Analyze the three replicates of both series of mixtures (raw and toasted) with the corresponding species-specific PCR system.
9. Construct the standard curve using a simple regression model by plotting the mean *Cp* values versus the log input DNA concentration ([ ]). The correlation between both variables is semilogarithmic where *b* is the slope and *a* is the intercept of the standard curve.
10. Calculate PCR efficiency (*E*) from the slope of the standard curve, according to the following formula:

$$E = \left(10^{(-1/\text{slope})} - 1\right) \times 100$$

Ideally the efficiency should be 100% (for each cycle the amount of product doubles the initial concentration), corresponding to a slope value of −3.32. Optimally, a real-time PCR reaction should have efficiency between 90% and 110%, which corresponds to a slope ranging between −3.58 and −3.10 values. Other parameters such as Cochran's test, regression analysis, or variance analysis with lack of fit can be evaluated following described validation protocols [14].

An example of species-specific Taqman real-time PCR assay developed for walnut detection [12] is shown in Fig. 1. The detection limit achieved for all the allergenic nut species described in this protocol is 0.1 mg/kg (*see* **Note 22**).

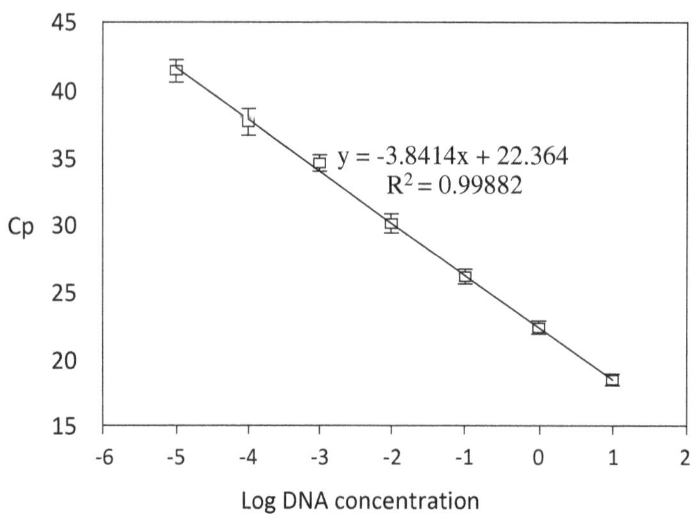

Total number of samples	42
"C" Cochran	0.046*
S^2 comb	0.596
Anova test "F" regresion (1)	5324.52**
Anova test "F" Lack of-Fit(2)	1.84***
Discriminating capacity	0.186*

* p<0.05
**p<0.01
***p>0.05
(1) P value = 0.000
(2) P value = 0.4186

Fig. 1 Linearity test, regression line, and sensitivity parameters of the walnut Taqman real-time PCR system. Three different DNA extractions at seven concentrations (100,000–0.1 mg/kg) for both binary mixtures of raw and heat roasted (160 °C/13′) walnut are used

4 Notes

1. Before and after use, all the flow laminar cabinets should be cleaned with Micro-90 (concentrated cleaning solution for critical cleaning applications, Cole-Parmer®, Illinois, United States), 70% ethanol and termi-DNA-Tor® (BioTools®, Madrid, Spain). To minimize the risk of contamination, we suggest to prepare all reagents in a cabinet (referred to as "reagents cabinet") different to the one employed for DNA manipulation (referred to as "DNA cabinet"). Also, different micropipettes for reagents and DNA samples, as well as different color tube racks (i.e. white for reagents and red for DNA solutions) are used. Use sterile filter pipette tips and microcentrifuge tubes RNase-, DNase-, and pyrogen-safe certified. Store tubes in closed sterile containers inside the reagents cabinet and use forceps for their manipulation to avoid hand contamination. Wear clean protective gloves during the entire procedure.
2. To avoid contaminations, these aliquots may be discarded among different extractions.
3. Thoroughly mix the Wizard® DNA Clean-Up Resin before removing an aliquot. If crystals or aggregates are present, dissolve by warming the resin to 37 °C for 10 min. Cool to 25–30 °C before using the 1 mL aliquot for the extraction.
4. The volume of the resulting Master Mix (5×) is sufficient for 64 reactions with a final volume of 10 μL per reaction.
5. This water is for exclusive use in PCR Mix preparation. Make 100 μL disposable aliquots into 200 μL microcentrifuge tubes.
6. Do not freeze lyophilized oligonucleotides (primers and probes). They must be stored at 4 °C until resuspended. Employ work solution A for the experiment unless PCR contamination is detected and this result is confirmed with the aliquots from this work solution. In this case, discard solution A and use B work solution from there on. The optimum concentrations of primers and probes for PCR are experimentally determined for each PCR system as those yielding the highest endpoint fluorescence and the lowest *Cp*.
7. Do not touch the surface of the capillaries. Always wear gloves when handling the capillaries.
8. The LightCycler® Centrifuge Adapters are designed to hold and protect the LightCycler® Capillaries during pipetting and centrifugation, ensuring that the entire volume of reaction mix is concentrated into the tip of the capillary. The cooling block maintains a low temperature environment during real-time PCR setup, significantly reducing the risk of primer-dimer formation.

9. If possible, sample digestion should be performed in a room different to the one used for the preparation of PCR reactions. Clean bench surface and scale plate with Micro-90, 70% ethanol, and termi-DNA-Tor. Work close to the sterile area around the Bunsen burner so that possible contaminants in the air are wafted away from your work area. After manipulation of each sample species, clean the bench again and move to a different one to avoid aerosol cross-contaminations within the different working species. Change your protective gloves between the different sample species.
10. Unless contrary indication, each DNA extraction is performed in duplicate. A negative DNA extraction control (NEC) is included for each DNA extraction. So, this control is handled in parallel, following the same procedure than the DNA samples: in the first step, add (in an empty vial) the extraction buffer, the guanidine hydrochloride, and the proteinase K. Then, follow the complete extraction procedure described.
11. During this 10 min interval, place a tube with the elution solvent (PCR water or TE buffer) in the thermoblock at 65 °C. For extraction of DNA >20 kb employ water or TE buffer pre-warmed to 80 °C. Also warm the Wizard® DNA Clean-Up Resin at 37 °C if crystals or aggregates are present.
12. Use this 10 min interval to prepare the vacuum manifold: attach the provided syringe barrel to the luer-lok extension of each mini-column (one per sample, do not re-use). Insert the tip of the minicolumn/syringe assembly into the one-way luer lock stop-cocks and connect the vacuum manifold to the vacuum pump.
13. The Nanodrop® spectrophotometer measures sample absorbance at three different wavelengths: 230, 260, and 280 nm. Absorbance at 260 nm provides dsDNA quantification following the conversion factor that one absorbance unit (1 A.U.) corresponds to 50 μg/mL of dsDNA, according to the Lambert–Beer law. Ratios of absorbance 260/280 and 260/230 are used to assess the purity of the DNA extract. A ratio of 260/280 ~ 1.8 is generally accepted as pure for DNA. If this ratio is appreciably lower, it may indicate the presence of protein, phenol, or other contaminants that absorb strongly at 280 nm. Expected 260/230 values are commonly in the range of 2.0–2.2. If the ratio is appreciably lower, it may indicate the presence of contaminants which absorb at 230 nm (EDTA, TRIzol, HCl, etc.).
14. Three different flow laminar cabinets will be used to perform real-time PCR assay: (1) "reagents cabinet" to prepare the master mix and other DNA-free solutions/reagents, (2) "DNA cabinet" for handling/pipetting DNA samples, and (3) a third cabinet to fill the capillaries. Before and after each use, switch

on the fan and UV for 10 min and clean all the cabinets with Micro-90, 70% ethanol, and termi-DNA-Tor.

15. Do not wear gloves or use new ones when handling computer and thermocycler equipment to prevent cross-contaminations.
16. We suggest the following steps to adjust the DNA concentration of the extracts in order to minimize the risk of contamination: (a) in the reagents cabinet and using forceps, place empty microcentrifuge tubes in the rack labeled as "PCR". Add the volume of water calculated for the dilution of each DNA extract employing micropipettes exclusive for reagents. (b) Thaw the DNA extracts, vortex and briefly spin the tubes. (c) In the DNA cabinet and employing micropipettes exclusive for handling DNA, add the necessary DNA volume for the calculated PCR concentration. Handle samples carefully and change gloves and clean surface and micropipettes when necessary.
17. All real-time PCR reactions are carried out in duplicate. The negative control of the PCR reaction (NC) and the negative control corresponding to each DNA extraction (NEC) must always be run in the same assay than the test DNA samples.
18. Although the required volume of PCR Mix will be prepared according to the number of reactions to be performed, it is advisable to calculate a little excess of PCR Mix volume to ensure enough amounts for all the tubes. Set the required number of PCR Mixes considering that each sample will be analyzed employing the species-specific PCR system for the allergens of interest and the universal positive amplification control (PAC) system.
19. We have observed that filling the capillaries with a certain speed minimizes the possibility of contamination.
20. If a *Cp* value is obtained for PCR negative control (NC), the result will not be valid, and the assay will be repeated. Similarly, if a *Cp* value is obtained for the negative extraction control (NEC), the assay can be firstly repeated. If the result is confirmed, repeat the sample DNA extraction before running again the PCR.
21. The close phylogenetic relationship among nuts, and the high number of plant and animal components that can be present in a commercial food, make it necessary to check the cross-reactivity of the PCR systems developed against a wide range of species.
22. As a further step, the applicability of the real-time PCR developed to detect the target species in foods is assessed by analyzing a range of commercial food products with different ingredients and label declarations.

References

1. Besler M (2001) Determination of allergens in food. TrAc Trends Analyt Chem 20:662–672
2. Scaravelli E, Brohee M, Marchelli R et al (2009) The effect of heat treatment on the detection of peanut allergens as determined by ELISA and real-time PCR. Anal Bioanal Chem 395:127–137
3. Stephan O, Vieths S (2004) Development of a real-time PCR and a sandwich ELISA for detection of potentially allergenic trace amounts of peanut (*Arachis hypogaea*) in processed foods. J Agric Food Chem 52:3754–3760
4. de la Cruz S, Cubillos-Zapata C, López-Calleja IM et al (2015) Isolation of recombinant antibody fragments (scFv) by phage display technology for detection of almond allergens in food products. Food Control 54:322–330
5. de la Cruz S, Alcocer M, Madrid R et al (2016) Production of *in vivo* biotinylated scFv specific to almond (*Prunus dulcis*) proteins by recombinant *Pichia pastoris*. J Biotechnol 227:112–119
6. Jothikumar P, Hill V, Narayanan J (2009) Design of FRET-TaqMan probes for multiplex real-time PCR using an internal positive control. Biotechniques 46:519–524
7. López-Calleja I, de la Cruz S, Pegels N et al (2013) Development of a real-time PCR assay for detection of allergenic trace amounts of peanut (*Arachis hypogaea*) in processed foods. Food Control 30:480–490
8. López-Calleja I, de la Cruz S, Pegels N et al (2013) High resolution Taqman real-time PCR approach to detect hazelnut DNA encoding for ITS rDNA in foods. Food Chem 141:1872–1880
9. López-Calleja I, de la Cruz S, González I et al (2013) Survey of undeclared allergenis pistachio (*Pistacia vera*) in comercial foods by hydrolysis probe real-time PCR. Food Control 39:49–55
10. López-Calleja I, de la Cruz S, Pegels N et al (2014) Sensitive and specific detection of allergenic almond (*Prunus dulcis*) in commercial food products by Taqman real-time polymerase chain reaction. Food Sci Technol 56:31–39
11. López-Calleja I, de la Cruz S, González I et al (2015) Development of real-time PCR assay to detect cashew (*Anacardium occidentale*) and macadamia (*Macadamia intergriofolia*) residues in market analysis of processed food products. Food Sci Technol 62:233–241
12. López-Calleja I, de la Cruz S, González I et al (2015) Market analysis of food products for detection of allergenic walnut (*Juglans regia*) and pecan (*Carya illinoinensis*) by real-time PCR. Food Chem 177:111–119
13. Official Journal of the European Union (2011) Regulation (EU) 1169/2011/EC of the European Parliament and of the Council of 25 October 2011 on the provision of food information to consumers, amending Regulations (EC) No 1924/2006 and (EC) No 1925/2006 of the European Parliament and of the Council, and repealing Commission Directive 87/250/EEC, Council Directive 90/496/EEC, Commission Directive 1999/10/EC, Directive 2000/13/EC of the European Parliament and of the Council, Commission Directives 2002/67/EC and 2008/5/EC and Commission Regulation (EC) No 608/2004, L304:18–43
14. Camacho MA, Torres AI, Gil-Alegre ME et al (1993) Validation protocol of analytical methods for finished pharmaceutical products. STP Pharma Prat 3:197–202

Chapter 9

Detection of Food Allergens by Phage-Displayed Produced Antibodies

Raquel Madrid, Silvia de la Cruz, Aina García, Rosario Martín, Isabel González, and Teresa García

Abstract

Phage display is a powerful tool to produce recombinant antibodies against a given antigen without animal immunization. This technology employs libraries of recombinant bacteriophages that display billions of different functional antibody fragments on their surface. They are selected by panning in vitro against the target antigen in search for specific binders. In this chapter, we describe the selection of single chain variable fragment (scFv) antibodies to be used for detection of allergenic proteins from nuts in food products. The artificial libraries TomLinson I+J (MRC Laboratory of Molecular Biology and MRC Centre for Protein Engineering) were employed that resulted in successful phage-ELISA systems for detection of almond and walnut proteins in commercial food products.

Key words Phage display, scFv, Biopanning, Allergen, ELISA

1 Introduction

Immunoassays used to detect allergenic ingredients in foodstuffs generally depend on the availability of antibodies raised in animals. However, current trends toward the replacement of live animals in procedures aim for alternatives not entailing their use, as an attempt to enforce the Three Rs principle [1].

Phage display technology relies on the expression of billions of different peptides or antibody fragments on the surface of filamentous phages [2, 3]. Best phage binders are selected by an in vitro selection procedure called biopanning, which is followed by the recovery of target-bound phage particles [4]. Once specific clones are isolated from the library and their specificity and sensitivity are assessed, antibody-codifying nucleotide sequences can be re-engineered by adding new domains that confer specific properties to the antibody–target complex.

Jing Lin and Marcos Alcocer (eds.), *Food Allergens: Methods and Protocols*, Methods in Molecular Biology, vol. 1592,
DOI 10.1007/978-1-4939-6925-8_9, © Springer Science+Business Media LLC 2017

In this work, TomLinson I+J commercial phage libraries were screened in search for phage-antibodies that would specifically recognize proteins from almond [5] and walnut. These synthetic libraries contain over 100 million different scFv fragments (V_H and V_K domains connected to one another by a flexible Glycine-Serine linker) cloned in an ampicillin-resistant phagemid vector pIT2 (HIS, MYC tag), and transformed into TG1 *E. coli* cells [6]. The antibody fragment (scFv) is displayed as a fusion with the terminal phage III protein [7]. TomLinson I+J repertories are based on a single human V_H framework (V3-23/D47 and J_H4b) paired with a single V_K (O12/O2/DPK9 and J_K1), with diversity introduced in the antigen-binding site [8]. The CDR3 of the heavy chains was designed to be as short as possible yet still able to form an antigen binding surface. It is recommended to use both repertories in parallel in order to obtain the maximum number of binders.

Specific phage-antibodies that bind to different target molecules can be isolated from the phagemid repertories following an affinity procedure called "panning". After each round of panning, the non-binders are washed away and the phagemids bound to the target molecules are eluted and amplified by infection into fresh TG1 cells. The process should be repeated twice or up to four times to ensure that more than half scFv selected bind specifically to the target antigen. The selected phage-scFvs can be screened for binding using a simple ELISA based protocol [5, 9, 10]. Finally, the proteins A and L can be used for detection, purification, or immobilization of the target-specific scFv selected from the TomLinson I+J repertoires [11]. The protocol described in this chapter is based on the work of Lee et al. 2007 [8], but includes some modifications to improve the selection of phage-antibodies specific for the target allergenic food, avoiding cross-reactions with non-target allergens.

2 Materials

Prepare all solutions with ultrapure water and reagents. Prepare and store all reagents at room temperature (RT) unless indicated otherwise.

2.1 Material

1. DynaBeads® M-280 Tosylactivated. Store at 6 °C.
2. Magnet (DynaMag™).
3. Mixer allowing tilting and rotation of tubes (e.g. Hulamixer® sample mixer).
4. Nunc™ MaxiSorb 96-well plates.
5. Nunc™ Immuno Stick.
6. Nunc™ Biobanking and Cell Culture Cryogenic Tubes.

7. 0.45 and 0.2 μM syringe filters.
8. UV-Vis spectrophotometer.
9. Sterile filter pipette tips.
10. Petri dishes of 90 mm and 140 mm diameter.
11. Incubators at 37 °C and 30 °C with shaker (250 rpm).
12. Centrifuge for conical tube and plate.
13. Water bath.

2.2 Reagents for the Library

1. Protein extraction buffer: 0.035 M Na_2HPO_4, 1 M NaCl, pH 7.5. Dissolve 12.54 g Na_2HPO_4 in 800 mL of deionized water. Adjust pH to 7.5, then add 58.4 g NaCl and water up to 1 L.
2. Pierce™ BCA Protein Assay Kit.
3. TomLinson I and J scFv libraries (distributed by MR Technology, Cambridge, UK). Check all libraries and stocks are frozen. Keep at −80 °C until needed. Freeze your own stocks at −80 °C.
4. Phagemid antibody libraries I and J.
5. Helper phage KM13.
6. Optimized antibody expression strain HB2151 and controls (anti-bovine serum albumin scFv in *E. coli* TG1TR).
7. Glycerol stocks of *E. coli* TG1 TR strain.
8. Glycerol stock of positive control clones (beta-galactosidase-specific dAb and anti-bovine serum albumin scFv in *E. coli* TG1 TR strain).
9. Glycerol stocks of negative control clone (phagemid).

2.3 General Reagents

1. TYE ampicillin agar plates: Dissolve 15 g Agar, 8 g NaCl, 10 g bacto-tryptone, and 5 g yeast extract for 1 L of double deionized water (ddH_2O). Autoclave. Cool down to 50 °C and add 1 mL of ampicillin solution (*see* **Note 1**). Pour plates. Plates can be stored at 4 °C for up to 4 weeks.
2. M9 minimal medium plates: Dissolve 15 g agar in 800 mL of ddH_2O. Autoclave. Cool down to 50 °C and add 200 mL 5xM9 salts, 10 mL 20% glucose, 1 mL of 1 M $MgSO_4$, 100 μL of 1 M $CaCl_2$, and 1 mL of 1 mg/mL VitB1. Pour plates. Plates can be stored at 4 °C for several months (*see* **Note 2**).
3. M9 salts (5× solution): Add 64 g Na_2HPO_4, 15 g KH_2PO_4, 5 g NH_4Cl, and 2.5 g of NaCl to 1 L of ddH_2O and autoclave.
4. 2xTY medium: Dissolve 16 g bacto-tryptone, 10 g yeast extract, and 5 g NaCl in 1 L of ddH_2O. Autoclave. Cool to RT (25 °C) and add antibiotic solutions and glucose solution as required. Can be stored at 4 °C for up to 4 weeks.

5. H-TOP Agar: Dissolve 10 g Tryptone, 8 g NaCl, 7 g Agar, 5 mM $MgCl_2$ (1 g of $MgCl_2 \cdot 6\ H_2O$) in 1 L ddH_2O. Autoclave (*see* **Note 3**).
6. Ampicillin solution: Dissolve ampicillin powder at 100 mg/mL in ddH_2O. Filter through 0.2 μM filter. Aliquot in 1 mL portions. Can be stored at −20 °C indefinitely. Thawed aliquots should be freshly diluted 1000-fold into medium or agar.
7. Kanamycin solution: Dissolve kanamycin powder at 50 mg/mL in ddH_2O. Filter through 0.2 μM filter. Aliquot in 1 mL portions. Can be stored at −20 °C indefinitely. Thawed aliquots should be freshly diluted 1000-fold into medium or agar.
8. PBS buffer: 1× phosphate buffer, pH 7.4. Dissolve 1.44 g Na_2HPO_4, 0.2 g KCl, 0.24 g KH_2PO_4, and 8 g NaCl in 1 L of ddH_2O. Adjust to pH 7.4 and autoclave. Can be stored at 4 °C for several months.
9. PBS buffer 10×: 2 g KCl, 2.4 g KH_2PO_4, 80 g NaCl, 14.4 g Na_2HPO_4. Dissolve in approximately 800 mL of ddH_2O, adjust pH to 7.4, then fill up to 1 L. Autoclave and store at RT. Dilute tenfold to be used for ELISA immunoassay.
10. MPBS: PBS buffer supplemented with 2% skimmed milk powder (w/v). Filter through 0.45 μM filter. Use directly and discard remaining buffer. Do not store.
11. Trypsin solution: Dissolve trypsin powder at 10 mg/mL in PBS (trypsin stock). Freeze in 20 μL aliquots at −80 °C. Can be stored in 100 μL at −20 °C for several months. For the experiment, dissolve 50 μL of trypsin stock in 450 μL of PBS.
12. Glucose solution 20%: Dissolve 100 g of glucose (dextrose) in 0.5 L of ddH_2O. Autoclave. Can be stored at 4 °C for several months (*see* **Note 4**).
13. PEG solution 20% PEG- 2.5 M NaCl: Dissolve 100 g of PEG 6000 and 73 g of NaCl in 500 mL of ddH_2O. Filter through 0.2 μM filter or autoclave. Can be stored at RT for up to a year.
14. BSA-PBS: PBS buffer supplemented with 3% (w/v) or 1% (w/v) bovine serum albumin depending on ELISA step. Use directly and discard remaining buffer. Do not store.
15. OVA-PBS: PBS buffer supplemented with 1% (w/v) ovalbumin. Use directly and discard remaining buffer.
16. Glycerol 70%: Add 70 mL glycerol and 30 mL of ddH_2O. Autoclave (*see* **Note 5**).
17. Buffer A: 0.1 M borate buffer, pH 9.5. Dissolve 6.18 g H_3BO_3 (MW 61.83) in 800 mL ddH_2O. Adjust pH to 9.5 using 5 M NaOH and adjust volume to 1 L with ddH_2O. Autoclave (*see* **Note 6**).

18. Buffer B: 0.1 M Na-phosphate buffer, pH 7.4. Dissolve 2.62 g NaH_2PO_4 H_2O and 14.42 g Na_2HPO4 2 H_2O. Adjust volume to 1 L with ddH_2O. Autoclave (*see* **Note 6**).
19. Buffer C: 3 M ammonium sulfate in Buffer A or B. Dissolve 39.64 g $(NH_4)_2$ SO_4 in Buffer A or B. Adjust pH with NaOH or HCl. Adjust up to 100 mL with Buffer A or B. Autoclave (*see* **Note 6**).
20. Buffer D or Blocking Buffer: PBS pH 7.4 with 0.5% (w/v) BSA. Add 0.88 g NaCl and 0.5 g BSA to 80 mL 0.01 M sodium-phosphate pH 7.4. Mix thoroughly and adjust volume to 100 mL with 0.01 M sodium-phosphate pH 7.4. Filter through 0.2 μM (*see* **Note 7**).
21. Buffer E or Washing and storage Buffer: PBS pH 7.4 with 0.1% (w/v) BSA. Add 0.88 g NaCl and 0.1 g BSA to 80 mL 0.01 M sodium phosphate pH 7.4. Mix thoroughly and adjust volume to 100 mL with 0.01 M sodium-phosphate pH 7.4. Filter through 0.2 μM (*see* **Note 7**).
22. Anti-M13 antibody horseradish-peroxidase (HRP) conjugate. Recognizes phage-antibodies through the M13 major coat protein (pVIII).
23. TMB solution (3,3′,5,5′-tetramethylbenzidine; Sigma cat. No. T0440-1L).
24. Stop solution for ELISA: Add 5.5 mL sulfuric acid (96%) to 200 mL of water.
25. My Taq™ Mix (Bioline cat n° 25042).

3 Methods

3.1 Protein Extraction

The same protocol is used to prepare extracts from reference allergenic nuts, and from unknown samples. To avoid cross-contamination, do not handle different allergenic nuts at the same time or in the same working surface. Clean bench thoroughly and change gloves between samples.

1. Grind the sample into small pieces (0.5 mm wide approximately) to facilitate the extraction, using a pestle.
2. Weigh 200 mg of ground sample to extract in a 2 mL tube.
3. Add 1800 μL of protein extraction buffer. Homogenize the mix with a disposable conical pestle (*see* **Note 8**).
4. Mix thoroughly for 10 min using Hula-Mixer, with vertical rotation, tilting, and vibration.
5. Centrifuge at 15,000 × *g* for 30 min.
6. Carefully take aqueous phase only (*see* **Note 9**).

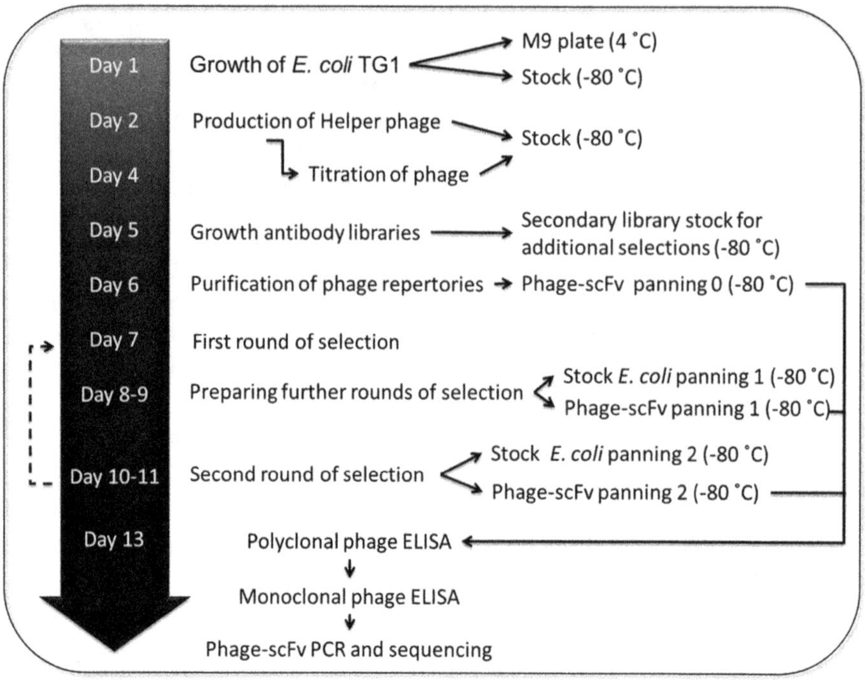

Fig. 1 Overall procedure

7. Filter the aqueous phase through 0.45 μM syringe filter.
8. Measure protein concentration employing Bicinchoninic acid assay (Pierce™ BCA Protein Assay Kit, Thermo Scientific™).
9. Store in 100 μL aliquots at −20 °C.

3.2 Isolation of Allergen-Specific Phage-scFv from the Libraries

The overall procedure can be completed in 2 weeks (Fig. 1).

DAY 1:

3.3 Growth of E. coli TG1 and Production of Large Quantities of Helper Phage

1. Streak *E. coli* TG1 from the glycerol stock on a M9 minimal medium and incubate overnight at 37 °C (Only grow *E. coli* 1 day to avoid cilia losing).
2. Pick a single colony from M9 minimal medium plate in a flask with 10 mL 2xTY medium (no antibiotics or glucose) and grow shaking at 37 °C 5 h, until OD = 1. (Use 2xTY medium as blank).
3. Plate 50 μL of the 2xTY culture in a plate of TYE with 100 μg/mL ampicillin and 50 μL in a plate with TYE with 50 μg/mL kanamycin. Incubate at 37 °C during 2–3 days to check for the absence of growth.

4. Streak the culture also in M9 minimal medium to have a stock plate with isolated colonies, incubate overnight at 37 °C only for 1 day, and then keep in the fridge.
5. Prepare stock vials of TG1 TR with the remaining 10 mL 2xTY culture, by adding 1.2 mL to a cryotube with 600 μL of glycerol 70%, and freeze at −80 °C.

DAY 2:

6. Pick a single colony from M9 minimal medium plate into 5 mL 2xTY medium, incubate at 37 °C, 250 rpm until OD600 = 0.4.
7. Prepare 14 tenfold serial dilutions of KM13 helper phage in PBS.
8. Add 10 μL of diluted KM13 helper phage to 200 μL TG1 culture each. Incubate in water bath at 37 °C for 30 min without shaking.
9. Take only the last nine phage dilutions in order to get well separated plaques and add 210 μL of each dilution into each vial with 3 mL pre-warmed H-top agar. Mix gently with culture and spread quickly over surface of pre-warmed TYE agar plates with 1% glucose (no antibiotics). H-top agar should be completely melted in microwave distributed in glass vials with 3 mL and cooled to 42 °C in a water bath before use. This step should be performed carefully, one vial at a time, to avoid H-top agar solidification.
10. Incubate overnight at 37 °C.

DAY 3:

11. Pick a single colony of *E. coli* TG1 from M9 minimal medium into 5 mL 2xTY and grow at 37 °C, until OD600 = 0.4.
12. Pick a small plaque with a sterile tip from TYE plates with H-top and place into 5 mL TG1 culture at OD600 = 0.4. Grow for 2 h at 37 °C, 250 rpm.
13. Dilute 100-fold into 500 mL of 2xTY medium. Shake in 2 L flask for 1 h at 250 rpm at 37 °C. Then, add kanamycin to a concentration of 50 μg/mL and grow overnight at 250 rpm at 30 °C.

DAY 4:

14. Spin the culture at 10,800 × *g* for 15 min at 4 °C in ten 50 mL conical centrifuge tubes.
15. To purify phage by PEG precipitation, add 400 mL supernatant to 100 mL of PEG solution, previously cooled. Incubate on ice for 1 h. In this step a kind of fog can be observed inside the tube corresponding to helper phage.
16. Spin at 10,800 × *g* for 30 min at 4 °C. Pour away supernatant with PEG. Resuspend the pellets in a total 8 mL PBS and add 2 mL PEG solution. Mix well and leave for 20 min on ice.

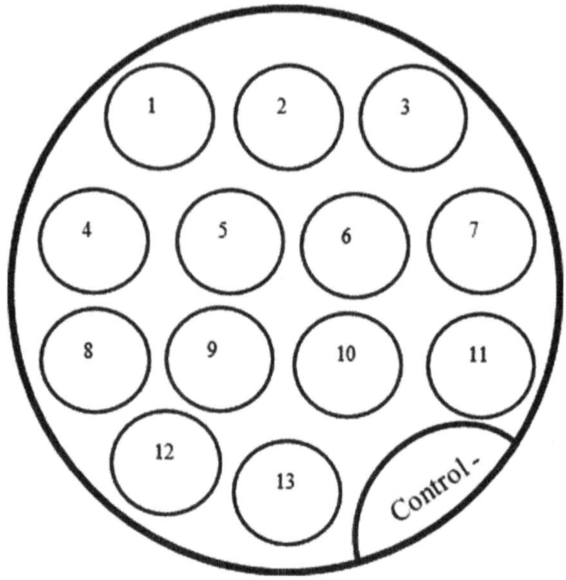

Fig. 2 Representative layout of a phage titration plate

17. Spin at 3300 × *g* for 30 min. Respin briefly and aspirate any remaining dregs of PEG/NaCl. Resuspend pellet in 5 mL PBS, distribute in microcentrifuge tubes and spin at 11,600 × *g* for 10 min in a microcentrifuge to remove any remaining bacterial debris. Be careful to take only the supernatant and transfer to a new tube.
18. Store the helper phage at 4 °C for short-term storage or in PBS with 15% glycerol for long-term storage at −80 °C.

3.4 Titration of the Helper Phage

1. Test trypsin cleavage: Add 5 μL of trypsin solution to 45 μL phage, and incubate for 30 min at 37 °C in a water bath.
2. Dilute 10 μL of trypsin-treated phage to 90 μL of PBS and make 100-fold serial dilutions of this in 1 mL aliquots of PBS. Perform the same dilution series using 10 μL of non-trypsin-treated phage.
3. Take 10 μL of each dilution series and infect 200 μL each of TG1 bacteria with OD600 = 0.4 (prepared as Subheading 3.3, **step 6**). Incubate in a water bath for 30 min at 37 °C.
4. Spot 10 μL from each phage dilution, treated and not treated with trypsin, on TYE plates supplemented with kanamycin 50 μg/mL and incubate at 37 °C overnight (Fig. 2). As negative control, plate 10 μL of not infected TG1. The number of colonies obtained from trypsin-treated phage should be at least 10^6-fold lower than that non-treated phage. If not, discard helper phage preparation and start from a different plaque.

5. To calculate the concentration of Helper phage:

$$\frac{PFU}{mL} = \frac{Colonies\ number \times Dilution\ factor}{Plated\ volume\ (mL)}$$

6. Phage can be frozen in liquid nitrogen (add 20% glycerol) and stored at −80 °C for many years.

DAY 5:

3.5 Growth of Phage-Antibody Libraries (See Note 10)

1. Add the frozen antibody library stock into 200 mL 2xTY medium supplemented with 1% glucose and 100 μg/mL ampicillin. The presence of 1% glucose allows the effective suppression of antibody expression during bacterial growth. Measure OD600 in a UV–Vis spectrophotometer. It should be approximately 0.1.
2. Grow culture at 37 °C, 250 rpm in a 2 L glass flask until OD600 = 0.4 (approximately 1–2 h).
3. Take 100 mL of this culture and add 2x10 [11] KM13 helper phages. Use the rest of the culture to make secondary bacterial stock of the library following Subheading 3.6.
4. Incubate in a water bath at 37 °C for 30 min.
5. Spin the culture at 3200 × *g* for 10 min. Resuspend in 200 mL of 2xTY medium with 0.1% glucose, 100 μg/mL ampicillin, and 50 μg/mL kanamycin.
6. Incubate at 30 °C with shaking overnight in a 2 L glass flask.

3.6 Make Secondary Stock of Libraries.

1. Grow the remaining 100 mL (from Subheading 3.5, **step 3**) for a further 2 h shaking at 37 °C.
2. Spin down the cells at 10,800 × *g* for 10 min. Resuspend in 10 mL of 2xTY containing 15% glycerol.
3. Store this secondary stock in 20× 500 μL aliquots at −80 °C. Use one aliquot for each phage preparation if you wish to perform additional selections.

DAY 6:

3.7 Purification of Phage Repertoire by PEG Precipitation

1. Spin the overnight culture from Subheading 3.5, **step 6** at 3200 × *g* for 30 min at 4 °C.
2. Add 20 mL PEG solution to 80 mL supernatant. Mix well and leave for 1 h on ice.
3. Spin 3200 × *g* for 30 min at 4 °C. Pour away supernatant with PEG/NaCl. Respin briefly and aspirate any remaining dregs of PEG/NaCl.
4. Resuspend the pellet in 1 mL PBS and spin at 12,000 × *g* for 10 min in a microcentrifuge to remove any remaining bacterial debris.

5. Store the phage at 4 °C for short-term storage or in PBS with 15% glycerol for long-term storage at −80 °C.
6. **To titer the phage stock** dilute 10 μL phage in 90 μL PBS, and repeat serial dilutions, until there are 13 dilutions in total. Add 200 μL of TG1 at an OD 600 of 0.4 to each tube and incubate at 37 °C in a water bath for 30 min. Spot 10 μL of each dilution on a TYE plate containing 100 μg/mL ampicillin and 1% glucose and grow overnight at 37 °C. Phage stock should be 10^{12}–10^{13}/mL, enough for at least ten selections. Store a part of this eluted phage (around 200 μL) to be used as "Panning 0" in ELISA, and use the remaining for panning 1.

3.8 First Round of Selection on Immuno Stick Paddles (See Note 11)

1. Coat Nunc™ Immuno Stick paddles overnight at 4 °C with 100 μg/mL of the required antigen in 1.5 mL PBS. The efficiency of coating can depend on the antigen concentration, the buffer, and the temperature. Usually, 10–100 μg/mL antigen in PBS is used (*see* **Note 12**).

DAY 7:

2. Wash paddles in the tube three times with PBS (fill the tube with PBS, screw and unscrew the paddle several times, and pour PBS out. Repeat three times).
3. Fill tubes with 3% BSA in PBS to block paddles. Incubate standing on the bench for 1 h at 37 °C.
4. Wash paddles in the tubes three times with PBS.
5. Add 1 mL phage (10^{12} phages) from Subheading 3.7, **step 5** (or from **step 6** stock) in 500 μL of 6% BSA in PBS. Add this mix to the tube containing the paddle coated with the non-target allergen. Incubate for 60 min at 25 °C rotating in the Hula-Mixer. Discard the paddle coated with non-target allergen and change it by the paddle coated with the target allergen. Incubate for 60 min at 25 °C rotating in the Hula-Mixer and for a further 60 min standing on the bench. Discard supernatant.
6. Wash paddle in the tube ten times with PBS.
7. Transfer the paddle to a new tube containing 500 μL of trypsin-PBS (50 μL of 10 mg/mL trypsin stock solution added to 450 μL PBS) and incubate rotating for 10 min at RT using Hula-mixer to elute the phage bound to the paddle.
8. Add 250 μL of the eluted phage to 1.75 mL of TG1 at an OD 600 of 0.4 (Prepared as in Subheading 3.3, **step 6**). The remaining eluted phage should be stored at 4 °C in case it is necessary to repeat infection. Incubate for 30 min at 37 °C in a water bath without shaking.
9. Take 10 μL of TG1 infected with eluted phage and dilute in 990 μL of PBS to obtain 10^2 dilution, and make two 100-fold serial dilutions of this to obtain 10^4 and 10^6 dilutions.

Pour 50 µL of each dilution on TYE plates containing 100 µg/mL ampicillin and 1% glucose and grow overnight at 37 °C to titer the phage. Incubate at 37 ° C overnight (*see* **Note 13**).

10. Spin the remaining TG1-infected culture at 11,600 × *g* in a microcentrifuge for 5 min. Resuspend the pelleted bacteria in 1 mL of 2xTY and plate 500 µL on two large Petri dishes (140 mm) containing TYE, 100 µg/mL ampicillin, and 1% glucose. Grow plates at 37 °C overnight.

DAY 8:

3.9 Preparing Further Rounds of Selection

1. After growing overnight culture in two large plates, add 1 mL of 2xTY medium to each one. Scrape cells from the agar using a glass spreader, and mix them thoroughly in a microcentrifuge tube.
2. Prepare 50 mL of 2xTY medium with 100 µg/mL ampicillin and 1% glucose and inoculate with 50 µL of the scraped TG1 culture. Grow shaking at 37 °C until OD600 = 0.4. Store the remaining bacteria at −80 °C making aliquots of 500 µL in 15% glycerol (stock *E. coli* panning 1).
3. Take 10 mL of this culture and add 5x10 [10] helper phage. Incubate without shaking in a 37 °C water bath for 30 min.
4. Centrifuge at 3200 × *g* for 10 min. Resuspend the pellet in 100 mL of 2xTY with 100 µg/mL ampicillin, 50 µg/mL kanamycin, and 0.1% glucose. Incubate overnight at 30 °C with shaking.

DAY 9:

5. Centrifuge the overnight culture at 3200 × *g* for 15 min.
6. Purify phage by PEG purification as described in Subheading 3.7 (Purification of phage repertoire by PEG precipitation).
7. Once resuspended in 1 mL PBS (Subheading 3.7, **step 4**), the precipitated phage can be stored at 4 °C for up to 1 week or used immediately for the second round of selection. Keep an aliquot (150 µL) of this precipitated phage, at −80 °C with 15% glycerol, labeled as "phage-scFv panning1", to be used in pools ELISA.

3.10 Preparation of Paramagnetic Beads for the Second Round of Selection

This protocol is based on use of 5 mg (165 µL) Dynabeads® M-280 Tosylactivated. It is not recommended to couple <5 mg beads at a time.

1. Wash of paramagnetic beads by resuspending the beads in a vial. Vortex for >30 s.
2. Transfer 165 µL of beads (5 mg) to a 2 mL screw cap tube.
3. Add the same volume of Buffer A or B and resuspend.
4. Place the tube in a magnet for 1 min and discard the supernatant.

5. Remove the tube from the magnet and resuspend the washed beads in the same volume of Buffer A or B as the initial volume of beads (**step 3**)
6. Transfer 165 μL of washed beads to a new screw cap tube. Place the tube in a magnet for 1 min and discard the supernatant.
7. Resuspend the beads in 100 μg of ligand for each 5 mg of beads (*see* **Note 14**). Add buffer A or B to a total volume of 150 μL. Mix thoroughly by vortex or pipetting. Add 100 μL Buffer C and mix by vortexing or pipetting.
8. Incubate in Hula-Mixer at 37 °C for 12–18 h (total volume = 250 μL).

DAY 10:

9. After incubation with the protein extract, place the tube on a magnet for 2 min and remove the supernatant.
10. Remove the tube from the magnet and add 1 mL Buffer D (blocking buffer), vortex 30 s and incubate at 37 °C for 2 h in Hula-mixer.
11. First spin the tube and then place it on a magnet for 2 min and remove the supernatant.
12. Remove the tube from the magnet and add 1 mL Buffer E (washing buffer), vortex for 5–10 s. Place the tube on a magnet for 2 min and remove the supernatant.
13. Repeat **step 12** once more.
14. Resuspend and dilute the beads in 1 mL of Buffer E. Vortex and split in two tubes (500 μL each). For the Panning it is enough to use 2.5 mg of beads. Store the remaining 2.5 mg of beads at 4 °C.

3.11 Second Round of Selection on Paramagnetic Beads

1. Take 500 μL (2.5 mg) of the beads coated with non-target allergen, place the tube on the magnet 2 min and remove the supernatant.
2. To perform the negative panning add 1 mL of eluted phage-antibodies from Subheading 3.9, **step 7** (10^{12} pfu) together with 500 μL BSA 6% to the tube. Incubate rotating in Hula-mixer for 1 h at 25 °C.
3. Place the tube on the magnet 5 min and collect the supernatant (from beads coated with non-target allergen or negative panning). The phage-antibodies not bound to these beads are used for positive panning in the tube containing beads coated with target allergen.
4. Place the tube containing 500 μL (2.5 mg) of beads coated with the target allergen on the magnet for 2 min, and remove the supernatant. Add the supernatant collected from

the previous step (negative panning) to the beads. Incubate in Hula-mixer for 1 h at 25 °C, and without shaking for a further hour at 25 °C.

5. Place the tube on the magnet 5 min and discard the supernatant.
6. Continue to wash with Buffer E. Repeat 20 times: Add 1 mL Buffer E, vortex the tube, place the tube on the magnet 1 min, discard supernatant.
7. Transfer the beads into a new tube to avoid eluting phage-antibodies stuck on the tube wall.
8. Add 500 μL of trypsin solution with PBS (50 μL of Trypsin with 450 μL of PBS). Incubate for 10 min in Hula-mixer at 25 °C.
9. Place the tube on the magnet 5 min and gather the supernatant with the target-specific phage-antibodies.
10. Repeat the same process with trypsin-eluted phages as described above for round 1 (from Subheading 3.10, **steps 8–10**).

DAY 11–12:

11. Obtain large quantities of phage-antibodies from round 2 using protocol described in Subheading 3.9, to continue with the third panning. Store infected bacteria (from Subheading 3.9, **step 2**) as "stock *E. coli* panning 2", and precipitated phage (from Subheading 3.9, **step 7**) as "phage-scFv panning 2".

3.12 Third Round of Selection on Immune Stick Paddles (Optional)

Exactly proceed again with the same protocol as is described in Subheading 3.8. After each round of selection, check the specificity of eluted phage-antibodies by ELISA.

DAY 13:

3.13 Screening Phage Particles by ELISA

Population of phage produced at each round of selection can be screened by ELISA for binding to the target and non-target allergen in order to identify "polyclonal" phage-antibodies with increased affinity to the target. Also, phages from single colonies can be screened by ELISA in order to identify "monoclonal" target-specific phage-antibodies. In general, we have found that 1% powder milk in PBS is best for blocking during monoclonal phage ELISA whereas 1% Ovalbumin in PBS is best for blocking in polyclonal phage ELISA.

3.13.1 Polyclonal Phage ELISA

1. Coat a Nunc™ MaxiSorb 96-well plate overnight with 100 μL per well of 1/200 protein extract in PBS (*see* **Note 15**). Incubate for 1 h at 37 °C.
2. Wash wells five times with PBS. You should check that all wells fill with wash solution (if they do not you may create false positives during further washes). Discard liquid by flipping plate

over and then shaking it. Add 200 μL per well of 1% MPBS (1% skimmed milk powder in PBS) or 1% OVA (1% ovalbumin in PBS) to block, and incubate for 2 h at RT, or 1 h at 37 °C, or overnight at 4 °C.

3. Wash wells five times with PBS. Add 1 μL PEG precipitated phage from the end of each round of selection in 100 μL 1% MPBS (or 1% OVA-PBS) to each well.
4. Incubate for 1 h at RT. Discard phage solution and wash ten times with PBS (*see* **Note 16**).
5. Add 1 in 5000 dilution of HRP-anti-M13 in 1% MPBS (or 1% OVA-PBS). Incubate for 1 h at RT. Wash 5 times with PBS.
6. Add 100 μL of TMB solution to each well and leave at RT for 2–15 min. A blue color should develop in positive wells.
7. Stop the reaction by adding 50 μL 1 M sulfuric acid. The blue color should turn yellow.
8. Read the absorbance at 450 nm.

Figure 3 shows representative polyclonal ELISA results for selection of almond-specific and walnut-specific phage-scFv.

3.13.2 Monoclonal Phage ELISA

1. Inoculate individual colonies from the titration plates from each round of selection (Subheading 3.8, **step 9**) into 200 μL 2xTY containing 100 μg/mL ampicillin and 1% glucose in 96 cell-well plates. Grow shaking (250 rpm) two or more hours at 37 °C.
2. Transfer a small inoculum (about 2 μL) from this plate to a second 96 cell-well plate containing 200 μL of 2xTY with 100 μg/mL ampicillin and 1% glucose per well. Grow shaking (250 rpm) at 37 °C for 2 h. (Make glycerol stocks of the original 96-well plate, by adding glycerol to a final concentration of 15%, and then storing the plates at −80 °C).
3. After 2 h incubation (of the second plate) add 25 μL 2xTY containing 100 μg/mL ampicillin, 1% glucose and 10^9 helper phage.
4. Shake (250 rpm) at 37 °C for 1 h. Spin 1800 × *g* for 10 min, then aspirate off the supernatant.
5. Resuspend pellet in 200 μL 2xTY containing 100 μg/mL ampicillin and 50 μg/mL kanamycin. Grow shaking (250 rpm) overnight at 30 °C.
6. Spin at 1800 × *g* for 10 min and use 50 μL of the supernatant (instead of the PEG precipitated polyclonal phage) in phage ELISA as detailed above.

Figure 4 shows the phage-ELISA results of individual clones after Planning 2 in the selection of walnut-specific phage-antibodies.

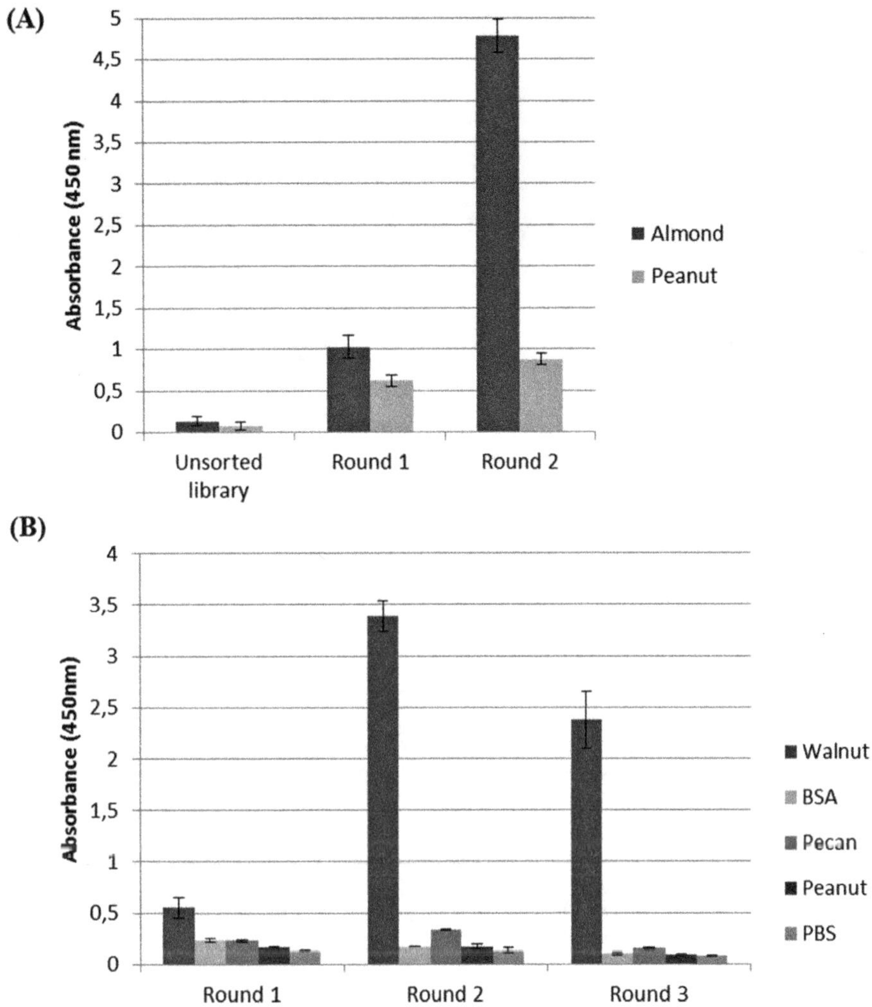

Fig. 3 Indirect phage-ELISA results obtained with polyclonal phages rescued at each round of selection against almond (**a**) and walnut (**b**) extract. Precipitated phages from each round of selection were analyzed by ELISA. Absorbance values are the mean of three independent determinations. Error bars show the standard deviation for each set of data

3.14 PCR Screening Selected Clones

Individual clones selected by ELISA can be further characterized through a PCR screening to check the presence of full length V_H and Vκ insert. Primers used and expected sizes depending on the fragments to be amplified are shown in Table 1.

To perform PCR analysis we used My Taq™ Mix (ready-to-use 2x mix for fast and highly-specific PCR) for a total volume of 25 μL per reaction (Table 2). All reactions must be set-up on ice and then subjected to temperature cycles for amplifications of the target sequences (Table 3).

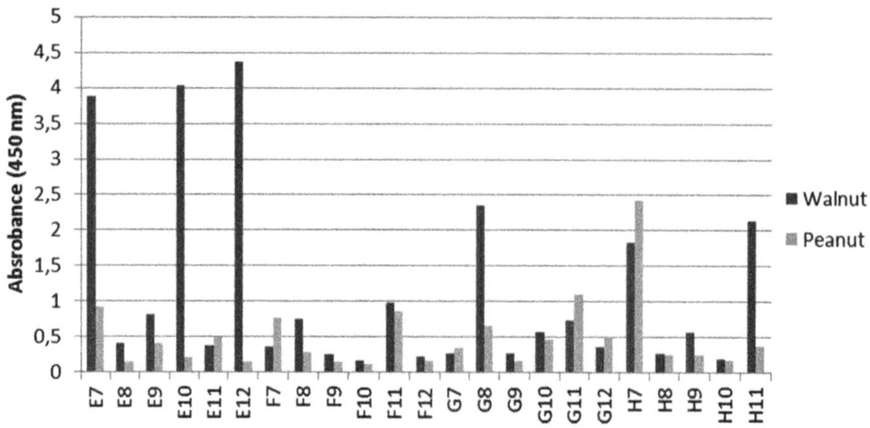

Fig. 4 Indirect phage-ELISA results obtained with monoclonal phages (phages obtained from individual colonies) against walnut extract after the second panning. Clone E12, later renamed as JR35, was selected after ELISA and sequencing characterization

Table 1
Primers used for PCR screening of individual clones

Fragment	Primers (5′-3′)	Expected size
Whole insert VH + Vκ	Fw- **LMB3:** CAG GAA ACA GCT ATG AC Rev.- **pHEN seq:** CTA TGC GGC CCC ATT CA	With whole insert: **935 bp** Without insert: **329 bp** With only V_H: **625 bp** With only V_k: **635 bp**
VH only	Fw- **LMB3:** CAG GAA ACA GCT ATG AC Rev.- **link seq new:** CGA CCC GCC ACC GCC GCT G	With insert: **527 bp** Without insert: **227 bp**
Vκ only	Fw-**DPK9 FR1:** CAT CTG TAG GAG ACA GAG TC Rev.- **pHEN seq:** CTA TGC GGC CCC ATT CA	With insert: **368 bp** Without insert: **no band**

Table 2
Preparation of PCR reactions for screening of individual clones

Component	Concentration	Volume per sample (μL)
Template	Culture from Subheading 3.13.2, **step 2** or pick a colony from Subheading 3.8, **step 9**	2
Primers (Fw and Rev)	20 nmol/mL each	0.5
My Taq™ Mix		12.5
Water (ddH2O)		Up to 25
Final volume PCR mix		25

Table 3
PCR cycling conditions for screening of individual clones

Step	Temperature	Time	Cycles
Initial denaturation	95 °C	1 min	1
Denaturation	95 °C	15 s	30
Annealing	User determined (usually 2–5 °C below the lower Tm of the primer pair)	15 s	
Extension	72 °C	10 s	

3.15 Sequencing-Selected Clones

For sequencing of selected clones, the following primers are recommended.

For VH use link seq new 5′-CGA CCC GCC ACC GCC GCT G-3′.

For Vκ use pHEN seq 5′-CTA TGC GGC CCC ATT CA-3′.

The nucleotide sequences obtained for the almond- and walnut-specific scFv (Fig. 5) are shown as an example, and also comparison of their deduced amino acid sequences (Fig. 6).

4 Notes

1. TYE plates are used in this protocol without, with 1%, and with 0.1% of glucose. For 1 L you must add 50 mL or 5 mL of glucose solution 20%, respectively. Add the glucose together with the antibiotic. Depending on required final volume, you must add the quantity of water necessary to maintain the glucose concentration. Plates should be dried in flow-bench before use.
2. $MgSO_4$, $CaCl_2$, and Vitamin B1 (Thiamine Hydrochloride) must be filtered through 0.2 μM filter in a laminar flow cabinet and used fresh that day.
3. Pour H-Top agar plates and store the excess for weeks at 4 °C. This medium solidifies very easily. It is important to warm up in a water bath (55 °C) before use.
4. It is advisable to separate the solution into smaller bottles before sterilization to avoid contamination.
5. To handle glycerol it is advisable to use a micropipette for viscous liquids.
6. Buffers A, B, and C are used for prewashing and coupling of Dynabeads® M-280 Tosylactivated. Buffer A is the recommended buffer for coupling. For pH labile ligands, use Buffer B. Do not add any protein (apart from your specific protein ligand), sugar, etc., to these buffers.

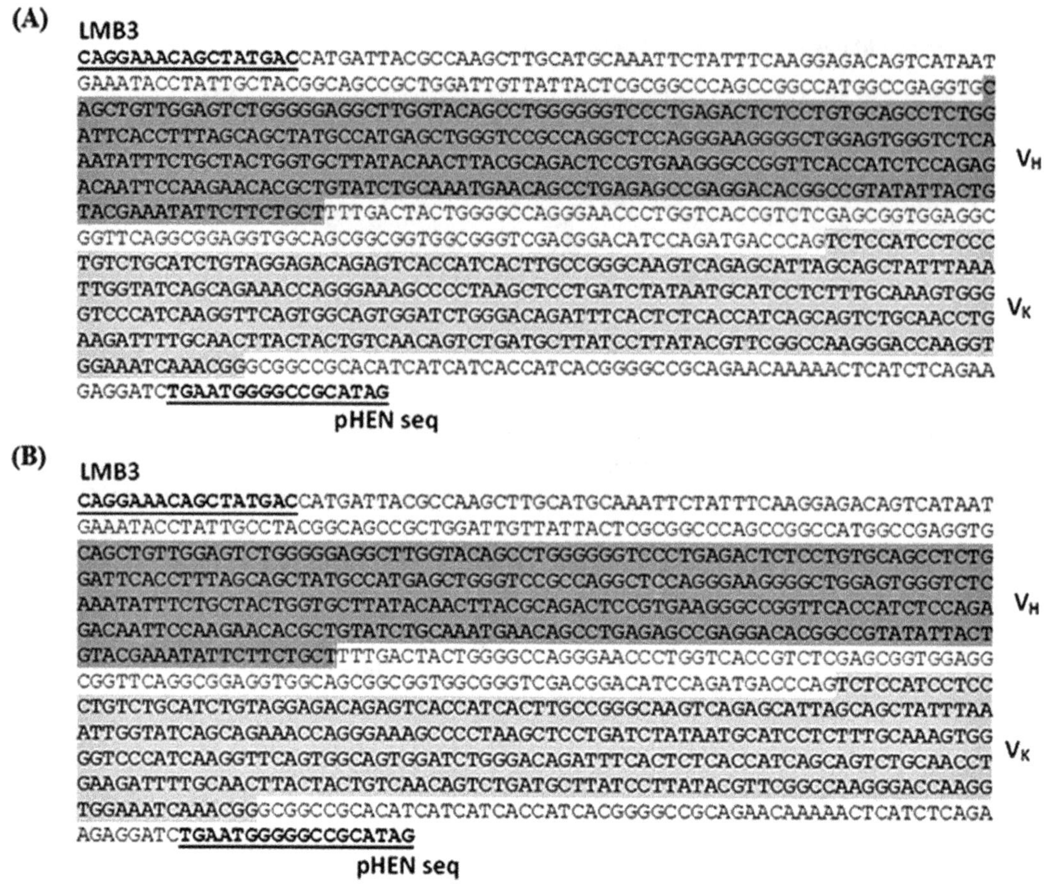

Fig. 5 Sequencing of pIT2 vector with primers LMB3 and pHEN. Sequence of V_H and V_K region specific to almond (**a**) and walnut (**b**). In *yellow* primers LMB3 and pHEN. In *pink* the sequence of V_H region and in grey V_K region

7. Buffers D and E are used for washing of all ligand-coupled beads. Buffer E can also be used for storage of ligand-coupled beads. Do not use these buffers or any buffer containing protein or aminogroups (e.g. glycine, Tris) for pre-washing or coupling to these beads. Protein blocking is recommended as it reduces aggregation and non-specific binding. If a preservative is needed for the coupled beads, a final concentration of <0.1% (w/v) sodium azide may be added to Buffer E.
8. The disposable pestle can be fabricated in the lab by sealing a glass Pasteur pipette or a micropipette tip with a flame.
9. Three layers are usually observed after centrifugation: a sediment, intermediate aqueous phase with proteins and DNA, and some floating particles.
10. It is advisable to run through the protocols using the control clones before you use the library: Streak the controls on TYE plates containing 100 μg/mL ampicillin and 1% glucose.

	H-CDR1 / H-CDR2
Almond	QPGGSLRLSCAAS**GFTFSSYA**MSWVRQAPGKGLEWVSA**ITSYGSDTY**YADSVKGRFTISR
Walnut	QPGGSLRLSCAAS**GFTFSSYA**MSWVRQAPGKGLEWVSN**ISATGAYTT**YADSVKGRFTISR
	H-CDR3 / Linker
Almond	DNSKNTLYLQMNSLRAEDTGVYYCA**KSAYDFD**YWGQGTLVTVS*SGGGGSGGGGSGGGGST*
Walnut	DNSKNTLYLQMNSLRAEDTAVYYCT**KYSSAFD**YWGQGTLVTVS*SGGGGSGGGGSGGGGST*
	L-CDR1 / L-CDR2
Almond	DIQMTQSPSSLSASVGDRVTIT**CRASQSISSYL**NWYQQKPGKAPKLLI**YSASALQS**GVPS
Walnut	DIQMTQSPSSLSASVGDRVTIT**CRASQSISSYL**NWYQQKPGKAPKLLI**YNASSLQS**GVPS
	L-CDR3 / Hys-Tag
Almond	RFSGSGSGTDFTLTISSLQPEDFATYY**CQQGASDPT**TFGQGTKVEIKRAAA*HHHHHH*GAA
Walnut	RFSGSGSGTDFTLTISSLQPEDFATYY**CQQSDAYPY**TFGQGTKVEIKRAAA*HHHHHH*GAA
Almond	EQKLISEEDLNGAA
Walnut	EQKLISEEDLNGAA

Fig. 6 Amino acid sequences of the almond [5] and walnut scFvs deduced from the nucleotide sequences by Expasy Website. Positions of the respective complementary determining regions for the variable domains of heavy (H-CDR 1-3) and light (L-CDR 1-3) chains are indicated

After overnight growth at 37 °C in an incubator pick a single colony from each and grow these overnight (shaking at 37 °C) in 5 mL 2xTY containing 100 μg/mL ampicillin and 1% glucose. Make phage for the positive and negative controls separately (use 500 μL of overnight in Subheading 3.9). Use a 1:100 mixture of phage produced from the positive and the negative controls and perform one round of selection (Subheading 3.8) using 100 μg/mL of BSA in PBS for coating. Check for enrichment of BSA binders (should be over 50% after one round of selection) by monoclonal phage ELISA (Subheading 3.12.2).

11. The first round of selection (enrichment of antigen-specific phage by binding to immobilized antigen) is the most important one. Any errors or loss of diversity made at this point will be amplified in subsequent rounds of selection.

12. To increase specificity of the phage selection for the target allergen, we first perform a negative panning with a non-target allergen. Thus, it is necessary to coat one immuno stick with the target allergen and a second one with a non-target allergen (e.g., for selection of phage-antibodies against almond, one immune stick is coated with 100 μg/mL of almond extract and the other with 100 μg/mL of peanut extract).

13. This method of phage titration allows recovery of isolated colonies to be analyzed by the monoclonal phage ELISA, after the second round of selection. After each round you should obtain at least 100 infective phages. If not, you must repeat the process, using the remaining 250 μL of eluted phage from

Subheading 3.8, **step 8**. If you obtain less than 100 phages again, repeat the selection starting at Subheading 3.8, **step 1**.

14. The concentration of protein extract must be calculated for each specific quantity of beads, for example, using 5 mg of beads, calculate the necessary volume of sample/protein extract to have a final concentration of 100 μg in a total volume of 150 μL with buffer A. To increase specificity of the phage selection for the target allergen, we perform a negative panning on paramagnetic beads in a similar way as explained in panning 1 with immuno sticks. Thus, it is necessary to prepare two different batches of coated beads, 5 mg of beads are coated with the target allergen in a screw cap tube (almond or walnut extract in our case) and 5 mg with the non-target allergen in a second tube (peanut extract).
15. To check specificity, include appropriate controls: wells coated with the target allergen, with non-target allergen(s), and without allergen (just PBS).
16. We do not recommend to include Tween 20 in phage ELISA, as we have observed a higher background.

References

1. Curzer HJ, Perry G, Wallace MC, Perry D (2016) The three rs of animal research: what they mean for the institutional animal care and use committee and why. Sci Eng Ethics 22:549–565. doi:10.1007/s11948-015-9659-8
2. Qi H, Lu H, Qiu H-J et al (2012) Phagemid vectors for phage display: properties, characteristics and construction. J Mol Biol 417:129–143. doi:10.1016/j.jmb.2012.01.038
3. McCafferty J, Griffiths AD, Winter G, Chiswell DJ (1990) Phage antibodies: filamentous phage displaying antibody variable domains. Nature 348:552–554. doi:10.1038/348552a0
4. Georgieva Y, Konthur Z (2011) Design and screening of M13 phage display cDNA libraries. Molecules 16:1667–1681. doi:10.3390/molecules16021667
5. de la Cruz S, Cubillos-Zapata C, López-Calleja IM et al (2015) Isolation of recombinant antibody fragments (scFv) by phage display technology for detection of almond allergens in food products. Food Control 54:322–330. doi:10.1016/j.foodcont.2015.02.011
6. Bird RE, Hardman KD, Jacobson JW et al (1988) Single-chain antigen-binding proteins. Science 242:423–426
7. Kristensen P, Winter G (1998) Proteolytic selection for protein folding using filamentous bacteriophages. Fold Des 3:321–328. doi:10.1016/S1359-0278(98)00044-3
8. Lee CMY, Iorno N, Sierro F, Christ D (2007) Selection of human antibody fragments by phage display. Nat Protoc 2:3001–3008. doi:10.1038/nprot.2007.448
9. Weber M, Bujak E, Putelli A et al (2014) A highly functional synthetic phage display library containing over 40 billion human antibody clones. PLoS One 9:e100000. doi:10.1371/journal.pone.0100000
10. de la Cruz S, López-Calleja IM, Alcocer M et al (2013) Selection of recombinant antibodies by phage display technology and application for detection of allergenic Brazil nut (*Bertholletia excelsa*) in processed foods. J Agric Food Chem 61:10310–10319. doi:10.1021/jf403347t
11. Rouet R, Lowe D, Dudgeon K et al (2012) Expression of high-affinity human antibody fragments in bacteria. Nat Protoc 7:364–373. doi:10.1038/nprot.2011.448

Chapter 10

Protein Microarray-Based IgE Immunoassay for Allergy Diagnosis

Nuzul N. Jambari, XiaoWei Wang, and Marcos Alcocer

Abstract

Protein microarray is a miniaturized multi-analyte, solid-phased immunoassay where thousands of immobilized individual protein spots on a microscopic slide bind are bound to specific antibodies (immunoglobulins) from serum samples, which are then detected by fluorescent labeling. The image processing and pattern recognition are then quantitatively analyzed using advanced algorithms. Here, we describe the use of an in-house-produced complex protein microarray containing extracts and pure proteins that has been probed with antibodies present in the horse sera and detection by fluorophore-conjugated antibody and data analysis. The flexibility of the number and types of proteins that can be printed on the microarray allows different set of specific IgE immunoassay analysis to be carried out.

Key words Protein microarray, Component-resolved diagnostics, Microarray-based allergy testing, Horse sera, IgE-binding assay, Partial Least Squares Discriminant Analysis (PLSDA), Variable influence on the projection (VIP)

1 Introduction

Protein microarray is a miniaturized multi-analyte, solid-phase immunoassay where proteins are immobilized or "spotted" onto a solid surface of a size of microscopic slide and hybridized or probed against microliters of serum samples. Any specifically bound immunoglobulins (Ig) from sera are then labeled with fluorophore-conjugated antibodies and detected under standard conditions.

Protein arrays of pure proteins and extracts have shown to be reproducible, sensitive, and very flexible regarding the different types of Igs that can be monitored simultaneously. Generally, the results are comparable to other standard laboratory methods such as UniCAP, ELISA, and immunoblot tests but with an improved efficiency in terms of quantities of the sample used.

Previously in our lab, we have developed protein microarray-based immunoassays for detection of food and environmental

Jing Lin and Marcos Alcocer (eds.), *Food Allergens: Methods and Protocols*, Methods in Molecular Biology, vol. 1592,
DOI 10.1007/978-1-4939-6925-8_10, © Springer Science+Business Media LLC 2017

allergens for humans [1–3] and more recently allergenic components from insect saliva used in equine allergy have been added [4].

The current array contains ca. 240 complex extracts and 120 pure proteins from food (fruit, dairy, seeds, fish, mollusks), environment (epithelium, pollen, fungi, and insects including recombinant *Culicoides* allergens) that are commercially available or in-house-produced. In these complex arrays, extracts and pure proteins are represented and a complex series of mathematical modeling procedures (discussed in [4]) has been developed and used to classify and guide the analysis.

The protein microarray used in this chapter was developed by spotting normalized purified protein solutions and extracts of interest onto 16-pad nitrocellulose FAST slide format using Marathon microarrayer, which was carried out by Arrayjet Ltd, Roslin, Scotland. The resulting 16-pad nitrocellulose FAST slide contains 12,288 spots per slide and each pad consists of 384 proteins, extracts, and controls spotted in duplicate at similar position (*see* Fig. 1c). Details of methodology for printing protein arrays will not be covered in this chapter.

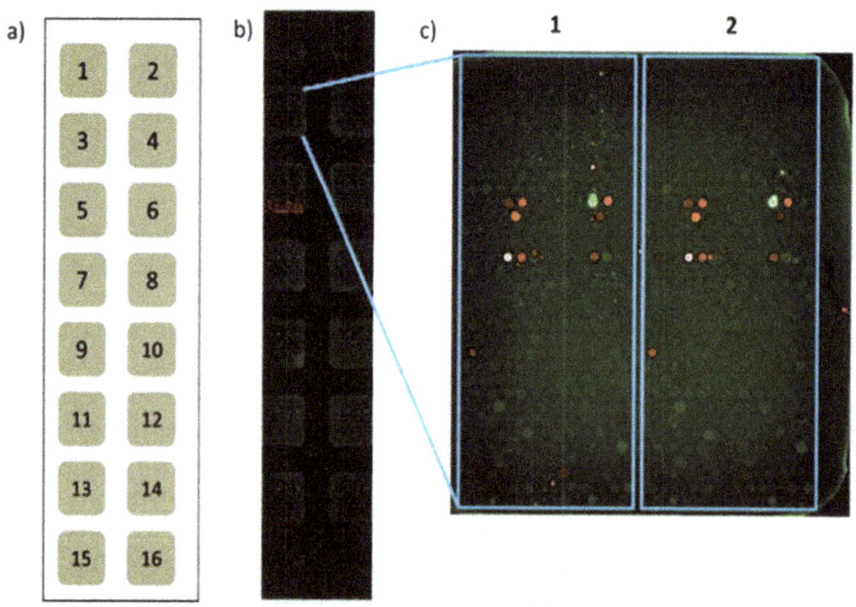

Fig. 1 (**a**) A diagram showing the 16-pad nitrocellulose FAST slide array that is printed with protein extracts and purified proteins from food, environment (including recombinant *Culicoides* allergens), and positive controls. The in-house assembled protein microarray slide contains 16 pads with a total of 12,288 proteins per slide printed in duplicate. (**b**) An image of a microarray after probing with 15 serum samples and a control, and detecting with DyLight647-labeled antibodies and visualized using GenePix 4000B scanner. (**c**) Pad '3' of the scanned microarray of a control (2% BSA in 0.2% PBST only) is shown with 384 protein spots printed in duplicate at similar positions in box '1' and box '2'. The array pad contains positive controls such as Cy5 and Cy3 conjugated proteins to help identify arrays while gridding the spotted antigens

2 Materials

2.1 Equipments

1. Printed 16-pad nitrocellulose slide arrays (*see* **Note 1**).
2. Corning® 5 slide Holder.
3. Mini slide boxes (25 slides).
4. Proplate slide module (Grace Bio-Labs, Inc.).
5. Proplate® Multi-Well Chambers with silicone gasket (Grace Bio-Labs, Inc.).
6. Proplate® adhesive seal strips with seal strip applicator (Grace Biolabs, Inc.).
7. Mistral 3000i centrifuge (4-place wind-shielded swing-out rotor (43124–708) with 2 × 96-well plate holders).
8. Mini Hybridization Oven with a rotator.
9. Thermo-Hypro 20 Hybridization Unit.
10. ELx50 Washer (BioTek Instruments, Inc., Winooski, VT, USA).
11. GenePix 4000B scanner (Molecular Devices, USA).

2.2 Buffers and Solutions (See Note 2)

1. 10 mM phosphate buffered saline, pH 7.4 (1× PBS): dissolve 8 g NaCl, 0.2 g KCl, 1.44 g Na_2HPO_4 and 0.24 g of KH_2PO_4in 800 ml deionized water, adjust to pH 7.4 with 2 N HCl and adjust volume to 1 L with deionized water.
2. 0.2% PBST: 0.2% (w/v) Tween 20 in 1× PBS.
3. 1% BSA: 1% (w/v) bovine serum albumin, low endotoxin, pH 7, ≥ 98% (BSA) in 0.2% PBST.
4. 2% BSA: 2% (w/v) BSA in 0.2% PBST.
5. 3% BSA: 3% (w/v) BSA in 0.2% PBST.
6. Wash buffer: 0.05% (w/v) Tween 20 in 1× PBS.

2.3 Sample

1. Horse sera (kept at −80 °C when not in use) (*see* **Note 3**).

2.4 Antibodies

1. Detection antibody: mouse anti-horse IgE mAb (1 mg/ml) [7].
2. Labeled secondary antibody: Dylight 649-labeled rabbit anti-mouse IgG Ab (Dylight 649,Rockland Inc., USA)(1 mg/ml).

2.5 Software

1. GenePix Pro software v6.0.1.27 (Axon Instruments).
2. Microsoft Excel software (Microsoft, USA).
3. Matlab (Version 9, The Mathworks Inc., USA).
4. Excellink toolbox (Mathworks) and Dataset Object (Version 5.0, Eigen-vector Research Inc., USA).

3 Methods

3.1 Sera Sample Preparation

1. Aliquot sera samples from horse patients/controls into smaller volume (100 μl/tube) and store aliquots at −80 °C until further use (*see* **Note 3**).
2. Thaw and keep sera samples on ice when in use.

3.2 Probing Protein Microarray

1. Label printed 16-pad array slides for identification.
2. Block the printed 16-pad array slides with 3% BSA. Place a maximum of three slides in each Corning® 5 slide holder and fill the slide holder with approximately 25 ml of 3% BSA in PBS without air bubbles.
3. Close the cap of the slide holder, sealed it with parafilm, and covered it with aluminum foil to prevent light exposure.
4. Incubate the slides for 3 h at 37 °C with rotation in a mini hybridizing oven and in the dark.
5. Wash the slides with 0.05% PBST three times for 2 min each. This is followed by 5 times washing with deionized water for 1 min each. Place slides in a slide holder box and place the box onto the 96-well plate holder. Dry slides by centrifugation (Mistral 3000i, rotor 43,124-708, with a 96-well holder) at 300 × *g* for 10 min at a room temperature (*see* **Note 4**).

3.3 Hybridization

1. Assemble the Proplate slide module (Grace Bio-Labs) by aligning edges of slides with the edges of upper structure (*see* **Note 5**).
2. Press gently on back side of the slide to adhere the slide to the gasket.
3. Slide clips until both ends are flush with the assembly. Make sure that the slide "star" position is at frame number 15.
4. Wet the 16-pad array membrane with 150 μl of 0.2% PBST per well.
5. Dilute horse sera in 1:2 with 2% BSA in a flow cabinet (*see* **Note 6**).
6. Aspirate 0.2% PBST from wells using multi-channel pipette without touching the surface of the slide.
7. Add 100 μl of diluted serum sample to each well. For each slide, dedicate a well (one of 16 pads) as a control by adding 100 μl of 2% BSA only.
8. Seal the Proplate slide module with Proplate adhesive seal strips (*see* **Note 7**).
9. Incubate slides in Proplate assembly in Thermo Hypro 20 hybridizer at 37 °C for 2 h with vibration (set to AVS 3).

3.4 Detection

1. Wash slides in Proplate assembly three times with 0.05% PBST using ELx50 Washer (*see* **Note 8**).
2. Dilute detection antibody, mouse anti-horse IgE mAb, in 1:400 in 1% BSA.
3. Add 100 μl of the diluted detection antibody to each well and incubate in Thermo Hypro 20 hybridizer at 37 °C for 1 h with vibration (set to AVS 3).
4. Wash slides in Proplate assembly three times with 0.05% PBST on ELx50 Washer.
5. Dilute labeled secondary antibody, DyLight 649 conjugated anti-Mouse IgG1, in 1:400 in 1% BSA.
6. Wash slides in Proplate assembly three times with 0.05% PBST and three times with deionized water using ELx50 Washer.
7. Carefully slide clips off and transfer the slide to a slide box with some tissue papers at the bottom.
8. Centrifuge slide at 300 × g (Mistral 3000i, rotor 43,124-708, with a 96-well holder) for 10 min at a room temperature to dry the slide (*see* **Note 4**).
9. Scan the slide on a dedicated scanner (GenePix 4000B) using the PMT parameter settings as 440 (645 nm) and 310 (532 nm). Save the image as tiff file.

3.5 Data Analysis

1. Create a gal (GenePixArrayList) file to indicate the position of each protein spotted on the array using GenePix Pro 6.1 software (Molecular Devices Corporation).
2. Grid the tiff image of scanned slide with the gal file using GenePix Pro 6.1 software (*see* **Note 9**).
3. Analyze the image to get the fluorescence intensity readings for each spot in the GenePix Result (gpr) file.
4. Subtract readings of a local background for each spot (around the diameter of the spot) from the fluorescence intensity reading of the spot.
5. In the gpr file, the fluorescence intensity of each spot is presented and annotated in a table where the mean, median standard error, and local background readings for each spot are tabulated and used for further calculation purposes.
6. Export gpr file into Microsoft Excel.
7. Average duplicate spot readings for each pad (both samples and a control).
8. Subtract averaged spot readings of control from averaged spot readings of samples to eliminate non-specific binding and inherent autofluorescence of some proteins using Visual Basic macros in-built into Microsoft Excel software (Microsoft, USA).

9. Comply normalized sera sample data and transfer them from Microsoft Excel to Matlab (Version Matlab (version 7.1 (R14SP3), The Mathworks Inc., USA) using Excel link toolbox (Mathworks) and the Dataset Object (Version 5.0, Eigenvector Research Inc., USA).
10. Perform Partial Least Squares regression (PLS) to establish the multivariate link between the array data sets and the results from standard IgE immunoassay (such as CAP) results.
11. Perform Partial Least Square Discrimination analysis (PLSDA) based on Partial Least Squares regression (PLS) model [5, 6] to construct predictive models (*see* **Note 10**). Use the threshold of >1 and scale the means of the data to unit standard deviation by auto-scale.
12. Employ internal cross-validation to assess the number of latent variables (data trends) to build model with minimal predictive error.
13. Confirm all the classification results by cross-validation where random subsets of the data are left out.
14. Build regression model with increasing number of latent variables and establish the prediction error for the left out samples for each model. The influence of individual features may be captured with variable influence on the projection (VIP) derived from the PLS coefficients for the optimal set of components from the PLS model (*see* Fig. 2).
15. Repeat **step 14** until all samples have been left-out once and establish an average prediction/classification error per number of latent variables. The result is an estimation of the most appropriate number of latent variables (with the lowest error) as well as an estimation of the prediction/classification error to be expected when applying the model to new data (*see* Fig. 3).

4 Notes

1. Printed microarray slides can be kept at room temperature for a long time but need to be stored in a dark and dry area.
2. It is better to prepare fresh buffers every time before the analysis. Buffers such as PBST may be kept at 4 °C for 7 days and 1× PBS may be kept at room temperature for a long time however, BSA in PBST has to be freshly prepared prior to the analysis.
3. To avoid repeated freeze–thawing of the sera used, aliquot sera into smaller quantities and store the aliquots at −80 °C. Keep thawed sera on ice when in use.

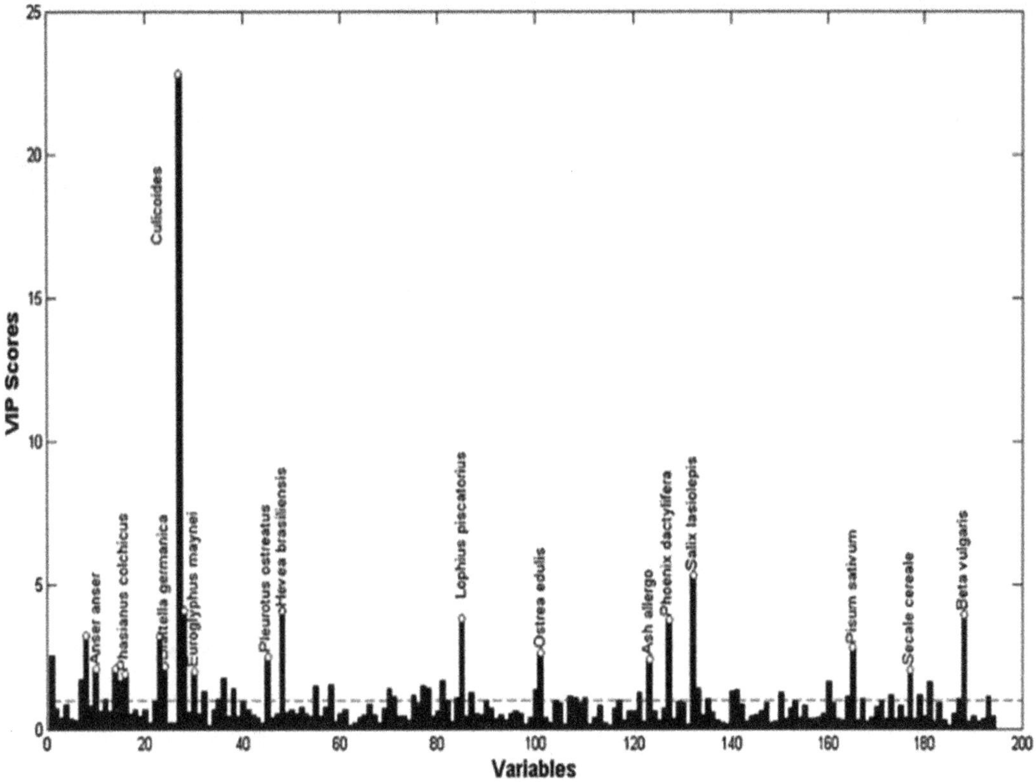

Fig. 2 An example of analyzed comparative result by determining the variable influence on projection (VIP) from insect-bite hypersensitive (IBH)-affected and healthy horses for each protein and extract. VIP is calculated by partial least square discrimination analysis software (PLSDA) from 35 insect-bite hypersensitive (IBH) affected and 37 healthy control horses using 200 averaged variables (extracts and pure proteins). The mean variable of *Culicoides nubeculosus* and *C. obsoletus* (extract and pure proteins) was the major variable identified as important for this classification. Some minor contributing variables are also shown. Graph is derived from a published data [4]

4. Tissues are placed at the base of the slide holder to quicken the drying process. Do not let the slide air-dry and the slide should be taken out quickly in the flat slide holder box for drying.
5. Place microscope slide (array side down) over silicone gasket, aligning edges with the edges of the upper structure and make sure that the slide properly adhere to the gasket. Improper assembly may cause the glass slide to be chipped or broken.
6. All works that involve the use of serum need to be performed in a flow cabinet. If human sera are used, please ensure that the preparation is performed in a designated area for human sample. Use of disposable gloves is mandatory. Any spillage should be wiped with Virkon and disposed in the clinical waste.
7. Proplate-assembled microarray slide need to be properly sealed between the wells. The solution tends to vaporize during the

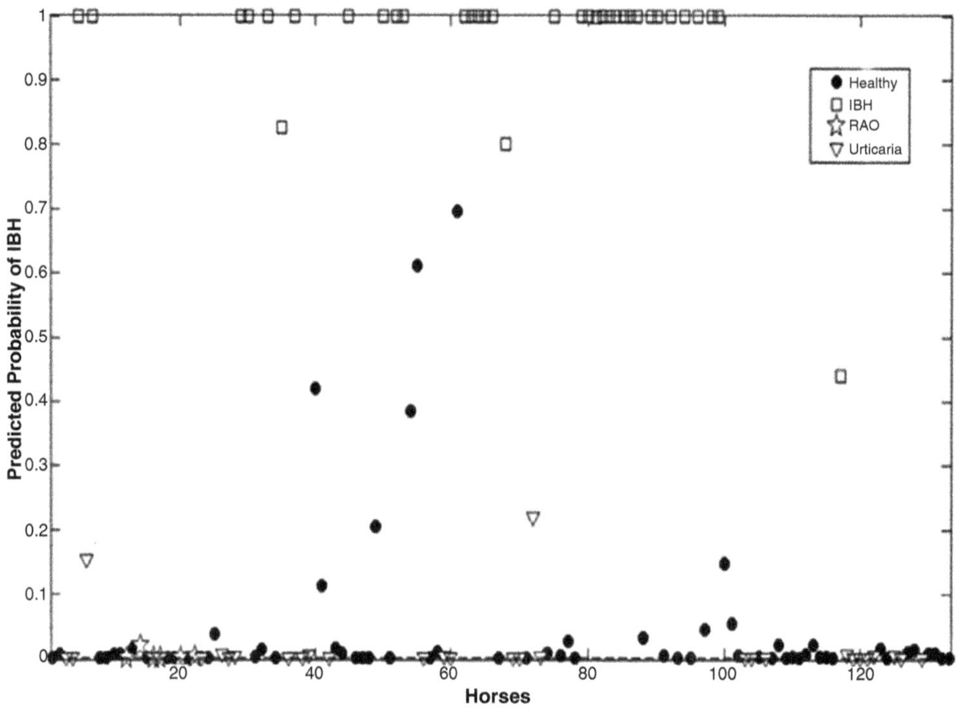

Fig. 3 Prediction probability of belonging to the IBH group of horses. Using the calibration parameters shown in Fig. 2, the predicted probability of each horse to belong to the IBH affected group ($n = 37$) when compared to control horses (healthy, recurrent airway obstruction (RAO) and urticaria; $n = 98$) is shown. The plot graph showed that 36 out of 37 IBH-affected horses had >70% probability of belonging to the IBH group, estimating that they are to be diagnosed as IBH. Image is derived from a published data [4]

hybridization process so improper sealing may cause the plate to dry. Avoid using parafilm.

8. For washing step, it is recommended to use an automated plate washer. ELx50 Washer used in our lab is an automated plate washer with 16-channel manifold for dual dispensing and aspirating solution that ensure a thorough washing of the array with low residuals. However, if the plate washer is not available, the washing step can be performed manually (but with a risk of remnant residuals).
9. The software to create the gal file that link the spot position with its protein identity is provided with the GenePix scanner but ultimately can also be created as tab delimited file in Microsoft Excel. Grid may need to be adjusted manually to fit the spot on the tiff image of the scanned slide.
10. PLSDA is suited for the analysis of protein microarray due to (a) its ability to handle data in which variables far out-number the number of samples and (b) in which features are correlated (multicollinearity).

Acknowledgements

Nuzul Jambari was sponsored by a full Ph.D. grant from the Ministry of Education of Malaysia.

References

1. Renault NK, Gaddipati SR, Wulfert F et al (2011) Multiple protein extract microarray for profiling human food-specific immunoglobulins A, M, G and E. J Immunol Methods 364(1–2):21–32
2. Renault NK, Mirotti L, Alcocer MJ (2007) Biotechnologies in new high-throughput food allergy tests: why we need them. Biotechnol Lett 29(3):333–339
3. Wulfert F, Sanyasi G, Tongen L et al (2012) Prediction of tolerance in children with IgE mediated cow's milk allergy by microarray profiling and chemometric approach. J Immunol Methods 382(1–2):48–57
4. Marti E, Wang X, Jambari NN et al (2015) Novel in vitro diagnosis of equine allergies using a protein array and mathematical modelling approach: a proof of concept using insect bite hypersensitivity. Vet Immunol Immunopathol 167(3–4):171–177
5. Eriksson L, Trygg J, Wold S (2014) A chemometrics toolbox based on projections and latent variables. J Chemometr 28(5): 332–346
6. Wold S, Sjostrom M, Eriksson L (2001) PLS-regression: a basic tool of chemometrics. Chemom Intel Lab Syst 58(2):109–130
7. Wilson, A. D., & Harwood, L. (2006) Production of monoclonal antibodies specific for native equine IgE and their application to monitor total serum IgE responses in Icelandic and non-Icelandic horses with insect bite dermal hypersensitivity. Vet Immunol Immunopathol, 112: 156–170

Chapter 11

Basophil Degranulation Assay

Madhan Masilamani, Mohanapriya Kamalakannan, and Hugh A. Sampson

Abstract

Basophil degranulation assay has gained importance over the last decade in both diagnosis of food allergy and evaluation of progression of immunotherapy. This assay involves the identification and quantification of the expression of CD63 molecule on basophil membrane. CD63 is a marker of multivesicular bodies that is exposed to cell membrane during the process of degranulation in which the contents of basophil granules are released. This chapter describes the methodology for performing this assay.

Key words Basophils, Degranulation, In vitro test, CD63, Flow cytometry

1 Introduction

Basophil degranulation assay, also called basophil activation test (BAT), is a powerful assay that mimics in vivo IgE-mediated reactions in a test tube. Basophils are granulocytes that represent lesser than 1% of peripheral blood leukocytes. The morphology of basophils is very similar to other granulocytes. However, the flow characteristics are like lymphocytes with moderate forward scatter and low side scatter. BAT is a flow cytometry–based assay that relies on detection of degranulation and activation markers on the surface of basophils upon IgE cross-linking. Allergen-specific IgE is bound to FcεRIa receptors on basophils and mast cells in sensitized individuals. Cross-linking of IgE with specific allergen induces a Fyn- and Lyn-mediated activation signaling cascade, which culminates in the release of mediators stored in the basophil granules. During the process of degranulation, the inner membrane of the granules fuses to the plasma membrane of the cell through SNARE complex formation and membrane fusion, thereby exposing the membrane proteins associated with the secretory vesicles. CD63 (also known as gp53) is a prototypic marker of such vesicular membrane along with a number of other proteins such as lysosomal-associated membrane glycoproteins (LAMPs, CD107a and -b).

Jing Lin and Marcos Alcocer (eds.), *Food Allergens: Methods and Protocols*, Methods in Molecular Biology, vol. 1592, DOI 10.1007/978-1-4939-6925-8_11, © Springer Science+Business Media LLC 2017

The expression of CD63 as a measure of vesicular fusion and degranulation was first discovered by Knol and colleagues in 1991 [1]. In addition to the presence of IgE on membrane, basophils are characterized by the expression of basophil-specific ecto-nucleotide pyrophosphatase/phosphodiesterase (CD203c), alpha-chain of the IL-3 receptor (IL-3Ra or CD123), C-C chemokine receptor type 3 (CD193 or CCR3), and low levels of MHC class II cell surface receptor HLA-DR. The lineage-specific marker CD203c is an ecto-enzyme, expressed on the cell membrane of basophils and mast cells. CD203c is upregulated upon cross-linking of FceRIa. CD123 is expressed in both dendritic cells and basophils. However, the expression of high HLA-DR in dendritic cells differentiates CD123 expressing basophils from dendritic cells. The expression of CD123 is relatively less variable compared to IgE expression on basophils and serves a definitive marker of basophil identification [2, 3]. Although some basophil subsets are known to express very low levels of MHC class II molecules (including HLA-DR), these molecules are incapable of antigen presentation [4]. Other molecules of interest that were tested are the inhibitory receptor CD300a, phosphorylation of p38 MAPK and STAT5, etc. [5, 6]. Although some of these proteins are also expressed on other cell types, the advances in multicolor flow cytometry and development of novel fluorophores in the last decade along with generation of monoclonal antibodies against distinct cellular markers have made the unequivocal identification and quantification of basophils possible.

The use of BAT has become widespread as a complementary in vitro diagnostic tool for food allergy caused by a number of foods. BAT has been found very helpful when other traditional measures (such as skin testing, allergen-specific IgE, and CRD) are limited or equivocal. Currently, the most important applications of BAT in food allergy are the following: (1) part of diagnostic evaluation, (2) determination of clinically relevant allergen, (3) discrimination between sensitization and clinical allergy, (4) evaluation of cross-reactivity, (5) monitoring the progress/outcome of allergen immunotherapy and tolerance induction, and (6) detection of trace allergens [7–10]. The biology of basophils and the clinical utility and applications of BAT have been extensively reviewed in the recent past [11–14]. A number of publications utilizing basophil activation tests in food allergy are available in literature. BAT has been applied for several foods such as peanut [15–18]; egg and milk [8, 10, 19–22]; and Bet v1-related food allergies (celery, carror, and apple) [23].

Several commercial basophil degranulation kits are available for diagnostic purposes using as few as two antibodies. However, it is preferable to use a full panel of antibodies to unambiguously gate-out the basophils [24]. Some of the commercial basophil activation kits for assessing basophil activation are (1) BASOTEST (OPREGEN Pharma/Glycotope Biotechnology, Inc.) contains a two-color antibody reagent for assessing the basophil degranulation such as anti-IgE-PE and anti-gp53 (CD63)-FITC; (2) BASOSTEP kit (Immunostep, Inc.) uses a cocktail of anti-CD63-FITC, anti-CD203c-PE, anti-HLA-DR-PerCP, and anti-CD123-APC antibodies for detection and determination of basophil activation and degranulation; (3) Flow2 CAST kit (Buehlmann, Inc.) uses anti-CD63-FITC and anti-CCR3-PE. As both eosinophils and basophils express CCR3, specific gating for basophils based on FSC/SSC profiles is warranted; and (4) BD FastImmune (BD BioSciences, Inc.) uses anti-CD63-FITC, anti-CD123-PE, and anti-HLA-DR-PerCP antibodies. A comparison study using BASOTEST and BD FastImmune test showed no significant differences between patient's basophil degranulation [25] suggesting the utility of commercial diagnostic test kits.

2 Materials

1. Heparinized whole blood.
2. Sodium heparin collection tubes for collecting whole blood.
3. RPMI-1640 medium (store at 4 °C in the dark).
4. Basophil reaction medium: 2 ng/ml IL-3 in RPMI-1640 medium.
5. Stop solution: Phosphate buffered saline (PBS), 20 mM EDTA, sterile filtered. Store at 4 °C and expires after 1 week.
6. 1× BD FACS lysing solution: made from 10× stock w/H_2O. Store at 4 °C and expires after 1 week.
7. Staining buffer: PBS, 2 mM EDTA, 0.5% BSA, sterile filtered. Aliquot in hood and store at 4 °C. Expires after 2 months.
8. Antibody staining cocktail: The following fluorescent-conjugated antibodies are used for staining: anti-CD63, anti-CD203c, anti-CD123, Lineage markers (anti-CD3, anti-CD14, anti-CD19, and anti-CD41a), anti-HLA-DR—all stored at 4 °C in the dark.
9. *N*-Formylmethionyl-leucyl-phenylalanine (FMLP) (1 μM final concentration): Prepare from stock fMLP (50 mg/ml) in dimethylformamide (DMF). Dilute in basophil reaction medium.
10. Rabbit anti-human IgE polyclonal antibody 1 μg/ml final concentration: Prepare from stock 20 μg/ml. Dilute in basophil reaction medium.
11. Polypropylene flow cytometry tubes.

3 Methods

3.1 Blood Collection, Stimulation, Staining, and FACS Acquisition

1. *Blood collection:* Whole blood should be obtained in sodium heparin collection tubes with corresponding participant labels. Blood collection in acid citrate dextrose or EDTA tubes is not recommended (*see* **Notes 1** and **2**)
2. *Basophil reaction medium:* 2 ng/ml IL-3 in RPMI-1640 medium. This medium can be prepared in 20× concentrations, and stored in −80 °C until used. Reconstituted 2× medium will be used to prepare allergen dilutions and incubation with equal volume of whole blood. Although IL-3 is routinely used to prime aliquoted basophils in degranulation assays, this practice has been under scrutiny [26].
3. *Allergen preparation:* A range allergen dilution should be prepared in basophil medium (*see* **Note 3**). Prepare several tenfold serial dilutions of allergen stimulant in 2× basophil medium.
4. *Controls:* The following controls are suggested to be included in every assay: (a) unstained cells—without stimulation, for cytometer set up; (b) RPMI medium alone; (c) Basophil reaction medium; (d) *N*-Formylmethionyl-leucyl-phenylalanine (FMLP, 1 μM); and (e) anti-IgE 1 μg/ml. Both FMLP and anti-IgE are diluted in basophil medium. FMLP is a potent chemotactic factor that binds to specific G-protein coupled receptors on cell surface and serves as positive control for non-IgE-mediated basophil degranulation.
5. *Basophil stimulation:* Transfer equal volume (250 μl) of whole blood to each allergen stimulant and control assay tube (except unstained cells tube), mix gently, and incubate for 30 min at 37 °C incubator at 5% CO_2 with no agitation. During incubation time, prepare antibody staining cocktail. The degranulation reaction is stopped by adding 50 μl of cold (4 ° C) stop solution. Immediately proceed to staining after this step.
6. *Antibody staining:* Stain cells with the Ab cocktail at 4 °C for 30 min in the dark. Wash the cells with 3 ml cold (4 °C) staining buffer. Centrifuge for 5 min at 300 × *g* at 4 °C. After spin, carefully aspirate supernatant without disturbing pellet (*see* **Note 4**).
7. *RBC lysis and fixation:* Add 4 ml of 1× FACS lysing solution to each tube with the cell pellet, mix thoroughly by inverting. Incubate at room temperature in the dark for 15 min. After incubation, spin tubes at 800 × *g* for 10 min. Aspirate the supernatants carefully, then resuspend pellet in 200 μl of staining buffer (*see* **Note 5**).
8. *Flow cytometric acquisition, gating, and analysis:* Acquire cells in a flow cytometer. Basophils are characterized as FSC^{med} SSC^{lo} $Lineage^{-}$ $HLA\text{-}DR^{-/lo}$ $CD203^{+}$ $CD123^{+}$ cells. About 150–2000 basophils can be measured in 100 μl whole blood (*see* **Note 6**).

3.2 Data Analysis

The most common data analysis procedure is the assessment of frequency of CD63+ basophils in allergen-stimulated cells in the appropriate basophil gate. At least 100 basophils should be analyzed to obtain accurate values. The individual basophil degranulation (i.e., CD63 expression) after FcεR stimulation varies widely in humans. Individuals who show 0–5% CD63 upregulation in basophils after FcεR stimulation are considered as nonresponders. Those who show response between 5 and 16% are low responders. The BAT assay will not be reliable in nonresponders, while the results from low responders should be interpreted with caution [17, 27]. The basophil allergen threshold sensitivity, also known as CD-sens, is another way of describing the patients' allergen sensitivity [28, 29]. CD-sens is defined as the inverted value for the lowest allergen concentration giving 50% (LC_{50}) of maximum CD63 upregulation multiplied by 100, i.e., ($1/LC_{50} \times 100$, where LC_{50} is half maximal effective concentration). The higher the value for CD-sens, the higher is the basophil allergen sensitivity. In addition, change in mean fluorescent intensities of basophil activation marker CD203 is also useful readout (*see* **Note 3**). Figure 1 shows a representative gating and histograms of BAT assays performed in whole blood from an egg allergic individual.

4 Notes

1. Blood collection in acid citrate dextrose or EDTA tubes is not recommended as these preservatives have been shown to diminish CD63 expression on basophils [30]. Basophil activation assay can be performed with either whole blood or isolated leukocytes. The use of whole blood simplifies the procedure, in spite of potential disadvantages such as low basophil recovery, sensitivity, and interference from other cell types in flow cytometry. Preferably, the assay should be performed within 4 h of blood collection as prolonged storage results in low sensitivities.
2. Basophils are known to exhibit variations depending on circadian clock activity [31, 32], which need to be taken into account when considering the expression of CD63 and CD203c as a biomarker for basophil degranulation in clinical research.
3. Optimal dilutions of each allergen to be tested need standardization prior to the experiment. BAT has been performed with commercial allergen extracts, recombinant allergens, or whole allergen extracts prepared in the lab following published methods [21, 23, 33–35].
4. Each antibody should be previously titrated for optimal dilutions. Optimal conjugated fluorophores are to be determined according to the availability of detectors in the flow cytometer.

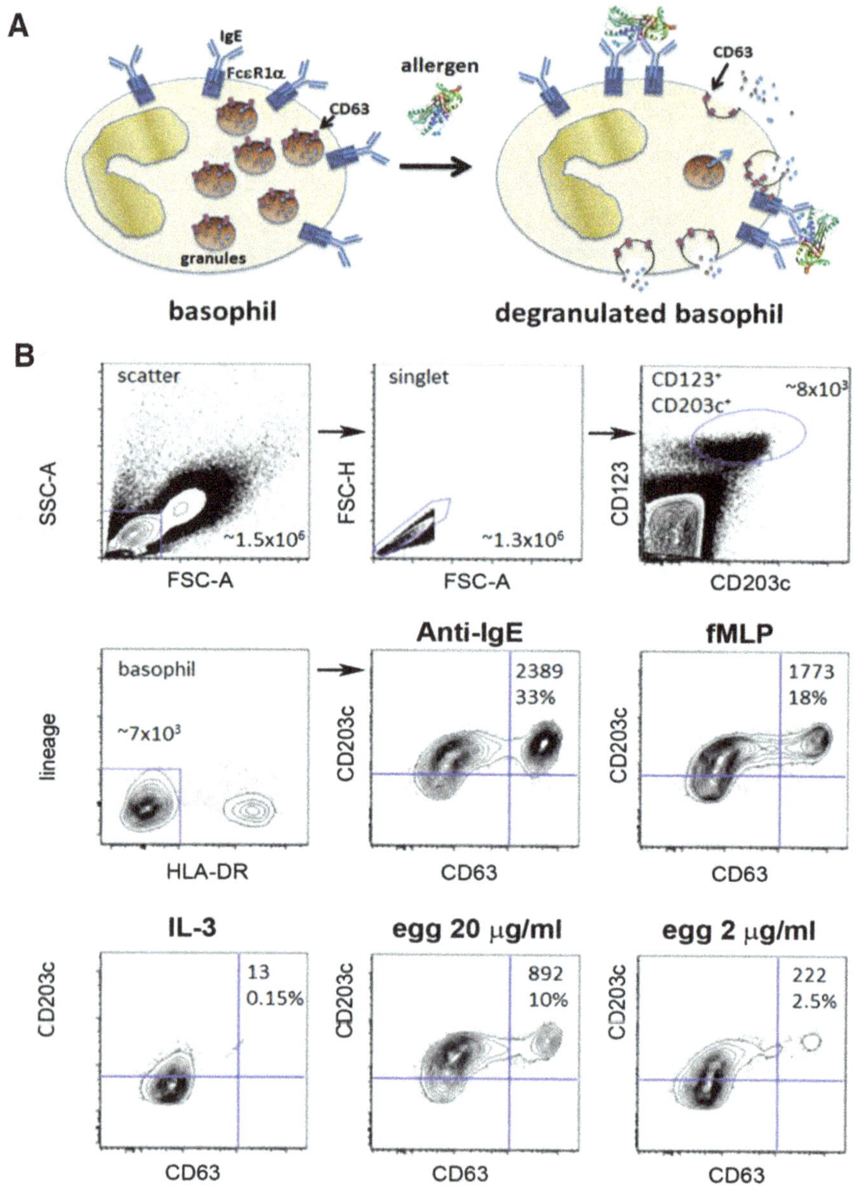

Fig. 1 (**a**) A schematic of allergen-induced basophil degranulation. (**b**) A representative gating and histograms of basophil degranulation assays performed in whole blood from an egg allergic individual. The *top* and *bottom numbers* within the quadrants represent the total number of cells within the gate and the frequency of cells, respectively

5. The use of BD FACS lysing solution enables simultaneous lysis of red blood cell and fixation of other cell types—reducing the assay time.
6. Optimal flow cytometer compensation settings should be determined prior to acquisition of samples using single-stained controls and fluorescent-minus-one controls. Basophils share

flow cytometric scatter characteristics of lymphocytes although they are highly granular due to their characteristic absorption of frequency of light used in cytometers. A number of alternative ways to gate basophils have been reported [36].

References

1. Knol EF, Mul FP, Jansen H, Calafat J, Roos D (1991) Monitoring human basophil activation via CD63 monoclonal antibody 435. J Allergy Clin Immunol 88:328–338
2. Han X, Jorgensen JL, Brahmandam A, Schlette E, Huh YO et al (2008) Immunophenotypic study of basophils by multiparameter flow cytometry. Arch Pathol Lab Med 132: 813–819
3. Varro R, Chen CH (2000) A no-wash 3-color basophil degranulation flow assay using the CD123 + HLA-DR-phenotype for basophil classification. Cytometry 10(Suppl):116
4. Voskamp AL, Prickett SR, Mackay F, Rolland JM, O'Hehir RE (2013) MHC class II expression in human basophils: induction and lack of functional significance. PLoS One 8:e81777
5. Gibbs BF, Sabato V, Bridts CH, Ebo DG, Ben-Zimra M et al (2012) Expressions and inhibitory functions of CD300a receptors on purified human basophils. Exp Dermatol 21:884–886
6. Sabato V, Verweij MM, Bridts CH, Levi Schaffer F, Gibbs BF et al (2012) CD300a is expressed on human basophils and seems to inhibit IgE/FcepsilonRI-dependent anaphylactic degranulation. Cytometry B Clin Cytom 82:132–138
7. Sabato V, van Hengel AJ, De Knop KJ, Verweij MM, Hagendorens MM et al (2011) Human basophils: a unique biological instrument to detect the allergenicity of food. J Investig Allergol Clin Immunol 21:179–184
8. Vila L, Moreno A, Gamboa PM, Martinez-Aranguren R, Sanz ML (2013) Decrease in antigen-specific CD63 basophil expression is associated with the development of tolerance to egg by SOTI in children. Pediatr Allergy Immunol 24:463–468
9. Faber M, Sabato V, De Witte L, Van Gasse A, Hagendorens MM et al (2014) State of the art and perspectives in food allergy (part I): diagnosis. Curr Pharm Des 20:954–963
10. Nucera E, Pecora V, Buonomo A, Rizzi A, Aruanno A et al (2015) Utility of Basophil Activation Test for monitoring the acquisition of clinical tolerance after oral desensitization to cow's milk: pilot study. United Eur Gastroenterol J 3:272–276
11. Uyttebroek AP, Sabato V, Faber MA, Cop N, Bridts CH et al (2014) Basophil activation tests: time for a reconsideration. Expert Rev Clin Immunol 10:1325–1335
12. Hoffmann HJ, Santos AF, Mayorga C, Nopp A, Eberlein B et al (2015) The clinical utility of basophil activation testing in diagnosis and monitoring of allergic disease. Allergy 70:1393–1405
13. Siracusa MC, Kim BS, Spergel JM, Artis D (2013) Basophils and allergic inflammation. J Allergy Clin Immunol 132:789–801 quiz 788
14. Ebo DG, Bridts CH, Hagendorens MM, Aerts NE, De Clerck LS et al (2008) Basophil activation test by flow cytometry: present and future applications in allergology. Cytometry B Clin Cytom 74:201–210
15. Rentzos G, Lundberg V, Lundqvist C, Rodrigues R, van Odijk J et al (2015) Use of a basophil activation test as a complementary diagnostic tool in the diagnosis of severe peanut allergy in adults. Clin Transl Allergy 5:22
16. McGowan EC, Savage JH, Courneya JP, Sterba PM, Parihar S et al (2014) Relationship of IgE to basophil phenotypes in peanut-sensitized adults. J Allergy Clin Immunol 134(746-749):e746
17. Glaumann S, Nopp A, Johansson SG, Rudengren M, Borres MP et al (2012) Basophil allergen threshold sensitivity, CD-sens, IgE-sensitization and DBPCFC in peanut-sensitized children. Allergy 67:242–247
18. Santos AF, Du Toit G, Douiri A, Radulovic S, Stephens A et al (2015) Distinct parameters of the basophil activation test reflect the severity and threshold of allergic reactions to peanut. J Allergy Clin Immunol 135:179–186
19. Sato S, Tachimoto H, Shukuya A, Ogata M, Komata T et al (2011) Utility of the peripheral blood basophil histamine release test in the diagnosis of hen's egg, cow's milk, and wheat allergy in children. Int Arch Allergy Immunol 155(Suppl 1):96–103
20. Sato S, Tachimoto H, Shukuya A, Kurosaka N, Yanagida N et al (2010) Basophil activation marker CD203c is useful in the diagnosis of hen's egg and cow's milk allergies in children.

Int Arch Allergy Immunol 152(Suppl 1):54–61

21. Ford LS, Bloom KA, Nowak-Wegrzyn AH, Shreffler WG, Masilamani M et al (2013) Basophil reactivity, wheal size, and immunoglobulin levels distinguish degrees of cow's milk tolerance. J Allergy Clin Immunol 131(180–186):e181–e183
22. Hochwallner H, Schulmeister U, Swoboda I, Spitzauer S, Valenta R (2014) Cow's milk allergy: from allergens to new forms of diagnosis, therapy and prevention. Methods 66:22–33
23. Erdmann SM, Sachs B, Schmidt A, Merk HF, Scheiner O et al (2005) In vitro analysis of birch-pollen-associated food allergy by use of recombinant allergens in the basophil activation test. Int Arch Allergy Immunol 136:230–238
24. Hamilton RG (2013) In vitro diagnostic methods in the evaluation of food hypersensitivity. In: Metcalfe DD, Sampson HA, Simon RA, Lack G (eds) Food allergy: adverse reaction to foods and food additives, 5th edn. Wiley-Blackwell, London
25. Michova A, Abugalia M, Ivanova T, Nikolov G, Taskov H et al (2006) Comparision of two-flow cytometry methods for basophil degranulation in patients sensitized to grass pollen. Allergy 61:1078–1083
26. Chirumbolo S (2011) The use of IL-3 in basophil activation tests is the real pitfall. Cytometry B Clin Cytom 80:137–138 author reply 139
27. Nilsson N, Nilsson C, Hedlin G, Johansson SG, Borres MP et al (2013) Combining analyses of basophil allergen threshold sensitivity, CD-sens, and IgE antibodies to hydrolyzed wheat, omega-5 gliadin and timothy grass enhances the prediction of wheat challenge outcome. Int Arch Allergy Immunol 162:50–57
28. Johansson SG, Nopp A, van Hage M, Olofsson N, Lundahl J et al (2005) Passive IgE-sensitization by blood transfusion. Allergy 60:1192–1199
29. Nopp A, Johansson SG, Ankerst J, Bylin G, Cardell LO et al (2006) Basophil allergen threshold sensitivity: a useful approach to anti-IgE treatment efficacy evaluation. Allergy 61:298–302
30. Sousa N, Martinez-Aranguren R, Fernandez-Benitez M, Ribeiro F, Sanz ML (2010) Comparison of basophil activation test results in blood preserved in acid citrate dextrose and EDTA. J Investig Allergol Clin Immunol 20:535–536
31. Baumann A, Skjold T, Hoffmann HJ, Lorentz A (2016) Diurnal variation of CD63 expression on activated blood basophils: a pilot study. Ann Allergy Asthma Immunol 116:77–78
32. Ando N, Nakamura Y, Ishimaru K, Ogawa H, Okumura K et al (2015) Allergen-specific basophil reactivity exhibits daily variations in seasonal allergic rhinitis. Allergy 70:319–322
33. Beyer K, Morrow E, Li XM, Bardina L, Bannon GA et al (2001) Effects of cooking methods on peanut allergenicity. J Allergy Clin Immunol 107:1077–1081
34. Garrido-Fernandez S, Garcia BE, Sanz ML, Echechipia S, Lizaso MT et al (2014) Are basophil activation and sulphidoleukotriene determination useful tests for monitoring patients with peach allergy receiving sublingual immunotherapy with a Pru p 3-enriched peach extract? J Investig Allergol Clin Immunol 24:106–113
35. Wallowitz ML, Chen RJ, Tzen JT, Teuber SS (2007) Ses i 6, the sesame 11S globulin, can activate basophils and shows cross-reactivity with walnut in vitro. Clin Exp Allergy 37:929–938
36. Chirumbolo S (2014) Major pitfalls in BAT performance may be caused by gating protocols and CD63% cut off evaluation. Cytometry A 85:382–385

Chapter 12

Use of Humanized RS-ATL8 Reporter System for Detection of Allergen-Specific IgE Sensitization in Human Food Allergy

Eman Ali Ali, Ryosuke Nakamura, and Franco H. Falcone

Abstract

Allergen-specific Immunoglobulin E (IgE) determination lies at the heart of diagnosis of sensitization to food and other allergens. In the past few years, reporter systems capable of detecting the presence of allergen-specific IgE have been developed by several labs. These rely on humanized rat basophil leukemia cell lines stably transfected with reporter genes such as firefly luciferase. In this chapter, we describe protocols for the use of the RS-ATL8 cell line (IgE cross-linking-induced luciferase expression; EXiLE) in 96-well and 384-well formats. We also describe optional treatment steps for enveloped virus and complement inactivation.

Key words Reporter system, Luciferase, Humanized RBL, IgE, Allergy, RS-ATL8, EXiLE

1 Introduction

Immunoglobulin E (IgE) is the antibody responsible for Type I allergic reactions via activation of the tetrameric high-affinity IgE receptor FcεRI, present on basophils and mast cells. Several cellular diagnostic techniques are used for the detection of specific IgE (sensitization) to suspected allergens. The most common diagnosis is the skin prick test (SPT), in which allergens are injected intradermally, and the subsequent wheal-and-flare reaction induced by the activation of resident mast cells measured against histamine and negative controls. While this method is simple, relatively safe, and cheap, as it requires no expensive instrumentation or reagents for detection, it is not amenable to the testing of large numbers of allergens. More importantly in the context of food allergy, skin prick testing, which is widely accepted in testing of environmental allergens such as tree or grass pollens, is more controversial for food allergens due to a high number of false positive reactions. Such false positive SPT tests may also occur in individuals who are tolerant

Jing Lin and Marcos Alcocer (eds.), *Food Allergens: Methods and Protocols*, Methods in Molecular Biology, vol. 1592,
DOI 10.1007/978-1-4939-6925-8_12, © Springer Science+Business Media LLC 2017

and thus cannot always be taken as an indication of clinical sensitivity to the offending allergen-containing food [1]. Furthermore, SPT does not reflect the more complex process of allergen degradation during transit through the gastrointestinal tract. The ability of proteins to resist conditions found in the GI tract (e.g., to withstand the actions of low pH, pepsin, bile acids, and trypsin) is of relevance to the ability of allergens to induce sensitization and, more importantly in the context of allergy testing, to trigger cell activation via the FcεRI receptor. Finally, false negative SPT test results can be obtained due to the intake of antihistamines by the patient. Patients to be tested should avoid taking antiallergic drugs before the test. For example, in Japan, 3–7 day-cessation is encouraged for histamine-release test of patients' basophils. However, such cessation of the drug may affect the patients' QOL.

A second cellular test method is based on measuring the activation of basophilic granulocytes in whole blood (Basophil Activation Test, BAT). BATs are more elaborate and expensive than SPT, as they require flow cytometry equipment; fluorescent antibodies for labeling of basophil surface activation markers, as well as trained personnel. About 10–20% percentage of individuals ("nonresponders") will not respond to IgE-dependent stimulation due to spleen tyrosine kinase (a.k.a. syk) deficiency [2], thus appear as negative, but this does not imply that these individuals are not atopic, as the nonresponder phenotype is not limited to nonatopics [3]. Due (at least in part) to the lack of standardization across laboratories, BATs are not widely used in allergy clinics.

An alternative technique, which is also currently not widely used due to a set of perceived limitations (discussed in detail in a recent review [4]), is the use of humanized rat basophilic leukemia (RBL) reporters. This system uses the RBL cell line, which as a minimum requirement needs to be stably transfected with the alpha chain of human FcεRI [5], for use with human blood samples. The requirement for the alpha chain is based on the fact that human IgE does not bind to the rat IgE receptor with high affinity [6]. Assessment of cell activation by allergens was in the past performed by measuring beta-hexosaminidase activity using fluorescent substrates, a method that is increasingly displaced by the use of more sensitive luciferase- [7, 8] or fluorescence-based [9] humanized reporter cell lines. Importantly, this system is not affected by the use of most antiallergic drugs. This is illustrated in Fig. 1, in which the luciferase-based RS-ATL8 reporter system (EXiLE), which is described in this chapter, is used in the presence of seven different drugs used for the treatment of allergic diseases.

As shown in Fig. 1, with the exception of Cyclosporin A, none of the tested drugs interferes with the use of the RS-ATL8 reporter cell line in concentrations achieved in vivo. The C_{max} value given for each drug represents the maximum (peak) achievable concentration in a specified compartment after one single administration.

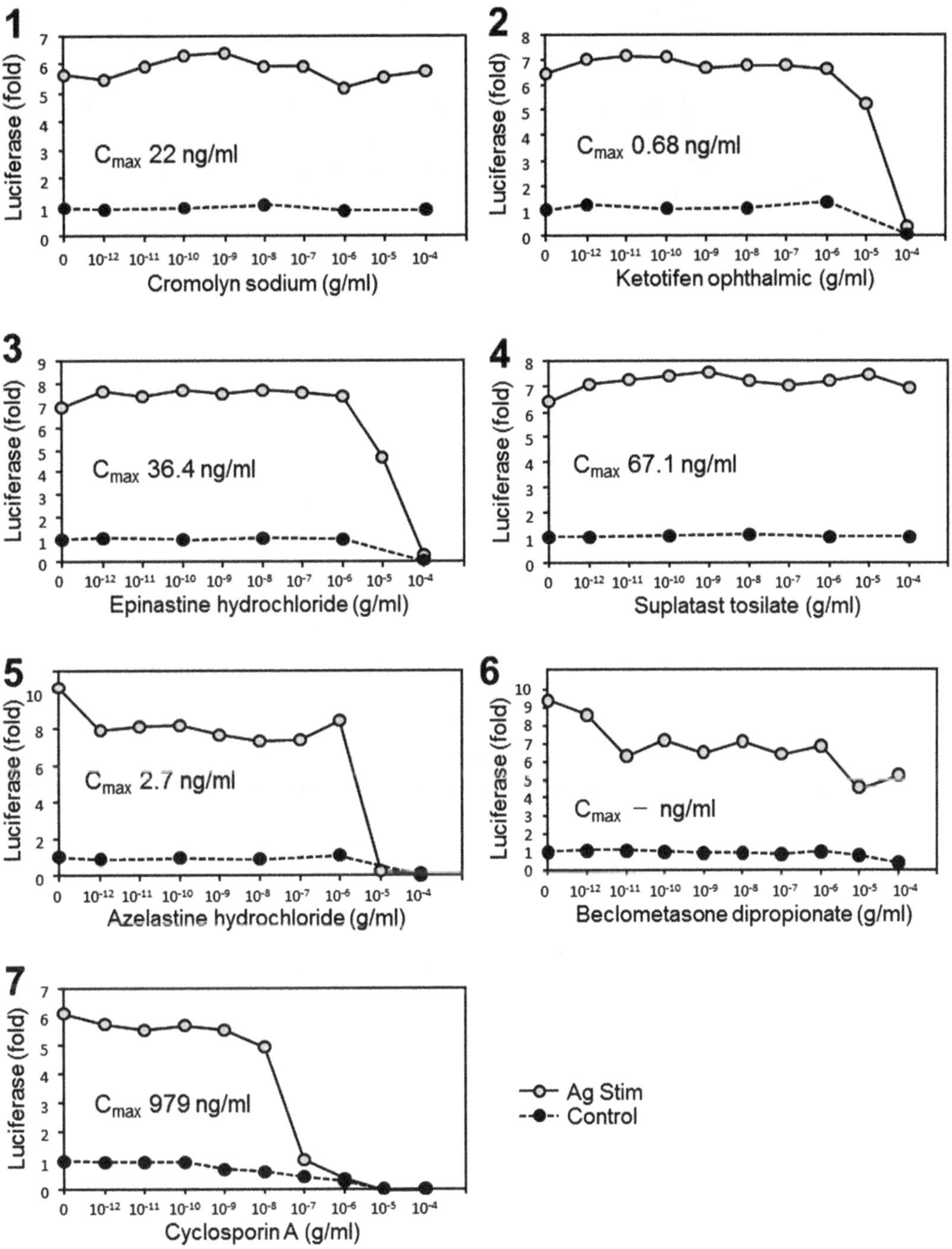

Fig. 1 Performance of the RS-ATL8 reporter system (EXiLE) in the presence of seven different drugs used for treatment of allergic symptoms. Shown is the n-fold increase in luciferase activity over unstimulated cells, using reporter cells sensitized with egg white allergic patient's serum (diluted 1:100) 3 h after stimulation with egg white extract (100 ng/mL), in the presence of different concentrations of the named drugs. (*1*) Cromolyn sodium; (*2*) Ketotifen ophthalmic; (*3*) Epinastine hydrochloride; (*4*) Suplatast tosilate; (*5*) Azelastine hydrochloride; (*6*) Beclometasone dipropionate; (*7*) Cyclosporin A. C_{max} values obtained from the package inserts of each drug

The sharp decrease seen for Ketotifen (2), Epinastine hydrochloride (3), and Azelastine hydrochloride (5) are due to direct cytotoxic effects on the cells at the highest concentrations (all well above the C_{max}, i.e., not normally achieved in vivo). Beclometasone dipropionate (6) does not have a C_{max} value, as it is used externally. The only drug that can exert an inhibitory effect at physiologically relevant concentrations is Cyclosporin A. This can be explained by its effects on calcineurin, which is an essential molecule in the signaling pathway used by the RS-ATL8 reporter system, as explained in the following text.

Due to their high sensitivity and their robustness, these newer reporter systems are amenable to high-throughput screening in different formats, either in 96-/384-well format or in the case of the NFAT-DsRed reporter, also in allergen array-based assays [9]. The best available reporter cell line is currently the RS-ATL8 reporter cell line [10], which reports IgE-dependent cytosolic NFAT dephosphorylation by Ca^{2+}- and calmodulin-dependent calcineurin activation and subsequent NFAT translocation to the nucleus, where it binds to a synthetic NF-AT promoter, inducing luciferase expression.

We have used RS-ATL8 cells in both 96- and 384-well formats. Using the latter format has the advantage of further reducing the amount of serum needed for assessment of allergen-specific IgE, which can be of particular advantage when dealing with small pediatric blood samples. However, due to the well-known bell-shaped dose dependency of FcεRI-mediated activation, some caution needs to be taken when adapting protocols from 96- to 384-well format. This is because transition affects the surface and volume to a different extent, and the plate geometries are different, as demonstrated in the following text.

As shown in Fig. 2a for a typical 96-well plate, D1 and D2 are not equal; hence to determine its volume, a **Conical Frustum Shape** needs to be used for general calculations. Accordingly, the top radius is 3.5 mm, while the bottom radius is 3.25 mm and the height is 11.2 mm. The total volume can be calculated as follows:

Volume of a conical frustum: $V = (1/3)\pi h(R_1^2 + R_2^2 + (R_1 R_2)) = 401\ mm^3 = 0.401\ cm^3$, where R_1 is $D_1/2$ and $R_2 = D_2/2$ and $h = H_3$, whereas the base surface can be calculated as

Base surface area of a conical frustum S (a circle) $= \pi \times R_2^2 = 38.5\ mm^2 = 0.38\ cm^2$, where $R_2 = D_2/2$. This is the total surface on which the reporter cell lines can grow as a cell monolayer in a 96-well plate in each well.

In contrast, the shape of a 384-well plate is an (inverted) **truncated square pyramid** with the square base surface area (Fig. 2b). Accordingly, the volume is determined as

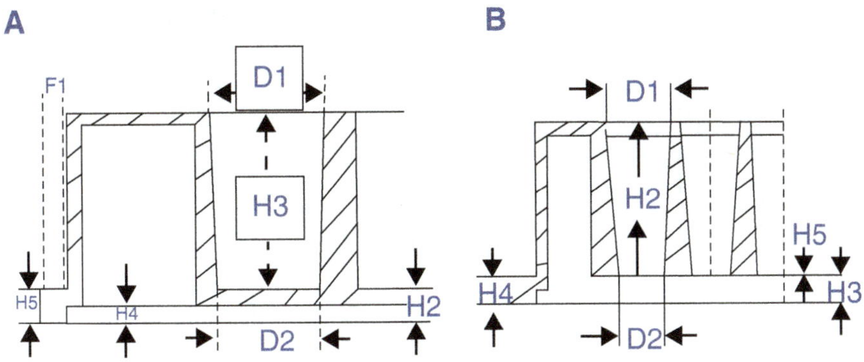

Fig. 2 (**a**) Dimensions of a typical 96-well plate. Total height of plate 14.5 ± 0.2 mm, *H2*: Vertical distance from inside well bottom to resting plane 3.2 mm, *H3*: Inside depth of well 11.2 mm, *H4*: Vertical distance from external well bottom to resting plane 2.1, *H5*: Height of flange 2.85 ± 0.15, *D1*: Well diameter, *top* 7.05 ± 0.2 mm, *D2*: Well diameter, *bottom* 6.5 mm. (**b**) Typical 384-well plate dimensions. *H1*: Plate total height 14.4 mm, *H2*: Vertical distance from inside well bottom to resting plane 2.7 mm, *H3*: Inside depth of well 11.6 mm, *H4*: Height of flange 2.5 mm, *H5*: Bottom thickness 0.25 mm, *D1*: Well diameter, *top* 3.7 mm, *D2* Well diameter, *bottom* 2.5 mm

Volume of a truncated square pyramid V = 1/3 (a2 + ab + b2)h, where $a = R_2 = D_2/2$, $b = R_1 = D_1/2$, and $h = H_2$. Accordingly, the volume is determined as $V = 1/3(R_2^2 + R_1R_2 + R_2^2)h$, giving 26.27 mm^3 or 0.026 cm^3, while the base surface area (square) is $S = R_2^2$, where $R_2 = D_2/\sqrt{2} = 3.13\ mm^2 = 0.031\ cm^2$.

So while the volume is reduced by a factor of 15.4 when transitioning from 96- to 384-well format, the surface is only decreased by 12.6-fold. Therefore, optimal conditions established for 96-well plates should take into account this difference when adapted to 384-well plates, for example, when deciding which concentration of optimal anti-IgE should be used as positive control in the assay. Without taking this into account, it is possible to reduce the efficiency of stimulation by entering the supraoptimal stimulation range. This is illustrated by a typical experiment shown in Fig. 3, in which RS-ATL8 cells sensitized overnight with the serum of a donor allergic to milk are stimulated with a wide range of allergen concentrations (1 pg/mL to 0.1 mg/mL). As can be seen, supraoptimal stimulations (leading to decreased measured reporter gene activation) are obtained with allergen concentrations higher than 100 ng/mL. The optimum stimulation conditions are therefore obtained in a relatively narrow range, although activation can also be measured outside this window. As could be expected and also shown in Fig. 3, the overall intensity of luciferase-induced chemiluminescence obtained is higher in 96-well plates, due to the higher cell numbers in each well. Also, the signal-to-noise ratio is slightly better in 96-well plates, but this may be offset by the advantage of using smaller volumes of serum and reagents when using 384-well plates.

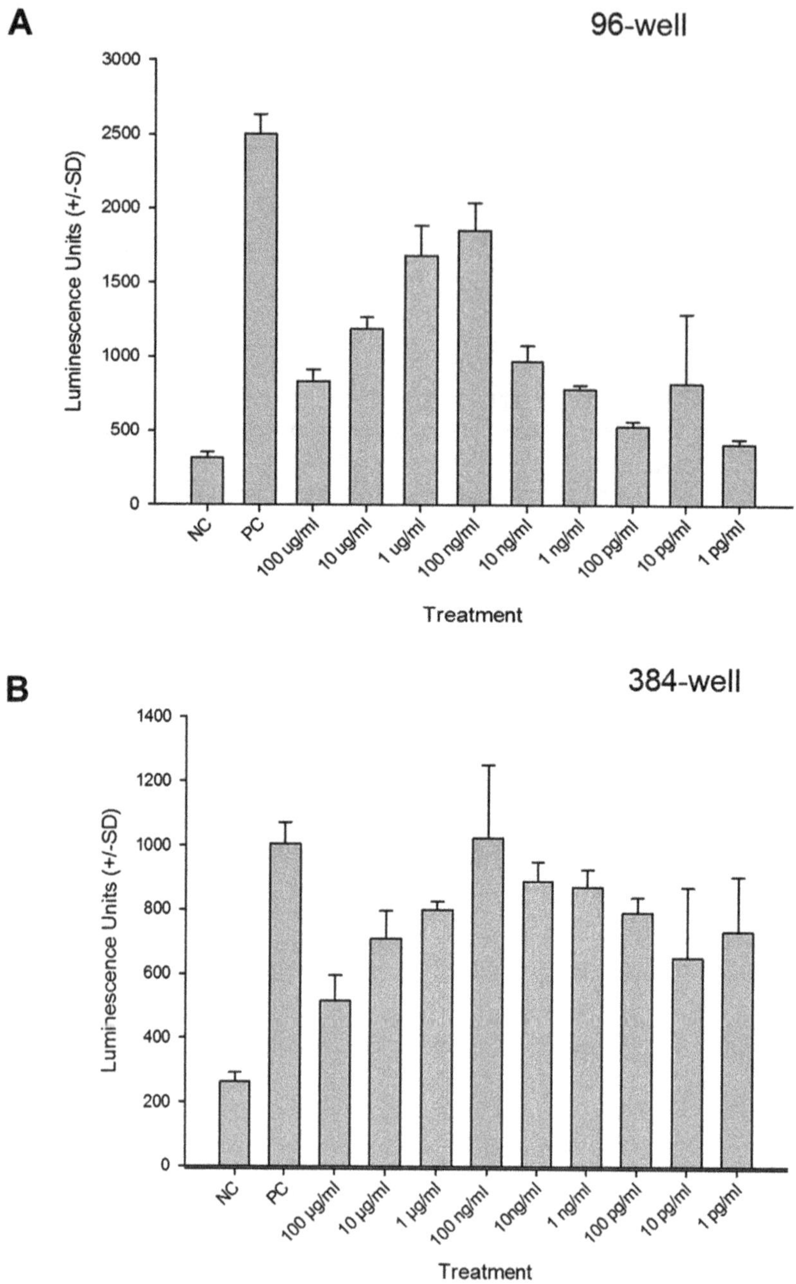

Fig. 3 RS-ATL8 cells were sensitized overnight with 1:50 diluted serum from a donor allergic to cow's milk for 16 h in a 96-well (**a**) or 384-well (**b**) plate. After one wash, cells were stimulated with a wide range of concentrations of fractionated allergen and activation measured as luminescence 4 h after stimulation. Data are shown as mean ± s.d. for triplicate determination

As pointed out by Dibbern and coauthors, who studied sera from peanut-sensitive patients [11], some sera can have toxic effects on RBL cells leading to apparently increased spontaneous (unstimulated) levels of beta-hexosaminidase. The cytotoxicity could be reduced by preabsorbing the sera on the parental RBL-2H3 cell line, which does not express the human FcεRI alpha chain and therefore does not reduce the availability of human IgE in the sample. An example of such treatment is shown in Fig. 4.

Figure 4 shows how pretreatment of cytotoxic sera can increase the stimulation levels obtained after allergen stimulation, as this allows the use of higher serum concentrations, achieving more efficient sensitization of the FcεRI receptor (and possibly also higher receptor surface expression) during overnight incubation. One important difference between the traditional use of beta-hexosaminidase for the assessment of activation compared with a reporter gene product such as luciferase is that cytotoxicity of sera can increase the background by damaging cells and releasing their granular content (including the measured beta-hexosaminidase), whereas it is much less likely to induce luciferase expression that is under the control of a synthetic NFAT promoter in the RS-ATL8

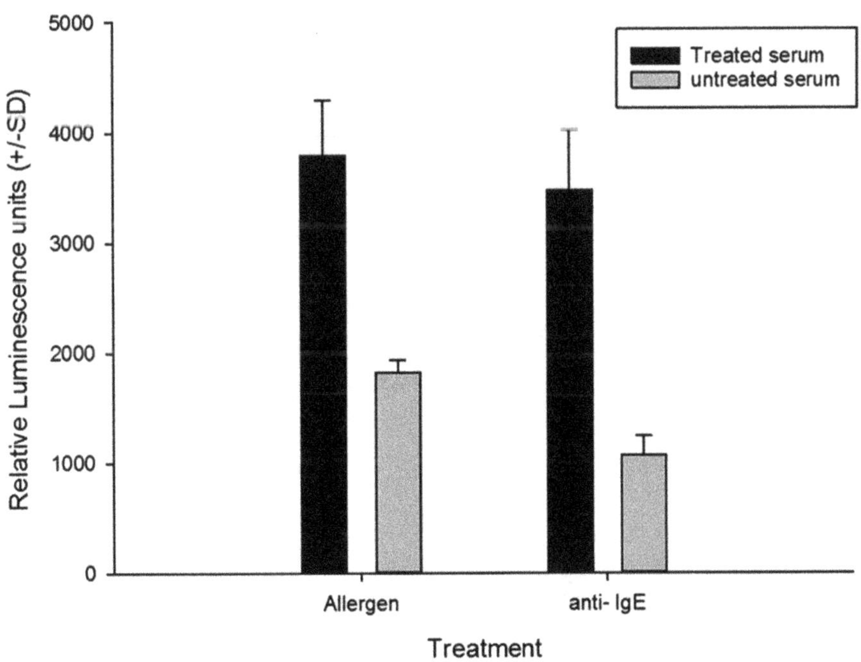

Fig. 4 Serum from a donor allergic to tufted grass was diluted 1:20 in cell culture medium and incubated for 1 h in a 96-well plate that had been coated with RBL-2H3 cells grown to full confluence. After 1 h, the supernatant was transferred to human FcεRI-expressing RS-ATL8 cells for 16 h for sensitization. After a wash, cells were stimulated with 10 ng/mL of *Holcus lanatus* pollen extract as the allergen. Luminescence was measured 4 h after stimulation. Shown is one experiment as mean ± s.d. for triplicate determination

cells. Thus, reporter cell lines, such as RS-ATL8 cells, are less prone to serum cytotoxicity-dependent artefacts than the traditional beta-hexosaminidase measurements with nonreporter, humanized RBL cell lines. However, also in the case of RS-ATL8, cytotoxicity will reduce signal strength as less viable cells will be available to produce luciferase upon stimulation.

Finally, in some cases, it may be necessary or desirable to treat sera in order to reduce the biohazard levels by neutralizing enveloped viruses such as HIV or Hepatitis B. This can be achieved by pretreating sera with a mixture of 0.3% (v/v) TNBP (tri-*N*-butylphosphate) and 1% (v/v) Tween-80 (polyoxyethyleneorbitan) [12]. However, we have previously shown that after this treatment, serum dilutions of less than 1:100 cannot be used for RS-ATL8 sensitization, as the detergents damage the cells [4]. Detergents can be removed after serum treatment using SDR HyperD® detergent removal resin as described in Subheading 3. An example of detergent removal is shown in Fig. 5.

Without detergent removal, any serum dilution lower than 1:50 would have completely destroyed the cells during overnight incubation, and 1:100 dilutions would have given reduced levels of activation compared with the nondetergent treated control (not shown).

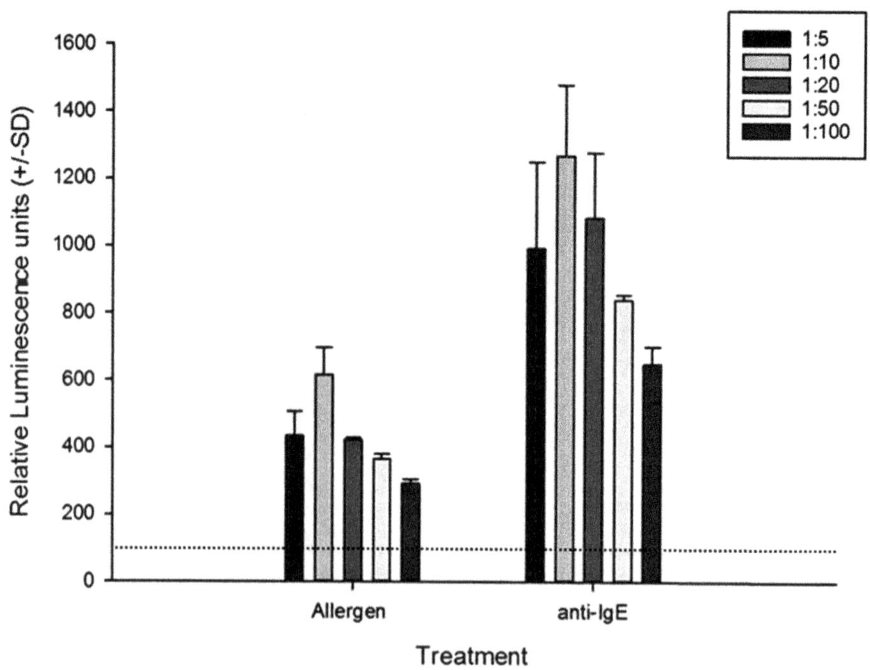

Fig. 5 Detergent removal effect. Serum from donor allergic to tufted grass was treated with detergents for 1 h and subsequently incubated using SDR HyperD® Detergent Removal resin for 30 min. RS-ATL8 cells were sensitized with different dilutions (1:5, 1:10, 1:20, 1:50, or 1:100) of the detergent- and resin-treated serum and stimulated with tufted grass pollen extract (allergen) or anti-IgE antibody (anti-IgE). Shown is one experiment as mean ± s.d. for triplicate determination. The *dotted line* indicates the negative control (=spontaneous activation) level

In this chapter, we describe the use of RS-ATL8 for the detection of allergen-specific IgE in human serum samples. We describe two slightly different protocols, one for 96-well and one for 384-well format, with optional treatment steps for the reduction of cytotoxicity by adsorption on parental RBL-2H3 cells and viral inactivation with detergents, with subsequent detergent removal via SDR HyperD® detergent removal resin.

2 Materials

2.1 Reagents

1. Humanized Rat basophilic leukemia cell line: RS-ATL8 can be obtained through an MTA from Ryosuke Nakamura (National Institute of Health Sciences, Tokyo, Japan) and RBL-2H3 cells, e.g., from the German Collection of Microorganisms and Cell Cultures, DSMZ, Germany (ACC312) or ATCC (ATCC® CRL-2256™).
2. Cell culture medium: Minimum Essential Medium (MEM), 10% fetal bovine serum (FBS), 2 mM L-glutamine (if not present in the MEM formulation). Also, it is recommended to add a standard antibiotic mixture such as 100 U/mL penicillin and 100 μg/mL streptomycin.
3. Washing buffer: Dulbecco's Phosphate Buffered Saline (DPBS) without Ca^{2+} and Mg^{2+}.
4. Freezing medium: DMSO (dimethyl sulfoxide, cell culture grade) 10% v/v and complete cell culture medium.
5. Cell dissociation reagents: Trypsin-EDTA or cell scraper (not highly recommended) (*see* **Note 1**).
6. Geneticin G418 (eukaryotic antibiotic to kill cells which may have lost the HsFcεRI transfected gene) (*see* **Note 2**).
7. Hygromycin B (eukaryotic antibiotic to kill the cells that have lost the transfected NFAT luciferase reporter gene) (*see* **Note 2**).
8. Sensitizing agents: Sera from allergic donors.
9. Stimulating agents: Allergens and anti-human IgE (control).
10. Reagents for luciferase activity detection: ONE-Glo Luciferase Assay System (Promega).
11. Detergent treatment: Add 44.5 μL 20% (v/v) Tween 80 (polyoxyethylene (20) sorbitan monooleate) in DPBS and 2.7 μL TNBP (tri(*n*-butyl)phosphate) to 1 mL of serum.
12. Resin: SDR HyperD® Detergent Removal resin.
13. 70% v/v industrial methylated spirits (IMS) in deionized water and tissue for aseptic cleaning.
14. Polyclonal anti-human IgE antibody to be used as positive control. We use goat anti-human IgE polyclonal IgG from Vector Labs, UK.

2.2 Supplies

1. Cell culture well plate: 96- and 384-well clear and white plates.
2. Electronic pipette.
3. Variable volume pipettes and tips.
4. 75 cm^2 cell culture flasks.
5. Sterile plastic centrifuge tubes (25, 50 mL tubes).
6. Visual counting method: Hemocytometer slide (e.g., improved Neubauer chamber).

2.3 Equipment

1. Microbiological safety cabinet (MSC) class II.
2. Incubator: Adjusted to a constant temperature of 37 °C and 5% CO_2 to maintain the required physiological pH (7.2–7.4).
3. Routine cell culture visualization: Inverted phase contrast microscope.
4. Centrifuge to spin down cells (suited for 50 mL centrifuge and 1.5 mL Eppendorf tubes).
5. Luminescence microplate reader.

3 Method

3.1 Cell Culture

Preserving a sterile environment is the most important aspect of the maintenance of cell culture in a laboratory. Work should be carried out in a clean and sterile class II Microbiological safety cabinet, by routinely wiping the cabinet with IMS before and after completion of work and the equipment, if necessary.

1. Cell defrosting: Defrost the cells using either the water bath or your hand to warm the cells until they begin defrosting. Then transfer the 1 mL cells to a centrifuge tube and add 9 mL of cell culture medium and centrifuge for 5 min with 300 × *g* to remove the supernatant that contains DMSO (*see* **Note 3**).
2. Remove the supernatant and resuspend the cell pellet in 10 mL prewarmed medium (*see* **Note 4**), then transfer to 25 cm^2 cell culture flask and place in the incubator.
3. Maintain transgene expression by including 1 mg/mL G418 and 600 μg/mL of Hygromycin in the medium every two weeks (*see* **Note 2**).
4. When cells are confluent, passaging (splitting) them requires the removal of the old medium and washing with 10 mL Ca^{2+}/Mg^{2+}-free DPBS (*see* **Note 5**), followed by addition of 2 mL of trypsin–EDTA and incubation in the incubator for 10 min (or until cells are detaching, which may happen earlier). After tapping the flask corners firmly but carefully with your knuckles, add 8 mL of warm medium. Then, transfer 9 mL to a centrifuge tube for further experiments (Subheading 3.3) and retain

1 mL of cells in the flask. Add 9 mL (*see* **Note 6**) of medium to the flask and keep in the incubator for further culture.

5. Cryopreservation: For long-term storage of cells, cryopreservation is needed. This requires harvesting of the cells, counting (*see* **Note** 7), resuspension in medium at a density of 5 × 10^6 cells/0.9 mL. After that, transfer 900 μL to each labeled vial and add also 100 μL of cell culture grade DMSO to obtain 10% v/v (*see* **Note 8**). Then, transfer the cryovials to Mr. Frosty (filled with isopropanol) freezing container (*see* **Note 8**). Store the container at −80 °C overnight and transfer to liquid nitrogen vapor phase the next day and store until required.

3.2 Serum Treatment (Optional)

From **step 4** in Subheading 3.1, either proceed directly to cell sensitization as described in Subheading 3.3 or follow the optional procedures for complement inactivation and enveloped virus removal described in this section.

1. Heat the sera for 5 min at 56 °C in a water bath.

   or

2. Incubate the sera in the desired (e.g., 1:50) dilution with RBL-2H3 cells for 1 h (*see* **Note 9**).
3. If removal of enveloped viruses is required, add Tween 80 and TNBP to serum as described in **item 11** Subheading 2.1, and mix carefully using a mixer for 1 h. If detergent has been used, it needs to be removed before the sensitization step as it will damage the cells otherwise. Prepare 5 mg/mL of the detergent removal resin in DBPS then mix 1:1 (v/v) with the serum. Then, incubate in a mixer at room temperature for 30 min. To remove the resin and the detergent bound to it, centrifuge for 5 min at 1000 × *g* and use the supernatant (*see* **Note 10**).

3.3 Cell Sensitization

To assess the presence of allergen-specific IgE in the tested serum, the reporter cells require to be sensitized overnight (or for a minimum of 8 h). This step will increase the levels of IgE receptor expression, thus sensitivity of the test will be increased. This is achieved by incubating the cells overnight with serum diluted 1:100 without pretreatment, or any other desired dilution (usually between 1:10 and 1:50) with pretreatment. Optimal dilution and the necessity to pretreat or not will depend on the cytotoxicity of the tested serum and the concentration of allergen-specific IgE, so will vary from sample to sample (*see* **Note 11**).

1. From Subheading 3.1, **step 4**, transfer the remaining cells to a centrifuge tube. Transfer 10 μL to the hemocytometer slide for cell counting and centrifuge the remaining cells at 300 × *g* for 5 min.

2. After calculating the number of cells in the tube, resuspend with the calculated amount of cell culture medium (*see* **Note 7**).
3. Mix the cells using the selected dilution of the serum (prepared in excess) and add 50 μL from each treatment in triplicate in a clear plate if using a 96-well plate, or 15.4 μL if using a 384-well plate using the optimum cell density (*see* **Note 7**).
4. Place the well plate in the cell culture incubator for 16–18 h.

3.4 Cell Stimulation

During the sensitization step, IgE will bind to the human FcεRI receptor and subsequent cross-linking by cognate allergen will reveal the presence of specific IgE in the serum during the cell stimulation step.

1. Prepare selected concentration of the allergen and control (anti-IgE) (*see* **Notes 12** and **13**).
2. Check the cell condition under a microscope (*see* **Note 14**).
3. Remove the old medium from the plate.
4. Add 15.4 or 50 μL of the allergen in the desired concentrations and the anti-IgE control to the cells in 384- and 96-well plates, respectively.

3.5 Luminescence Measurement

1. Add 15.4 or 50 μL of ONE-Glo Luciferase Assay System (Promega) to each well in a 384-well plate or in a 96-well plate, respectively (*see* **Note 15**).
2. Transfer 30.6 or 100 μL of the mixture from the clear plates to a 384- or 96-white well plate, respectively, and measure the luminescence response using the plate reader.

3.6 Waste Disposal

Cell culture contaminated plastics, tissues, tips, and tubes must be autoclaved before disposal. Also, contaminated liquid can be treated with disinfectant overnight and then disposed of in accordance with legislation and/or local regulations for safe disposal of genetically modified organisms (GMOs).

4 Notes

1. The use of cell scraper is not recommended, because it can cause more cell death than Trypsin-EDTA. Also, the cells tend to clump and so, it is not easy to count them under the microscope.
2. G418 stock = 1 g/mL. Final = 0.5 mg/mL (1:2000 dilution), Hygromycin stock = 50 g/mL. Final = 200 μg/mL (1:250 dilution). These antibiotics are relatively expensive but have to be used to prevent loss of transgene expression in the long term.

There is no need to include these antibiotics during washes or splitting of the cells, but they should be included at least twice a month. We have cultured the cells in the absence of antibiotics for 3 months without noticing any effects on their performance.

3. Freezing medium contains 10% DMSO, which is toxic to cells when they are defrosting. It is therefore important to rapidly reduce the DMSO concentration to 1% (where toxicity is less pronounced) by diluting the cells 1:10 in cell culture medium immediately after defrosting.
4. It is important to ensure that no air bubbles are generated during resuspension of the cells. It is best to flick the tube containing the cell pellet *before* adding the medium to loosen the pellet. When adding the medium, carefully pipette up and down a few times without sucking in or expelling all the liquid. This will avoid air bubbles that damage the cells.
5. The wash is intended to remove most of the culture medium for two reasons; the bovine serum in the medium contains serum trypsin inhibitor that would inactivate the trypsin used for detachment; furthermore, as cell attachment requires Ca^{2+} and Mg^{2+}, the use of Ca^{2+}/Mg^{2+}-free DPBS followed by inclusion of EDTA (a divalent metal ion chelator) further supports cell detachment.
6. RS-ATL8 cells grow in a monolayer at the bottom of the flask. Perform 1/5 split for 2 days, 1/10 for 3 days, and 1/20 for 4 days for when you want the cells to be confluent again.
7. To calculate the needed amount of the medium to be resuspended,

$$\textit{Number of the cells in the flask} = \textit{Number of cells counted} \times 10^4 \times \textit{volume of cells in the flask}\ (\text{e.g.,}10\ mL). \quad (1)$$

$$\textit{Cell density needed}\ (100{,}000\ \textit{in}\ 96\text{-}\textit{well or}\ 50{,}000\ \textit{in}\ 384\text{-}\textit{well}) \times 1000\ (\textit{in}\ 1\ mL)/50\ (\textit{in}\ 96)\ 15.4\ (\textit{in}\ 384). \quad (2)$$

Divide Eq. 1 by Eq. 2 to obtain the volume needed.

8. DMSO is added to reduce the formation of ice crystals inside the cells, and Mr. Frosty (filled with isopropanol) freezing container allows controlled cooling down at a rate of approximately 1 °C/min from room temperature to −80 °C.
9. After incubating the RBL-2H3 with the serum in a well plate, to sensitize the RS-ATL8 simply transfer the supernatant to the wells containing the RS-ATL8. This can be on the same plate if numbers allow.

10. Use of a sterile syringe filter for resin/detergent removal is not recommended due to the small volume of the serum and the incurred volume loss during filtration.
11. Ideally the optimal serum dilution would be assessed in preliminary experiments; some sera can be used in 1:10 or 1:20 dilution without affecting cell viability. In practice, such experiments may not be possible due to lack of serum. In this case, we found it safest to use a 1:100 dilution without pretreating the serum.
12. Activation via the high-affinity IgE receptor follows a bell-shaped dose-dependent curve. Lower levels of activation will be obtained by either suboptimal or supraoptimal levels of allergen (or anti-IgE). The optimum will depend on issues such as the number and distance of IgE epitopes on the allergen, the binding affinity of the IgE antibodies, and other factors that are usually unknown. Ideally, the allergen concentration would be optimized using a fixed amount of serum during sensitization and challenging the cells with different dilutions of allergen (and anti-IgE antibody as a positive control). However, in most cases, either there will be not sufficient serum or reactivity will be unknown, so in practice, at least three different concentrations of allergen should be used (over at least three orders of magnitude). The assay is very sensitive, and we regularly see optimal allergen concentrations of 100 pg/mL or 1 ng/mL.
13. Optimum polyclonal anti-IgE concentration is 1 μg/mL when using goat anti-human IgE polyclonal IgG from Vector Labs. If using a different antibody, the optimal concentration needs to be determined experimentally.
14. Healthy cells have elongated shape and are attached to the bottom (flask or plate) or a more rounded shape if confluent. Dead cells have abnormal smaller shape and detach from the surface.
15. For a maximum response after adding the Luciferase reagent, the measurements should be carried out within 30 min.

Acknowledgments

E.A.A. was funded by a University of Nottingham Vice-Chancellor's Scholarship for Research Excellence (International) and the Gordon Memorial College Trust Fund. Sera from milk allergic individuals and fractionated milk allergens were kindly provided by M. Alcocer, University of Nottingham. Our thanks to Colin Fitzsimmons (University of Cambridge), who introduced us to the use of the resin for detergent removal.

References

1. Hill DJ, Heine RG, Hosking CS (2004) The diagnostic value of skin prick testing in children with food allergy. Pediatr Allergy Immunol 15:435–441
2. Kepley CL, Youssef L, Andrews RP et al (1999) Syk deficiency in nonreleaser basophils. J Allergy Clin Immunol 104:279–284
3. Küster H, von Manstein S, Ruocchio-Wiglinghaus S et al (2005) Mutations in the high-affinity IgE receptor beta-chain are not associated with nonresponder status. Allergy 60:1040–1045
4. Wan D, Wang X, Nakamura R et al (2014) Use of humanized rat basophil leukemia (RBL) reporter systems for detection of allergen-specific IgE sensitization in human serum. Methods Mol Biol 1192:177–184
5. Taudou G, Varin-Blank N, Jouin H et al (1993) Expression of the alpha chain of human Fc epsilon RI in transfected rat basophilic leukemia cells: functional activation after sensitization with human mite-specific IgE. Int Arch Allergy Immunol 100:344–350
6. Miller L, Blank U, Metzger H, Kinet JP (1989) Expression of high-affinity binding of human immunoglobulin E by transfected cells. Science 244:334–337
7. Wan D, Ludolf F, Alanine DGW et al (2014) Use of humanised rat basophilic leukaemia cell line RS-ATL8 for the assessment of allergenicity of *Schistosoma mansoni* proteins. PLoS Negl Trop Dis 8:e3124
8. Nakamura R, Ishiwatari A, Higuchi M et al (2012) Evaluation of the luciferase assay-based in vitro elicitation test for serum IgE. Allergol Int 61:431–437
9. Wang X, Cato P, Lin H-C et al (2013) Optimisation and use of humanised RBL NF-AT-GFP and NF-AT-DsRed reporter cell lines suitable for high-throughput scale detection of allergic sensitisation in array format and identification of the ECM-integrin interaction as critical factor. Mol Biotechnol 56:136–146
10. Nakamura R, Uchida Y, Higuchi M et al (2010) A convenient and sensitive allergy test: IgE crosslinking-induced luciferase expression in cultured mast cells. Allergy 65:1266–1273
11. Dibbern DA, Palmer GW, Williams PB et al (2003) RBL cells expressing human Fc epsilon RI are a sensitive tool for exploring functional IgE-allergen interactions: studies with sera from peanut-sensitive patients. J Immunol Methods 274:37–45
12. Poulsen LK, Sørensen TB (1993) Elimination of viral infection risk from blood samples for allergy testing. Allergy 48:207–208

Part III

Allergenic Epitope Mapping

Chapter 13

Assessment of IgE Reactivity of β-Casein by Western Blotting After Digestion with Simulated Gastric Fluid

Sara Benedé, Rosina López-Fandiño, and Elena Molina

Abstract

Cow's milk allergy is defined as an immunologically mediated adverse reaction to cow's milk proteins and it is usually, along with hen's egg allergy, the first food allergy identified in childhood.

One of the main aspects to consider when evaluating the allergenic potential of food proteins is the effect of gastric digestion. It is known that allergens are usually able to survive the harsh acidic environment of the stomach, tolerate the presence of surfactants, and resist digestion by pepsin. They might also be digested into high molecular weight peptide fragments, which retain the same, or sometimes increased, IgE-binding. In this respect, western blotting is a highly sensitive and efficient technique that we have used to detect IgE-binding to the digests of milk and egg proteins. Given the importance of the resistance of food proteins to gastric digestion in their capacity to modulate the immune response, we describe in this chapter the assessment of IgE reactivity of a relevant cow's milk allergen, β-casein, by western blotting after simulated digestion under relevant physiological conditions.

Key words Digestibility, Food allergy, Gastric digestion, Immunoassay, SDS-PAGE, Simulated gastric fluid, Western blotting

1 Introduction

A food allergy reaction arises when the immune system overreacts reproducibly to a food (usually to the proteins of the food), leading to an adverse health effect. Some allergies are cell mediated, but IgE-mediated food allergy is believed to be responsible for the most of the food-induced hypersensitivity reactions [1]. IgE binds to high-affinity receptors present on mast cells and basophils. Crosslinking of receptor-bound IgE by an allergen triggers cell activation and degranulation, resulting in the release of histamine and other mediators of the allergic response.

Studies in Western countries have indicated that cow's milk, followed by hen's egg, are the most prevalent allergens during infancy and early childhood, causing serious problems for the allergic individuals, their families and caregivers, and the public health [2, 3].

Jing Lin and Marcos Alcocer (eds.), *Food Allergens: Methods and Protocols*, Methods in Molecular Biology, vol. 1592, DOI 10.1007/978-1-4939-6925-8_13, © Springer Science+Business Media LLC 2017

Cow's milk contains between 3 and 3.5% proteins and includes approximately 20 different proteins that may be involved in allergic sensitization [4]. Caseins (up to 80% of the total milk protein content) are one of the most critical milk allergens accounting for the highest circulating IgE levels [5]. Among them, β-casein (Bos d8) (approximately 27% of the total milk proteins) represents a severe health risk to patients with cow's milk allergy, since 75% of the sera from patients with allergy to cow's milk have IgE directed against β-casein [6]. Whey proteins account for the remaining 20%, being β-lactoglobulin (Bos d5) and α-lactalbumin (Bos d4) the major allergens of this fraction [7].

In the hen's egg, egg white is the main source of allergens. Four proteins, ovalbumin (55% of the protein content), ovomucoid (11%), ovotransferrin (12%), and lysozyme (3%), named from Gal d1 to Gal d4, have been identified as the major ones [8]. Ovalbumin is considered one of the dominant allergens [9], although ovomucoid has been stressed as an important cause of egg hypersensitivity [10].

Although there are no molecular properties common to all food allergens, resistance to digestion is regarded as a shared feature that, together with factors such as the food matrix and the processing conditions, could contribute to the maintenance of the allergenic structures or reveal formerly hidden sites during their passage through the gastrointestinal tract [11].

We have investigated in previous studies the residual IgE-binding in the digestion products of β-casein [12], β-lactoglobulin [13], ovalbumin [14], ovomucoid [15], and lysozyme [16]. Gastric digestion of main milk and egg allergens was simulated using a relevant digestion model mimicking the physiological process. Pepsin-to-protein ratio was taken into account, as well as the pH and the presence of phospholipids. Immunoreactivity retained after gastric digestion against IgE from sera of allergic patients was evaluated by western blotting. Following the separation of the mixture of intact (if not fully digested) and hydrolyzed protein by PAGE-SDS, proteins and peptides were transferred from the polyacrylamide gel onto a nitrocellulose paper that was incubated with allergic patients' sera containing human IgE. Immunodetection was carried out with anti-human IgE and the biotin-streptavidin amplification system (the mouse anti-human IgE conjugated to biotin interacts with the conjugated streptavidin-horseradish peroxidase). Finally, a chemiluminescent substrate was used to obtain a highly precise detection of proteins or their digests from western blots by an image analyzer.

2 Materials

Prepare all solutions using deionized water and analytical grade reagents. Prepare and store all reagents at room temperature (unless indicated otherwise). Diligently follow all waste disposal regulations when disposing waste materials.

2.1 Simulated Gastric Digestion

1. Phosphatidylcholine.
2. Porcine pepsin (EC 3.4.23.1, 3640 U/mg β-casein).
3. Simulated gastric fluid: 35 mM NaCl, pH 2. Weigh 1 g of NaCl. Add 400 mL of water. Mix and adjust pH with 1 N HCl and add water to a final volume of 500 mL. Store at 4 °C.

2.2 SDS Polyacrylamide Gel

1. Sample buffer: 0.5 M Tris–HCl, pH 6.8, containing 1.6% SDS, 8% glycerol, 4% 2-β-mercaptoethanol, and 0.002% bromophenol blue. Prepare by mixing 5 mL of 1 M Tris–HCl pH 6.8, 160 mg of SDS, 0.8 mL of 100% glycerol, 0.4 mL of 100% β-mercaptoethanol, and 0.2 mL of 0.1% bromophenol blue. Adjust the final volume to 10 mL with water.
2. 4–12% Criterion™ XT Bis-Tris Gel, 12 + 2 well (Bio-Rad).
3. Running buffer: XT-MES running buffer (Bio-Rad). Prepare a 1× running buffer by diluting 100 mL of 20× stock buffer in 1.9 L of water (*see* **Note 1**). Store at 4 °C.
4. Criterion cell tank (Bio-Rad).
5. Gel-loading tips.
6. Precision plus protein standards, molecular mass marker ranging in molecular mass from 10 to 250 kDa (Bio-Rad). Store at −20 °C.
7. Fixation solution: 40% ethanol (v/v), 10% acetic acid (v/v). Prepare by mixing 400 mL of ethanol, 100 mL of acetic acid, and 500 mL of water.

2.3 Immunoblotting

1. Nitrocellulose membranes, precut, 0.45 μm, 15 × 15 cm (Bio-Rad).
2. Extra thick blot filter paper, precut, 14 × 16 cm (Bio-Rad).
3. Western blot transfer buffer: 0.048 M Tris, 0.039 M glycine, 20% methanol. Dissolve 5.8 g of Trizma (Sigma-Aldrich) and 2.9 g of glycine in 200 mL of water. Add 200 mL of methanol and water to a final volume of 1 L (*see* **Note 2**). Store at 4 °C.
4. Tris buffered saline (TBS, 10×): 1.5 M NaCl, 0.5 M Tris, pH 7.6. Dissolve 60.5 g of Trizma and 88 g of NaCl in 500 mL of water. Mix and adjust pH with 1 N HCl. Add water to a final volume of 1 L.
5. TBS containing 0.05% Tween-20 (TBST). Dilute 100 mL of TBS 10× in 900 mL of water. Add 0.5 mL of Tween 20 (*see* **Note 3**).

6. Blocking solution: 1% bovine serum albumin (BSA) in TBST. Dissolve 1 g of bovine serum albumin in 100 mL of TBST. Store at 4 °C.
7. Diluent solution: 0.1% BSA in TBST. Dilute 10 mL of blocking solution in 90 mL of water. Store at 4 °C.
8. Trans-blot® SD semidry transfer cell (Bio-Rad).
9. Plastic container.
10. Ponceau S solution: 0.1% Ponceau S bioReagent in 5% acetic acid. Dissolve 0.2 g of Ponceau S bioReagent in 190 mL of water. Add 10 mL of acetic acid and mix. Store at 4 °C and protected from light to prevent degradation.
11. Membrane washed-out solution: 0.1 M NaOH.
12. Imaging system: Molecular Imager VersaDoc™ MP 4000 System (Bio-Rad).
13. Image acquisition software: Quantity One® 1-D analysis software (Bio-Rad).

2.4 Proteins, Antibodies and Conjugates

1. β-casein from bovine milk.
2. Human sera from milk allergic patients.
3. Mouse anti-human IgE Fc-biotin antibody, clone HP6029.
4. Streptavidin-horseradish peroxidase conjugate.
5. Amersham ECL prime western blotting detection reagent (GE Healthcare).

3 Methods

3.1 *In Vitro* Digestion Model (See Fig. 1)

3.1.1 Preparation of the Phospholipid Vesicles Solution

1. Dissolve 0.1 g of phosphatidylcholine in 10.4 mL of simulated gastric fluid to obtain a final concentration of 9.58 mg/mL.
2. Sonicate the solution until clear to the eye (for a total of 5 min) (*see* **Note 4**).
3. After sonication, filter the sample through a 0.22 μm nylon filter to remove any titanium particle deposited by the sonication.

3.1.2 Simulated Gastric Digestion

1. Dissolve 43 mg of β-casein in 3 mL of simulated gastric fluid and incubate for 10 min at 37 °C.
2. Adjust to pH 2 with 1 N HCl.
3. Complete with simulated gastric fluid until a final volume of 3.416 mL.
4. Take an aliquot of 316 μL (4 mg of β-casein) in a tube label as CP (control protein) containing 78 μL of 1 M $NaHCO_3$ and add 406 μL of water to obtain a final sample volume of 4 mg/mL.

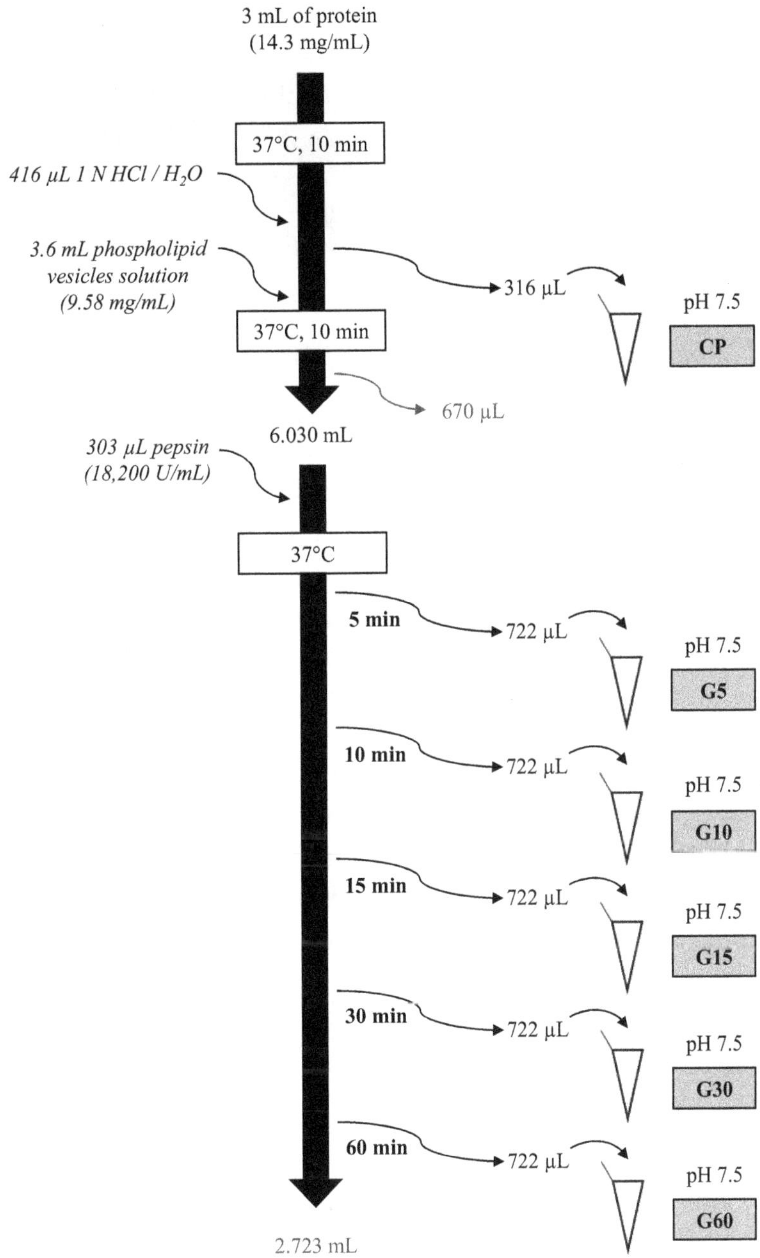

Fig. 1 Diagram of protein digestion with simulated gastric fluid

5. Add 3.6 mL of phospholipid vesicles solution and incubate for 5 min at 37 °C.
6. Prepare a solution of pepsin in simulated gastric fluid at 18,200 U/mL. Prepare immediately before use it to avoid degradation.
7. Take 6.030 mL of the mix β-casein-phospholipid vesicles solution and add 303 μL of pepsin solution (18,200 U/mL)

to obtain a physiological ratio of 182 U of pepsin per mg of β-casein.

8. Gastric digestion is performed in a shaking incubator at 37 °C.
9. After 5 min since addition of pepsin, take an aliquot of 722 μL in a tube label as G5 containing 78 μL of 1 M $NaHCO_3$ (increasing the pH to 7.5 stops pepsinolysis) and add 200 μL of water (*see* **Note 5**).
10. After 10, 15, 30, and 60 min since addition of pepsin, repeat **step 9** and take aliquots in labeled tubes as G10, G15, G30, and G60 respectively (*see* **Note 5**).

3.2 Electrophoresis SDS-PAGE

1. Dilute all samples (CP, G5, G10, G15, G30, and G60), 1:4 (v:v) in sample buffer.
2. Heat the diluted samples at 90–95 °C for 5 min.
3. Remove the gel from the package.
4. Remove the combs by pulling them upward firmly and smoothly and rinse the wells with running buffer (*see* **Note 6**).
5. Remove the tape from the bottom of the cassette.
6. Insert the cassette into the slot in the Criterion cell tank. The criterion cell tank allows running two gels at once.
7. Fill the upper chamber with running buffer.
8. Fill the lower buffer tank with running buffer to the marked fill line.
9. Load 30 μL of the sample or 10 μL of molecular mass marker using a pipet with gel-loading tips (*see* **Note 7**).
10. Place the lid on the tank, aligning the color-coded plugs with corresponding jacks on the lid.
11. Turn on power supply and run the gels at 150 V. Check for bubbles at the cathode side to ensure that gel rig is running.
12. After electrophoresis is complete (*see* **Note 8**), turn off the power supply, disconnect the electrical leads, and remove the lid.
13. Remove the gels from the cell and break the seals on both sides of the cassette using the Criterion cell lid (see instruction from manufacturer) or a spatula.
14. Pull the two halves of the cassette apart and remove the gel by floating the gel into deionized water.
15. Rinse the gel carefully in deionized water for 1 min to remove the traces of running buffer.
16. Cut the gel in two parts (*see* Fig. 2) and proceed to Subheadings 3.3 or 3.4.

3.3 Visualizing the Gel

1. Wash the right half of the gel for 5 min in water (*see* **Note 9**).
2. Discard all the water and add the fixative solution to completely cover the gel.

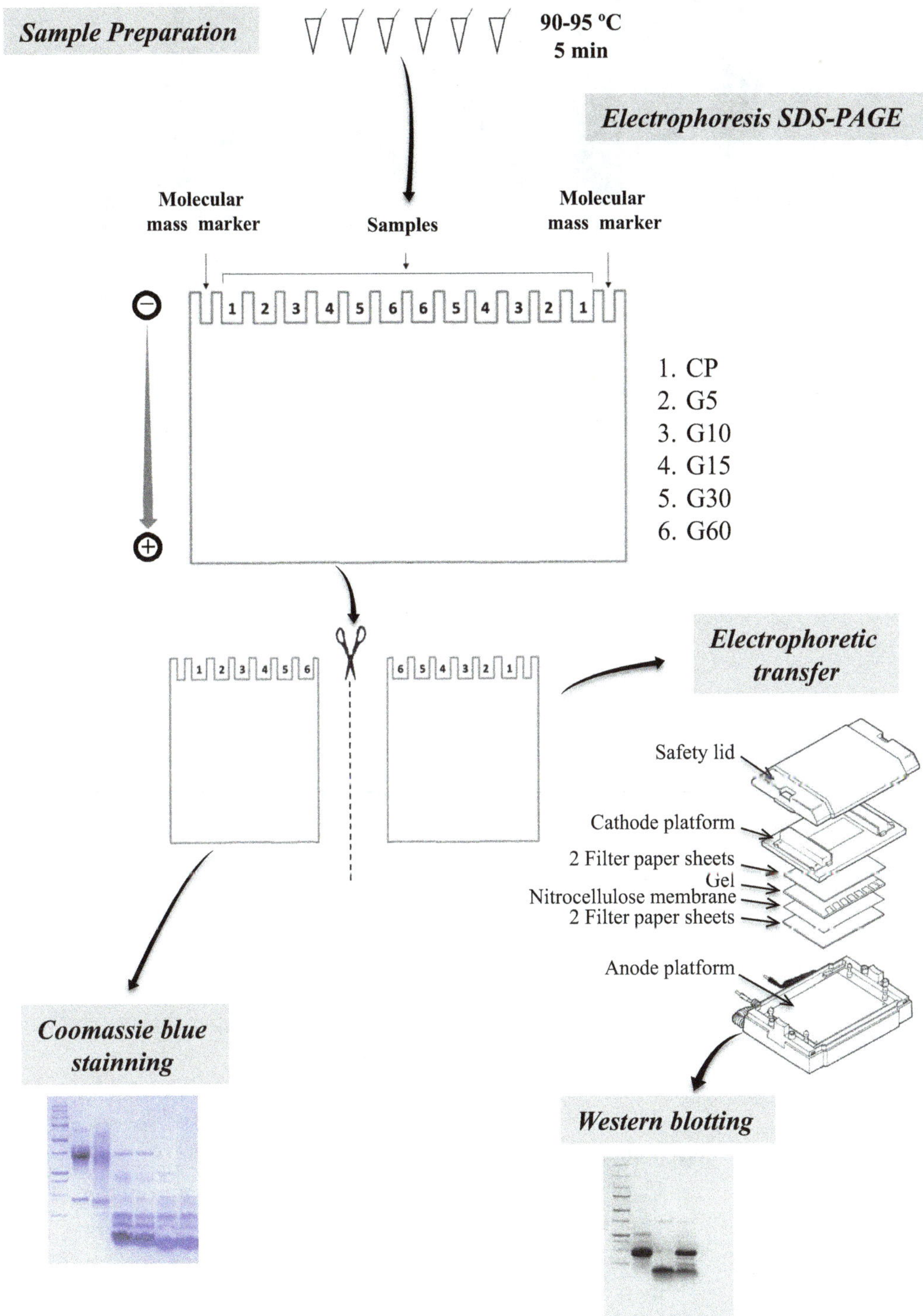

Fig. 2 Schematic of the western blotting workflow for assessment of IgE reactivity of milk and egg allergens after digestion with simulated gastric fluid

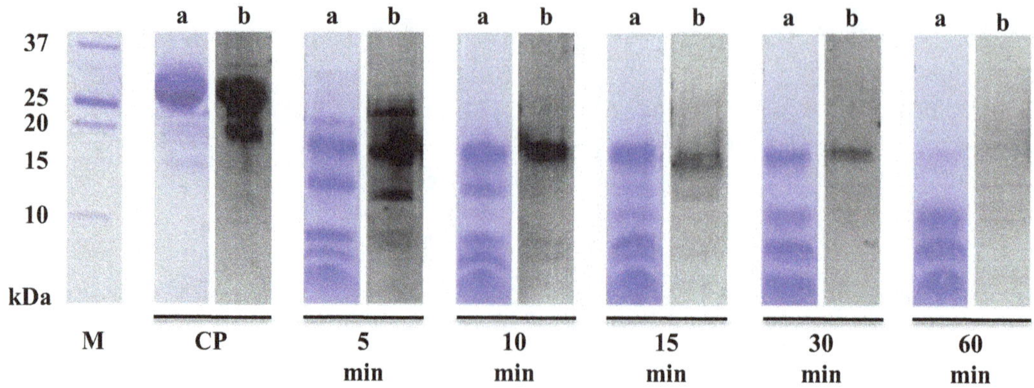

Fig. 3 SDS-PAGE patterns (**a**) and subsequent western blotting (**b**) of β-casein after 5, 10, 15, 30, and 60 min of in vitro gastric digestion with simulated gastric fluid. Electrophoresis was performed using bis-tris 12% acrylamide gels with reducing agents. *M* molecular mass marker, *CP* control protein

3. Gently shake on an orbital shaker for 30 min.
4. Remove all the fixation solution and rinse the gel in deionized water for 1 min.
5. Add enough Coomassie blue G-250 stain (Bio-Rad) to completely cover the gel.
6. Gently shake on an orbital shaker for 1 h (*see* **Note 10**).
7. Rinse the gel in deionized water for at least 1 h (*see* **Note 11**).
8. Acquire the image immediately using the Gel Doc system (*see* Fig. 3).

3.4 Electrophoretic Transfer

1. Wash the left half of the gel for 5 min in water (*see* **Note 12**).
2. Cut the nitrocellulose membrane and four pieces of filter paper to the exact shape of the left half of the gel (*see* **Note 13**).
3. Soak the left half of the gel (*see* **Note 14**), the nitrocellulose membrane (*see* **Note 15**), and the filter paper sheets in western blot transfer buffer for 20 min.
4. Remove the safety cover and the stainless-steel cathode assembly from the transfer cell and place two presoaked sheets of filter paper onto the platinum anode (*see* **Note 16**).
5. Place the pre-wetted nitrocellulose membrane on top of the filter paper.
6. Carefully place the equilibrated gel on top of the nitrocellulose membrane, aligning the gel on the center of the membrane (*see* **Note 17**).
7. Place the other two sheets of presoaked filter paper on the top of the gel.
8. Carefully place the cathode onto the stack. Press to engage the latches with the guideposts without disturbing the filter paper stack.

9. Place the safety cover on the unit and plug the unit into the power supply.
10. Turn on the power supply and transfer the gel for 30 min at 18 V.

3.5 Transfer Effectiveness Assessment

1. Following transfer, turn the power supply off, and disconnect the unit from the power supply.
2. Remove the safety cover and the cathode assembly. Discard the filter paper and the gel and take the nitrocellulose membrane. Do not allow the membrane to dry out.
3. Immerse the nitrocellulose membrane into Ponceau S solution and place it on an orbital shaker for 5 min at room temperature (*see* **Note 18**).
4. Rinse membrane with deionized water for 2 min to remove the background staining.
5. After seeing the protein bands to verify that the transfer is successful, wash the nitrocellulose membrane with the membrane washed-out solution for 10–20 s until the membrane is clean.
6. Rinse the nitrocellulose membrane in deionized water for 5 min.

3.6 Western Blotting

1. Block the membrane with blocking solution for 1 h at room temperature.
2. Wash with TBST for 5 min.
3. Add appropriate amount of sera from milk allergic patients to cover the membrane (usually 1:100 dilution but depends on the IgE levels in the sera. Diluted in diluent solution) and incubate overnight at 4 °C on an orbital shaker.
4. Wash 5× with TBST, 5 min each time.
5. Add anti-human IgE Fc biotin conjugate antibody (1:500 dilution, diluted in diluent solution) and incubate overnight at 4 °C on an orbital shaker.
6. Wash 5× with TBST, 5 min each time.
7. Add streptavidin-horseradish peroxidase conjugate (1:3000 dilution, diluted in diluent solution) and incubate 1 h at room temperature on an orbital shaker.
8. Wash 5× with TBST, 5 min each time.
9. Drain excess liquid by lightly blotting the membrane on dry filter paper.
10. Add Amersham ECL prime western blotting detection reagent (*see* **Note 19**) onto the membrane and make sure it completely covers the membrane and incubate 5 min at room temperature, protected from exposure to the light.
14. Drain off excess detection reagent by holding the membrane edge gently against a filter paper and using the image acquisition system, acquire the image immediately to avoid fluorescence degradation (*see* Fig. 3).

4 Notes

1. We routinely reuse the running buffer at least twice or thrice.
2. The final pH should be around 9.2. Do not use salts to adjust the pH because they could modify the conductivity of the buffer.
3. Tween 20 has a high density. Use a syringe, instead of a pipette, to ensure the addition of the right volume.
4. Sonication will reduce the crude lecithin solution into a suspension of single shelled liposomes. Place the container with the solution of phosphatidylcholine in an ice bath to cool the solution if it becomes hot during sonication.
5. Addition of water adjusts the final volume in all samples to 1 mL. The amount of digested protein in 1 mL of all samples (G5, G10, G15, G30, and G60) corresponds to the digestion of 4 mg of β-casein.
6. Do not pull comb out too quickly as wells will form holes, resulting in the loss of your sample.
7. Work as fast as you can without sacrificing accuracy and safety. The longer your samples sit in the buffer, the more diffuse your bands will be when you visualize the gel.
8. Electrophoresis is complete when the dye front has reached the anode.
9. Washing removes remaining SDS, which will interfere with the staining.
10. Protein bands will be visible within 20 min and reach maximum intensity within 1 h. Longer incubations will increase background.
11. Rinsing the gel overnight in water after staining will further reduce background. Stained gels can be stored in water.
12. Washing removes the remaining salts. Salts will increase the conductivity of the transfer buffer and the amount of heat generated during the transfer.
13. Transfer will be incomplete if any portion of the gel is outside the membrane and paper filters.
14. Do not soak for more than 20 min. Low molecular weight macromolecules (10,000 Da) may diffuse out of gels more readily. Twenty minutes will help to limit diffusion of low molecular weight macromolecules while providing efficient salt reduction.
15. To avoid membrane contamination, always use forceps or wear gloves when handling membranes.
16. Roll a pipet or test tube over the surface of the filter paper (like a rolling pin) to exclude all air bubbles. These air bubbles can block transfer of molecules.

17. Remember the orientation of the gel in the transfer cell when put in the chamber.
18. Since Ponceau S staining is reversible, it allows further immunological detection. This stain does not produce a deleterious effect on the sequencing of blotted polypeptides.
19. Allow the detection solutions to equilibrate to room temperature for 20 min. Mix detection solutions A (luminol) and B (peroxide) in a ratio of 1:1 to a working solution. Protect the mix reagent from exposure to the light.

References

1. Burks AW, Tang M, Sicherer S et al (2012) ICON: food allergy. J Allergy Clin Immunol 129:906–920
2. Schoemaker AA, Sprikkelman AB, Grimshaw KE et al (2015) Incidence and natural history of challenge-prov en cow's milk allergy in European children—EuroPrevall birthcohort. Allergy 70:963–972
3. Nwaru BI, Hickstein L, Panesar SS et al (2014) The epidemiology of food allergy in Europe: a systematic review and meta-analysis. Allergy 69:62–75
4. Herz U (2008) Immunological basis and management of food allergy. J Ped Gastroenterol Nutr 47:S54–S57
5. Restani P, Ballabio C, Di Lorenzo C et al (2009) Molecular aspects of milk allergens and their role in clinical events. Anal Bioanal Chem 395:47–56
6. Shek LP, Bardina L, Castro R et al (2005) Humoral and cellular responses to cow milk proteins in patients with milk-induced IgE-mediated and non-IgE-mediated disorders. Allergy 60:912–919
7. Monaci L, Tregoat V, van Hengel AJ et al (2006) Milk allergens, their characteristics and their detection in food: a review. Eur Food Res Technol 223:149–179
8. Benedé S, López-Expósito I, Molina E et al (2015) Egg proteins as allergens and the effects of the food matrix and processing. Food Funct 6:694–713
9. Mine Y, Zhang M (2008) Recent advances in the understanding of egg allergens: basic, industrial, and clinical perspectives. J Agric Food Chem 56:4874–4900
10. Cooke SK, Sampson HA (1997) Allergenic properties of ovomucoid in man. J Immunol 159:2026–2032
11. Verhoeckx KC, Vissers YM, Baumert JL et al (2015) Food processing and allergenicity. Food Chem Toxicol 80:223–240
12. Benedé S, López-Expósito I, Giménez G et al (2014a) In vitro digestibility of bovine β-casein with simulated and human oral and gastrointestinal fluids. Identification and IgE-reactivity of the resultant peptides. Food Chem 143:514–521
13. Benedé S, López-Expósito I, Giménez G et al (2014b) Mapping of IgE epitopes in in vitro gastroduodenal digests of β-lactoglobulin produced with human and simulated fluids. Food Res Int 62:1127 1133
14. Benedé S, López-Expósito I, López-Fandiño R et al (2014c) Identification of IgE binding peptides in hen egg ovalbumin digested in vitro with human and simulated gastroduodenal fluids. J Agric Food Chem 62:152–158
15. Benedé S, López-Fandiño R, Reche M et al (2013) Influence of the carbohydrate moieties on the immunoreactivity and digestibility of the egg allergen ovomucoid. PLoS One 8(11):e80810
16. Jiménez-Saiz R, Benedé S, Miralles B et al (2014) Immunological behavior of in vitro digested egg-white lysozyme. Mol Nutr Food Res 58:614–624

Chapter 14

IgE Epitope Mapping Using Peptide Microarray Immunoassay

Jing Lin and Hugh A. Sampson

Abstract

IgE epitope mapping has the potential to become an additional tool for food allergy diagnosis/prognosis and to lead to a better understanding of the pathogenesis and tolerance induction of food allergy. Due to its ability to screen thousands of targets in parallel using small volumes of sample, peptide microarray has greatly facilitated large-scale IgE epitope mapping. In the past 10 years, we have developed and optimized a reliable and sensitive peptide microarray immunoassay, which has been successfully applied for IgE epitope mapping of many food allergens in our lab. Here, we describe the method of performing the peptide microarray immunoassay for IgE epitope mapping. In addition, we have upgraded the microarray platform to measure antibody affinity by adding one additional competition step, which is also described in this chapter.

Key words IgE, Food allergy, Epitope mapping, Peptide microarray , Antibody affinity, Immunoassay

1 Introduction

Food allergy has emerged as an important public health problem in many countries [1]. The most common type of food allergy is mediated by immunoglobulin E (IgE) antibodies through their bindings to specific allergens. The groups of amino acids within allergenic proteins that are bound by IgE antibodies are called IgE-binding epitopes or B-cell epitopes. Identification of IgE-binding epitopes in food allergens will contribute to the design of safe immunotherapeutic agents and a better understanding of the pathogenesis and tolerance induction of food allergy. In addition, studies have suggested a role for sequential IgE-binding epitopes as biomarkers for characterizing various phenotypes of food allergy and may be used for clinical allergy diagnosis and prognosis [2].

Due to its ability to screen thousands of targets in parallel using small volumes of sample, the peptide microarray immunoassay has been applied in our laboratory for large-scale epitope mapping of IgE antibodies [3, 4]. In the past 10 years, we have developed and

Jing Lin and Marcos Alcocer (eds.), *Food Allergens: Methods and Protocols*, Methods in Molecular Biology, vol. 1592,
DOI 10.1007/978-1-4939-6925-8_14, © Springer Science+Business Media LLC 2017

optimized a reliable and sensitive peptide microarray immunoassay. Our optimized peptide microarray platform is capable of generating reproducible data with high correlation coefficients ($r > 0.9$) [4], and detecting IgE binding from diluted serum samples with whole food protein-specific IgE levels as low as 0.068 kU_A/L [5]. Using our peptide microarray, we have successfully mapped the sequential IgE-binding epitopes for a variety of food allergens, such as allergens from peanut/tree nuts, milk, egg, lentil, shrimp, soybean, etc. [6–9], and identified several IgE epitopes as candidate biomarkers for allergy diagnosis/prognosis or tolerance prediction [5, 8].

Using the peptide microarray immunoassay, we are able to measure in one single assay the concentration and diversity of a patient's IgE antibodies toward different allergenic epitopes, but it does not provide information about the affinity of IgE antibodies. Two important steps in the progressive differentiation of antigen-specific B cells are clonal expansion and affinity maturation in which antibody clones with higher affinity expand and further diversify [10]. In allergy, it may lead to IgE antibody clones with higher diversity and affinity. Thus, characterization (i.e., concentration, diversity, and affinity) of antibody clones in the IgE repertoire may reveal a patient's allergic history and/or current status. So far most studies on IgE epitopes focused on the concentration and diversity of IgE antibodies, but not the affinity of IgE antibodies due to the difficulty in measuring antibody affinity.

One method to measure antibody affinity is to use surface plasmon resonance (SPR)-based biosensors, which measure the binding affinity and kinetics of antigen and antibody interaction. Christensen et al. [11] demonstrated that higher affinity IgE binding to Der p 2, as measured using SRP technology, was associated with allergy effector cell degranulation. But this requires specific equipment that is not commonly available in most laboratories. Another method is to use thiocyanate, a chaotropic agent that interferes with non-covalent binding, to remove low affinity IgE bound to an allergen. Using a thiocyanate ELISA elution assay, El-Khouly et al. [12] found a weak correlation between the affinity of peanut-specific IgE to Ara h 2 and the severity of peanut allergy.

Compared with thiocyanate elution, which works by nonspecifically dissociating antigen–antibody complexes, the use of competing proteins to specifically elute IgE antibodies with lower affinity binding to the epitopes of the same protein may be a more relevant indicator of antibody affinity. We therefore included one additional competition step to enable our peptide microarray immunoassay to measure antibody affinity. Using the competitive peptide microarray assay, we were able to show that higher IgE affinity was associated with more severe allergic reactions to milk allergens [8].

In this chapter, we provide the detailed protocol of IgE epitope mapping using the peptide microarray immunoassay. This method is not only useful for epitope mapping of IgE antibodies, but can also be applied to other immunoglobulin subclasses (e.g.,

IgG4) by switching to the corresponding secondary antibody. In addition, we describe the additional competition step that can be added to the regular protocol to measure the affinity of peptide-bound antibodies.

2 Materials

1. Microarray printing slides: SuperEpoxy 2 (SME2) glass slides from ArrayIt. Store the slides under vacuum before printing and use within 6 months of the manufacturing date. The notch on the upper right corner of the slide indicates that samples should be printed on the side facing upward.
2. Peptides: A library of overlapping peptides (*see* **Note 1**), consisting of 20 amino acids, overlapping by 17 (3-offset), corresponding to the primary sequence of the target protein(s), are commercially synthesized by JPT Peptide Technologies GmbH (*see* **Note 2**). The synthesized peptides are supplied as lyophilized powder with high purity (QC control by HPLC and mass spectrometry).
3. 384-well, round-bottom, non-sterile assay plates with lids.
4. Ultrasonic bath.
5. Microarray printer: NanoPrint 60 with 2 × 4 Stealth Micro Spotting Pins (SMP3B), controlled by the NanoPrint Microarray Manager Software (ArrayIt).
6. Slide Staintray that can fit up to 10 or 20 slides and hold water to maintain proper humidity. The staintray should be protected from light during immunolabeling.
7. Pap pen.
8. High-throughput slide wash station (ArrayIt) that is equipped with a magnetic stir bar and a slide rack to wash up to 25 slides at the same time. Slides can be washed inside this wash station on a magnetic stir plate.
9. Dimethyl Sulfoxide (DMSO), 99.7 + %, Extra Dry over Molecular Sieve, from Acros.
10. Phosphate-Buffered Saline (PBS): 10× stock solution. 1×, 0.1×, and 0.05× solutions are prepared by diluting the stock solution in distilled water 1:10, 1:100, and 1:200, respectively.
11. Phosphate-Buffered Saline-Tween (PBST): 0.5% Tween-20 in PBS. Add 1 mL of Tween 20 to 2 L of 1× PBS.
12. 1 mM EDTA in PBST: Prepare a 0.5 M stock solution of EDTA by dissolving 186.12 g in 800 mL dH_2O, adjusting pH to 8.0 with NaOH or HCl, and top up to 1 L with dH_2O. Prepare the 1 mM solution by diluting 100 μL of 0.5 M EDTA with PBST to a final volume of 50 mL.

13. 15 mM Tris–HCl buffer, pH 8.0: Prepare 1 M Tris–HCl buffer, pH 8.0 by dissolving 121 g Tris base in 1 L distilled water and adjusting pH to 8.0 with concentrated HCl. Dilute 15 mL of 1 M Tris–HCl buffer, pH 8.0 with 985 mL of distilled water to make 15 mM Tris–HCl buffer, pH 8.0.
14. Protein Printing Buffer (PPB): 2× solution, from ArrayIt. 2× PPB is used to dilute the peptides before printing.
15. Blocking Buffer: 1% human serum albumin (HSA) in PBST. It is used to block all unbound sites on the slide surface prior to incubation with serum samples, and as the diluent for both serum and detection antibodies.
16. Dendrimer Buffer: UltraAmp Binding Buffer II from Genisphere.
17. A serum pool of several patients allergic to the specific food/allergen is served as positive control and a pooled serum sample of non-allergic, non-atopic patients, or individual non-allergic patient's serum sample is served as negative control (*see* **Note 3**).
18. Competition mixture: The competition mixture is derived from the same food proteins that the printed peptide sequences are derived. For example, if the printed peptides are based on the amino acid sequence of milk allergens, use the same milk allergens for competition. Prepare a stock solution of the proteins in PBS, then dilute to the appropriate concentration using blocking buffer and mix with other proteins.
19. Anti-Human IgE cocktail containing several Biotin conjugated monoclonal mouse Anti-Human IgE antibodies in blocking buffer (*see* **Note 4**). The antibody cocktail must be prepared freshly right before use. A few antibodies that we have been using are Biotin conjugated monoclonal Mouse Anti-Human IgE from BD Biosciences, Biotin conjugated monoclonal Mouse Anti-Human IgE (ε-chain specific) from Molecular Probes by Life Technologies.
20. Dendrimer signal amplification system: UltraAmp Anti-Biotin oyster 550, from Genisphere.
21. Salmon Sperm DNA.
22. ScanArray Gx Microarray Scanner from PerkinElmer.

3 Methods

3.1 Printing and Preprocessing of Peptide Microarray Slides

1. Preparation of printing plate: The lyophilized peptides are resuspended in DMSO at 1 mg/mL, diluted 1/2 in 2× protein printing buffer (PPB) (*see* **Note 5**), and transferred (10–15 μL/well) into the printing plate with lid. The printing plate is centrifuged at 300 rcf for 5 min to remove any bubbles that may

affect printing, and stored in a sealed plastic bag at −80 °C until use. The printing plate can be used for up to five printings.

2. Before peptide printing, the printing plate containing peptides in printing buffer is left at room temperature for 10–15 min, placed on a pedestal in an ultrasonic bath, sonicated for 60 s, and centrifuged at 300 rcf for 3 min at room temperature.
3. Peptides are printed from the printing plate onto the SME2 slides using the NanoPrint 60 microarray printer loaded with the Stealth Micro Spotting Pins (SMP3B) (*see* **Note 6**). The peptides are printed in two sets of triplicate spots. In addition to peptides, 20% of the printed spots are "blanks" composed of 50% v/v DMSO in PPB as negative control for background normalization. It is recommended to print some fluorescent-labeled protein at specific location to facilitate grid alignment. Other proteins, such as different concentrations of purified human IgE, may be printed to serve as positive controls. In order to save slide space and serum volume used for immunolabeling, two arrays can be printed on a single slide.
4. During printing, the humidity is maintained at 55–65% to avoid sample evaporation. Once completed, humidity is turned off and slides are dried overnight in the printer to ensure peptide binding to the slide substrate.
5. Following overnight drying, take out the slides from the microarray printer and scan the printed slides using the microarray scanner to monitor the quality of printed spots. Any slide with missing spots should be discarded or marked.
6. Use pap pen to make hydrophobic barrier around the printed area to create a rectangular incubation area for immunolabeling. Make sure there is enough space between the barrier and the printed spots to allow for proper hybridization. The two arrays on each slide can be separated using pap pen. Leave the slides at room temperature for at least 2 h to let the ink dry.
7. Wash the slides twice, each for 20 min, with PBST and 0.05× PBS respectively, in the high-throughput wash station with stirring to remove unbound peptides. This prewash can reduce nonspecific binding and background noise. Slides are then dried by centrifugation at 130 rcf for 3 min. Following centrifugation, the slides can be immunolabeled right away or stored in a vacuum container for up to 3 weeks.

3.2 Immunolabeling of Microarray Slides

All the incubation steps in immunolabeling are performed in a slide staintray/humidity chamber protected from light on a rotating platform with gentle agitation/rotation. It is very important to add water into the humidity chamber to maintain proper humidity and keep the slide covered with solutions/buffers at all times; never let the slide dry during immunolabeling. All solutions/buffers should be removed by aspiration at the corner of each array (without touching the printed spots) unless otherwise stated.

3.2.1 Blocking

1. Place the slides on the hybridization chamber, and add 250 μL of blocking buffer onto each array. Incubate for 1 h at 31 °C with gentle rotation.
2. Carefully remove the blocking buffer by aspiration.

3.2.2 Serum Incubation

1. Patient serum samples (*see* **Note 3**), diluted 1:5 in blocking buffer, are added to the arrays (250 μL/array) and gently rotated overnight at 4 °C (*see* **Note 7**).
2. Following overnight incubation, serum is removed by gently tapping the slides on tissue paper. If there are more than two arrays per slide, avoid contamination between arrays.
3. The slides are transferred onto a slide rack, dipped two times in PBST, and washed in the high-throughput wash station containing fresh PBST 2 × 5 min at room temperature.
4. Place the slides back into the hybridization chamber and the remaining PBST is removed by aspiration.

If the purpose of the experiment is to measure the amount of IgE antibodies to each peptide, skip Subheading 3.2.3 and continue with Subheading 3.2.4. If the purpose of the experiment is to measure the affinity of peptide specific IgE antibody, continue with Subheading 3.2.3.

3.2.3 Competition with Allergen

The conditions (e.g., temperature, competitor concentration, and incubation time) for performing the competition vary depending on the patient population and the allergens, and should be optimized before applying onto individual serum samples. We use a scatter plot to evaluate the effect of competition by plotting the standard conditions (standard protocol without the competition step) vs. the competition, or competition with blocking buffer which contains human serum albumin as a negative control vs. competition with the specific allergen. When optimizing using a serum pool, which contains a mixture of high and low affinity antibodies, the conditions resulting in more scattered points in the scatter plots are usually selected as it reflects the different affinity of IgE antibodies to different epitopes (*see* **Note 8**).

As an example, Fig. 1 compares different competition temperatures using a serum pool of five patients highly sensitive to milk. Competition at 31 °C seems to be too harsh because IgE binding to most peptides is competed off. Competition at 16 °C is selected because the points are more scattered.

1. The competition mixture is derived from the same food proteins that the printed peptide sequences are derived and is added to the arrays (250 μL/array) and gently rotated for 1 h at 16 °C.

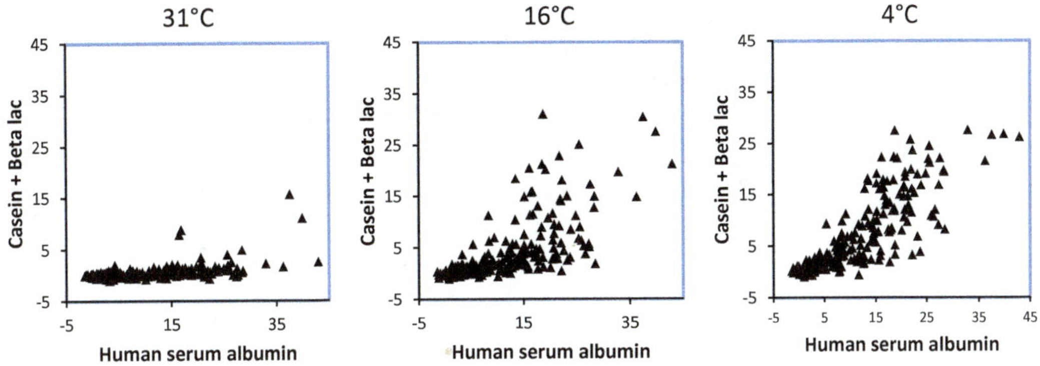

Fig. 1 Scatter plot comparing IgE binding between competition with a negative control (blocking buffer containing human serum albumin, *x*-axis) and competition with a mixture of 2 mg/mL caseins and 3 mg/mL beta-lactoglobulin (*y*-axis) at different temperatures for 4 h. Each spot represents IgE binding (represented as a *z* score) to 1 peptide of milk allergens

2. Gently tap the slides on tissue paper to remove the competition mixture, then wash the slides 2 × 5 min in the high-throughput wash station containing fresh PBST at room temperature.
3. Place the slides back into the hybridization chamber and the remaining PBST is removed by aspiration.

3.2.4 Secondary Antibody Incubation

1. Prepare the secondary antibody, which is a cocktail of several Biotin-conjugated monoclonal mouse Anti-Human IgE antibodies right before the incubation. The antibodies are each diluted 1:250 in blocking buffer. The concentration of each antibody needs to be optimized using a serial dilution of the antibody and choose the dilution that gives the strongest signal versus low background.
2. Add 250 μL of the antibody cocktail onto each array, and incubate for 4 h. If possible, incubate at a slightly higher temperature (e.g., 31 °C for 4 h) to increase sensitivity (*see* **Note 7**).
3. Following incubation, quickly wash the slides (remain in the humidity chamber) with PBST from a squeeze bottle and remove the remaining PBST by aspiration. Add 300 μL of 1 mM EDTA in PBST to each array and leave on a rotating platform for 5 min at room temperature.
4. Quickly wash the slides again with PBST from a squeeze bottle. Remove the remaining PBST by aspiration.

3.2.5 Dendrimer Amplification

This step is to amplify the signal using dendrimers to increase the sensitivity of the assay.

1. Add 200 μL of Dendrimer Buffer onto each array, and leave for 1 min before removing by aspiration.

2. Prepare the dendrimer cocktail (200 μL/array: 12 μL anti-Biotin dendrimer, 4 μL salmon sperm DNA, and 184 μL dendrimer buffer) right before adding them onto the slide. If possible, incubate at a slightly higher temperature (e.g., 31 °C for 4 h) to increase sensitivity (*see* **Note 7**).
3. Following incubation, quickly wash the slides (in the humidity chamber) with PBST from a squeeze bottle. Transfer the slides onto a slide rack. Dip ten times in 15 mM Tris–HCl and dry the slides by centrifugation. Dip five times in 0.1× PBS and dry by centrifugation. Dip five times in 0.05× PBS and dry again (*see* **Note 9**). Scan the slides or store in vacuum.

3.3 Slide Scanning

1. Scan the immunolabeled slides using a ScanArray®Gx microarray scanner. Save the scanned images as TIF files.
2. Align the image with a gal file that contains information on sample location and ID and is generated by the NanoPrint Microarray Manager Software (ArrayIt) for each printing. The fluorescent signals of all spots are digitized with ScanArray Express software (Perkin Elmer) and exported as comma-delimited text (.csv) files, which contains mean and median fluorescent signal (expressed as digital fluorescence units [DFUs]) of each spot and its local background.

3.4 Data Analysis

The following calculation can be performed using R programming language (http://www.r-project.org/), or other software that does not require programming, such as Microsoft Excel.

1. Calculate the readout (S_i) for each spot, including the replicates for peptides and blanks (PPB + DMSO), by using the equation below.

$$S_i = Log_2 \frac{Median(Spot)}{Median\ (Local\ background)}$$

2. Transform the S_i for each spot into a Z score (Z_i) by using the equation below.

$$Z_i = \frac{S_i - Median(S_{Blank})}{MAD(S_{Blank})}$$

Median (S_{Blank}) and MAD (S_{Blank}) are the Median and, the Median Absolute Deviation (MAD) of all the readouts of the blanks spots, respectively. MAD is a robust version of the standard deviation.

An index Z value of each peptide is generated by taking the Median of Z scores of the replicate spots. An individual peptide sample is considered positive if its index Z exceeds 3, meaning that the signal is above the background noise plus three times the MAD. As MAD is a robust version of the standard deviation, this means the signal is significantly above the background with p value less than 0.003.

3. (Optional) In order to eliminate nonspecific background noise, single-positive peptides with negative binding by four adjacent peptides (with overlapping amino acid sequence) are filtered out by replacement with the median of itself and the four adjacent peptides.
4. Further data analysis (e.g., Wilcoxon test, clustering) and presentation (e.g., Heat map) can be performed using R programming or other software such as Microsoft Excel, GraphPad Prism, and TIGR Multiexperiment Viewer (TMeV).

4 Notes

1. The use of overlapping peptides facilitates both the mapping of epitope sequences and the identification of key amino acids based on IgE-binding intensity. In addition, peptides can form secondary structures and solid phase bound peptides may not always be exposed and available for binding with IgE antibodies. By using overlapping probes, we increase the chances of detecting all epitopes.
2. Currently, there are quite a lot of companies in the market providing custom peptide synthesis service. We have also used the peptide synthesized by Chinapeptides Co., Ltd. (Shanghai, China) who supplies lyophilized peptide with purity >90%.
3. In addition to individual patient samples being tested, a positive and a negative control are required to run together with the serum samples being tested in each peptide microarray experiment to ensure that the assay is working properly and for data normalization. A serum pool of several patients allergic to the specific food/allergen can serve as a positive control and a pooled serum sample of nonallergic, non-atopic patients, or individual non-allergic patient's serum sample can serve as a negative control. These control serum pools are very important as they can be used for optimization of the experimental conditions, validation of antibodies, and controls run in each experiment for data normalization.
4. We recommend using a cocktail of more than one monoclonal antibody (higher specificity than polyclonal antibody), and the specificity of the antibody needs to be validated before incorporating them into the cocktail.

5. Sometimes, some peptides tend to form smaller spots after printing. This may be improved by adding Sarkosyl. We have tried to improve spot morphology using 0.02% of Sarkosyl.
6. We have tested the printing consistency of the SMP3B printing pins by printing fluorescent labeled proteins without reloading and found that the pin can deposit the same amount of samples and print at least 250 consistent spots. Therefore, the pins are usually used to print no more than 200 spots from each sample loading. In addition, the first two printed spots after each sample loading are usually very large and should not be used. We usually place two microscope glass slides on the first two printing positions and then discard them after printing. It is better to keep the microarray printing facility in a clean room to avoid any dirt or dust that gets into the printing plate or onto the slide surface during printing. In addition, it is important to clean the pins properly between loading different peptides to prevent cross-contamination. This can be done by washing the pins for 2 min between each loading of peptides in the sonicating bath station (filled with 10% ethanol) in the microarray printer.
7. The current experimental protocol (e.g., overnight serum incubation at 4 °C and secondary antibody incubation for 4 h at 31 °C) has been optimized based on our current peptide library and other experimental conditions, and may be affected by many factors, such as peptide purity, temperature and humidity in the lab, secondary antibody batch, etc. When setting up the peptide microarray facility, it is recommended to test different printing and immunolabeling conditions using the positive and negative control sera and find the optimal conditions that give maximum binding without compromising specificity. If any of the factors is changed, it is better to test the relevant conditions again to ensure optimal conditions.
8. The optimization of the competition condition is the key step in the measurement of antibody affinity using the microarray. The optimal conditions are the conditions that can differentiate antibodies with low and high affinity: Low affinity antibodies are competed off while high affinity antibodies remain bound. As noted above, this will result in more scattered points in scatter lots.
9. The final wash aims to remove unbound dendrimer molecules and reduce excess salt deposits on the array surface that will give high background noise. It is not recommended to wash the slides with water because this will remove bound dendrimer.

References

1. Sicherer SH, Sampson HA (2014) Food allergy: epidemiology, pathogenesis, diagnosis, and treatment. J Allergy Clin Immunol 133(2):291–307
2. Lin J, Sampson HA (2009) The role of immunoglobulin E-binding epitopes in the characterization of food allergy. Curr Opin Allergy Clin Immunol 9(4):357–363
3. Shreffler WG, Lencer DA, Bardina L et al (2005) IgE and IgG(4) epitope mapping by microarray immunoassay reveals the diversity of immune response to the peanut allergen, Ara h 2. J Allergy Clin Immunol 116(4):893–899
4. Lin J, Bardina L, Shreffler WG et al (2009) Development of a novel peptide microarray for large-scale epitope mapping of food allergens. J Allergy Clin Immunol 124(2):315–322
5. Lin J, Bruni FM, Fu ZY et al (2012) A bioinformatics approach to identify patients with symptomatic peanut allergy using peptide microarray immunoassay. J Allergy Clin Immunol 129(5):1321–1328
6. Ayuso R, Sanchez-Garcia S, Lin J et al (2010) Greater epitope recognition of shrimp allergens by children than by adults suggests that shrimp sensitization decreases with age. J Allergy Clin Immunol 125(6):1286–1293
7. Flinterman AE, Knol EF, Lencer DA et al (2008) Peanut epitopes for IgE and IgG4 in peanut-sensitized children in relation to severity of peanut allergy. J Allergy Clin Immunol 121(3):737–743
8. Wang J, Lin J, Bardina L et al (2010) Correlation of IgE/IgG4 milk epitopes and affinity of milk-specific IgE antibodies with different phenotypes of clinical milk allergy. J Allergy Clin Immunol 125(3):695–702
9. Han Y, Lin J, Bardina L et al (2016) What characteristics confer proteins the ability to induce allergic responses? IgE epitope mapping and comparison of the structure of soybean 2S albumins and Ara h 2. Molecules 21(5):622
10. McHeyzer-Williams MG, McHeyzer-Williams LJ (2005) Antigen-specific memory B cell development. Annu Rev Immunol 23:487–513
11. Christensen LH, Holm J, Lund G et al (2008) Several distinct properties of the IgE repertoire determine effector cell degranulation in response to allergen challenge. J Allergy Clin Immunol 122(2):298–304
12. El-Khouly F, Lewis SA, Pons L et al (2007) IgG and IgE avidity characteristics of peanut allergic individuals. Pediatr Allergy Immunol 18:607–613

Chapter 15

T-Cell Proliferation Assay: Determination of Immunodominant T-Cell Epitopes of Food Allergens

Madhan Masilamani, Mariona Pascal, and Hugh A. Sampson

Abstract

Characterization of allergen-specific T cells is critical to understand their contribution to disease pathogenesis. The identification of immunodominant T-cell epitopes is crucial for development of T-cell-based vaccines. Peptide-specific T-cell proliferation studies are usually performed in a library of short synthetic peptides (15mer or 20mer) with 3 or 5 offset spanning the entire length of the allergen. T-cell peptide epitopes lack the primary and tertiary structure of the native protein to cross-link IgE, but retain the ability to stimulate T cells. The peptides sequences can also be obtained either by in silico approaches and in vitro binding assays. The efficacy of T-cell epitope-based peptide immunotherapy has been proven in certain allergies. The present methodology describes T-cell proliferation assays using whole blood sample from allergic subjects.

Key words T cell, T cell proliferation, Peptides, Epitopes, Thymidine incorporation

1 Introduction

Allergen-specific IgE production and activation of mast cells, basophils, and eosinophils are the hallmarks of type I allergic immune response. Both branches of the immune system, innate and adaptive, participate in establishing the TH2 immune response that characterizes the allergic diseases [1]. Dominant TH2 responses to allergens during the sensitization phase lead to immunoglobulin (Ig) class switching to IgE as well as recruitment and activation of pro-inflammatory effector cells such as mast cells, basophils, and eosinophils [2–5]. Allergen-specific T cells are crucial in this inflammatory cascade [5]. Although different types of T lymphocytes (e.g., CD4+, CD8+, and natural killer T cells) have the capacity to respond to allergens, CD4+ T cells are the predominant effector population, which recognize peptides derived from allergens presented by antigen presenting cells (APCs) in the context of major histocompatibility complex (MHC) class II molecules. These cells exert their effects through the production of TH2 cytokines, mainly IL-4, IL-5, and IL-13. IL-4 is critical in

Jing Lin and Marcos Alcocer (eds.), *Food Allergens: Methods and Protocols*, Methods in Molecular Biology, vol. 1592,
DOI 10.1007/978-1-4939-6925-8_15, © Springer Science+Business Media LLC 2017

both the development of TH2 cells and antibody isotype switching to IgE [6].

Natural allergens drive diverse T-cell lineages that secrete multiple cytokines. It seems that different allergic phenotypes are linked to various combinations of CD4+ subsets, which include not only the well-established TH2 and TH1 lineages, but also the TH9, TH17, TH22, Treg, TR1, and TFH lineages that have been more recently discovered. Their cytokines have different functional roles in allergy [5]. Regulatory subsets, Treg and TR1, antagonize the activity of TH2 cells. Skewing allergen-specific T-cell responses toward a regulatory phenotype seems to be crucial for the beneficial effects of allergen-specific immunotherapy (ASIT) [7].

The specific immune response to allergens is decisive in the development of clinically healthy or allergic states [8]. In non-allergic subjects, a substantial fraction of allergen-specific T cells have a memory phenotype, but at lower frequencies than in allergic subjects. However, differentiated Th2 cells are present only in allergic subjects and their disappearance correlates with successful immunotherapy and tolerance [7, 8]. However, the T-cell receptor (TCR) of allergen-specific memory T cells from allergic subjects shows higher avidity compared to those of non-allergic subjects; even at a naive stage, suggesting that differences in T-cell repertoire development could exist. Moreover, in non-allergic subjects, the antibody response varies between having no response and the production of allergen-specific IgG_4- or IgG_1 with or without low amounts of allergen-specific IgE. In healthy individuals, during an immune response toward common environmental allergens, antigen-specific TR1 cells have been found to be the dominant subset along with a high concentration of specific IgG_4 and detectable IgE. Similarly, the major components of an immune response after ASIT are IL-10- and TGF-β-producing TR1 cells, IgG_4 antibodies, and suppressed effector cells (i.e., mast cells, basophils, and eosinophils) [7, 8].

Identification of precise T-cell epitopes within allergens is an important step toward elucidating mechanisms of disease pathogenesis and for the design of T-cell vaccines. Peptide-immunotherapy relies on the well-established role of T cells in food and environmental allergies, but with the substantial advantage of surpassing the high rate of adverse reactions caused by traditional immunotherapeutics based on whole proteins or extracts of allergenic sources [9]. Synthetic short peptides lack the primary and tertiary structures of the native protein to cross-link IgE, but retain the ability to stimulate T cells. The efficacy of T-cell epitope-based peptide immunotherapy (IT) has been proven in both bee venom [10] and cat dander allergies [11, 12]. Administration of synthetic peptides that contain the immuno-regulatory epitopes of Fel d 1, the major allergen in cat allergy, has been shown to induce both short-term [12] and long-term [11] beneficial effects (i.e., clinically relevant reduction in rhinoconjunctivitis symptoms).

In food allergy, the T-cell response toward several food allergens has been studied [5, 13]. Multiple T-cell epitopes have been described for a broad range of food allergens, from milk [14], egg [15], celery [16], peanut [17], peach [18–20], beef [21], shrimp [22] to Brazil nuts [5, 13]. The role of T-cell epitopes in cross-reactivity issues, such as the birch pollen associated food allergy, has been demonstrated [16]. Bet v $1_{142\text{-}152}$, the dominant T-cell epitope of birch pollen allergen, is important for the cross-reactivity with Bet v 1 related food allergens [23]. Nevertheless, evidence for a relevant T-cell epitope not cross reactive with homologous pollen allergens has been also demonstrated for the hazelnut allergen Cor a 1.04, a Bet v 1 homologue protein [24]. These findings suggest that T cells specific for food epitopes but nonreactive to pollen do exist which is suggestive of the ineffectiveness of pollen-specific IT to induce tolerance on concomitant food allergy [25].

Several allergenic proteins in peanut have been identified including Ara h 1, Ara h 2, Ara h 3, Ara h 6, Ara h 8, and Ara h 9. Most patients are sensitized to Ara h 1, Ara h 2, or Ara h 3 [26]. One of the major obstacles in identification of T-cell epitopes is the low frequency of allergen peptide-specific $CD4^+$ T cells in the circulation, even in sensitized individuals. It has been estimated that the frequency of Ara h 1 specific T cells in a sensitized individual will be around 9 cells per million [27]. Ara h 1 epitopes had been mapped in two previous studies, assaying peptide pools in 12 and 22 patients respectively [27, 28], and using two different approaches: tetramer-guided epitope mapping and CFSE-based proliferation assays using T-cell clones generated from allergic individuals. These methods have high specificity, but low sensitivity, thus requiring external validation with patient samples at the end [29]. The amino acid sequence of Ara h 1 is more than twice that of Ara h 2 and this limits experimental assays with/using overlapping peptides for the entire length of the protein in human blood samples. We have recently utilized an in silico epitope discovery algorithm (NetMHCIIpan [30, 31]) combined with an in vitro HLA binding assay to prospectively preselect Ara h 1 and 2 peptides that can be evaluated by T-cell stimulation assays [32, 33]. This approach has been also successfully used in other food allergens such as shrimp [22].

Here, we provide the T-cell proliferation assay methodology for the determination of immunodominant T-cell epitopes. This assay is based on the principle that soluble short synthetic peptides from allergens will be taken up by the antigen presenting cells, loaded onto MHC class II compartments and presented to CD4+ T cells. Only the peptide-specific T cells will be able to interact with the peptide-MHC class II complex leading to proliferation and clonal expansion (Fig. 1). The proliferating T cells can be quantified by tritiated thymidine incorporation followed by DNA harvesting and radioactive scintillation. In this assay, tritiated

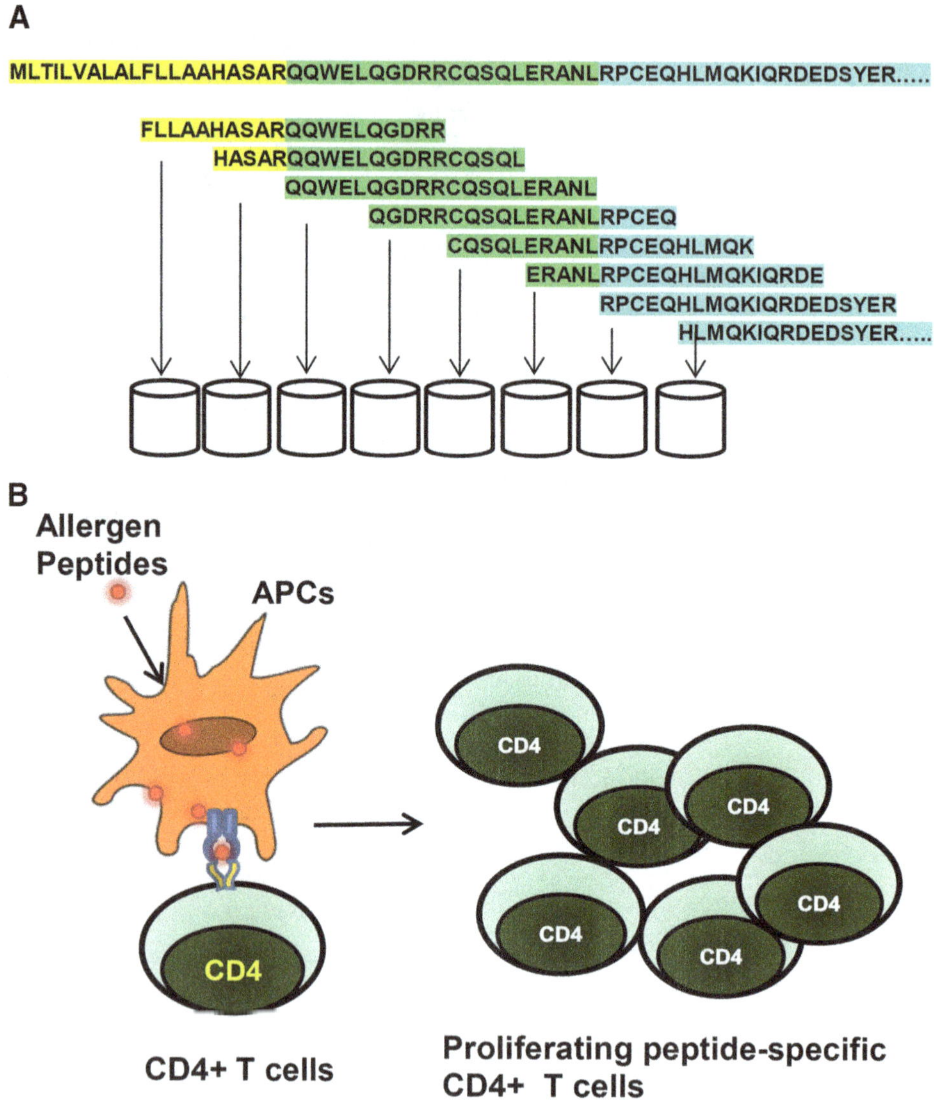

Fig. 1 Schematic representation of T-cell epitope discovery. (**a**) Overlapping peptides of candidate antigen are generated and plated in multi-well tissue culture plate. (**b**) Peripheral blood mononuclear cells from allergic subjects were isolated and cultured for 5–7 days. The proliferating T cells were quantified by either tritiated thymidine incorporation or CFSE dilution

thymidine, a radioactive nucleoside, is added during in vitro culture of PBMCs with allergenic peptides. During peptide-specific proliferation of T cells, thymidine is incorporated in the newly synthesized strands of chromosomal DNA. The incorporated radioactivity is measured using a scintillation beta-counter to determine the extent of cell division.

Thymidine incorporation assays have been widely used methodology for the detection of antigen-specific T-cell proliferation. Recent development of flow cytometry-based assays had largely replaced thymidine incorporation assays due to the versatility of simultaneous detection of multiple markers and other phenotypic characterization of T cells. However, in conditions where the frequency of individual peptide-specific T cells is very low (as in most food allergies) [27], the utilization of flow cytometry (*see* **Note 1**: Alternate methodologies) is limited because of poor resolution of proliferating T cells. In such cases, a large number of PBMCs are required and must be obtained by leukapheresis [34]. The detection of incorporated radioactive (tritiated) thymidine still proves to be sensitive in this case as it requires relatively less volume of blood compared to flow cytometry.

2 Materials

1. Heparinized whole blood.
2. Ficoll Paque Plus.
3. Serum-free AIM-V medium (store at 4 °C in the dark).
4. Sterile phosphate-buffered saline (PBS).
5. Allergen extracts (Final concentrations: 50 and 100 μg/mL).
6. Allergen peptides (Final concentrations ~20 μg/mL) (*see* **Note 2**).
7. Anti-CD3-CD28 beads (Dynabeads® Human T-activator CD3/CD28, Life Technologies).
8. 96-U-well plates.
9. Thymidine, [Methyl-3H] (Perkin Elmer) (*see* **Note 3**).
10. Glass fiber filters.
11. DNA harvestor (Tomtech).
12. Scintillation liquid (Scintisafe 30% cocktail, Fisher Scientific).
13. Scintillation counter (Wallach, Perkin Elmer).
14. Genomic DNA extraction kit (QIAamp DNA Mini Kit—Qiagen).
15. LIFECODES HLA-DRB1*/-DQB/-DPB Typing Kits for use with Luminex (Immuncor Trasplant Diagnostics Inc).
16. Luminex xMAP™ Technology equipment.
17. Thermocycler.

3 Methods

3.1 Experimental Procedure

1. *Blood collection:* Whole blood should be obtained with sodium heparin collection tubes. Preferably, the assay should be performed within 24 h of blood collection as prolonged storage results in low sensitivities.

2. *Isolation of peripheral blood mononuclear cells (PBMC):* Aseptically transfer the blood from each subject into a 50 mL sterile tube. Dilute blood with twice the original volume with sterile PBS. Mix gently. Carefully layer of blood on the top of 15 mL Ficoll in a 50 mL tube. Centrifuge 800 × g for 20 min at 20 °C with no acceleration and with breaks off. Isolate the PBMC layer with a sterile transfer pipette and transfer it to a new 50 mL sterile tube. Resuspend PBMC with sterile PBS (up to 50 mL) and centrifuge 500 × g for 15 min at room temperature, with maximum acceleration and with breaks on. Aspirate the supernatant with a sterile pipette and disturb the pellet by gently tapping the tube. Add 1 mL sterile AIM-V medium. Make sure the pellet is completely resuspended and perform cell count.
3. *Peptide and stimulant plate preparation:* Aliquot peptides in triplicates on a 96-well plate at desired concentration. Leave sufficient empty wells in between to prevent cross-contamination. Include the following control wells: Positive controls: whole allergen extracts (at least two different concentrations); anti-CD3/CD28 beads (T-cell expander) (0.5 μL/well). Negative controls: Medium-only control (no peptides or allergens); Nonspecific allergen extract control. For peanut whole extract stimulation use a 50 or 100 μg/mL final concentration.
4. *Peptide-PBMC culture:* Plate 200 μL of PBMCs (0.5 to 1 million cells) to each well of the peptide and control stimulants. Culture at 37 °C in a humidified 5% CO_2 incubator for 4 days.
5. On day 4 of culture, in the hood, gently resuspend the cells resting at the bottom of the well with multi-channel pipette. Centrifuge the plate at 300 × g for 7 min at room temperature with the centrifuge with maximum acceleration and break on. Aseptically transfer 100 μL of the supernatant to another 96-round bottom well plate stored at −80 °C for further use (for cytokine analysis). Add 100 μL of AIM-V to each well and gently resuspend the cell pellet.
6. Add 20 μL (10 μCi) of 3H-Thymidine (diluted working solution) to each well. (Tritiated thymidine working stock: 250 μL stock 3H-Thymidine (1 mCi/mL) + 4750 μL AIM-V sterile medium (final volume 5 mL). Culture for another 48 h at 37 °C in a humidified 5% CO_2 incubator.
7. On day 6 of culture, extract DNA from the cells onto a glass fiber filter using DNA harvester. Follow the manufacturer's recommended procedure.
8. Dry the filter paper under infra-red lamp, place it in appropriately sized plastic bag, add scintillation liquid gently to completely wet the filter (do not add excess fluid); remove the extra liquid

by pressing or rolling a cylinder on the surface. Seal all the sides of the filter mat and cut the sides to fit the scintillation cassette.

9. Obtain scintillation counts (counts-per-minute, CPM) on a scintillation counter by following manufacturers' procedures.
10. HLA-Typing: Isolate genomic DNA from venous blood. Perform HLA typing of loci DRB1, DPB1, and DQB1 with the PCR-SSO technique, in which a locus-specific DNA amplification is done using the polymerase chain reaction technique (PCR) and sequence-specific oligonucleotides (SSO) and the automatized system with Luminex® technology following manufacturers' procedure [35].

3.2 Data Analysis

1. The average CPMs for each peptide, whole allergen extracts, and anti-CD3/CD28 beads culture wells are compared with those containing medium alone (unstimulated cells). Calculate within subject variability of CPMs and estimate per-individual coefficient of variation (CV). Calculate stimulation index for each peptide.
2. *Stimulation Index (SI):* CPM of peptide/antigen-stimulated T cells (test) divided by CPM of unstimulated cells (negative control). If SI exceeds the estimated maximum coefficient of variation [CV = Standard Deviation (σ) /Mean (μ)] (>1+CVmax), the T-cell responses are considered positive. SI that equals or less than estimated maximum CV (>1 + CVmax) is considered negligible. Peptides inducing positive proliferative responses (SI $\geq$ 1.5) in at least 25% of the recruited subjects were considered significant.
3. *Population Coverage:* One of the major pitfalls in the characterization of immunodominant peptides for food allergens is the diversity of MHC class II molecules (HLA-DR, -DQ, and -DP). Given the extensive polymorphisms of these molecules, a single T-cell epitope may or may not bind a specific MHC class II molecule. In other cases, the peptide can bind more than one MHC molecule. Therefore, for clinical applications, any meaningful characterization of food allergen T-cell epitopes must recognize the MHC diversity and must include appropriate population coverage. This calculation can be done when the HLA genotype frequencies and the existing MHC/peptide recognition patterns are known utilizing tools available at the immuno epitope database (www.iedb.org) [36].

4 Notes

1. *Alternate method to investigate peptide-specific T-cell responses:* Carboxyfluorescein succinimidyl ester (CFSE) dilution assay can be used as an alternative to H^3-thymidine incorporation

assay (provided the frequency of peptide-specific T cells is high and detectable). T-cell proliferation assay using CFSE dilution followed by flow cytometry [37] has been described for peanut allergy [38]. CFSE (or its analogues such as Oregon Green (OG), SNARF-1, etc.) [39] is a membrane-permeable dye that binds to cytoplasmic proteins. Following each cell division, the intensity of CFSE fluorescence is roughly halved in daughter cells. Thus, $CFSE^{low}$ cells represent cells that are proliferating. The advantage of this methodology is the use of nonradioactive reagents for the experimentation. In addition, it is possible to further characterize the functional subsets of T cells (such as Th2, Treg, etc.) and to follow the changes in T-cell phenotype over a course of time. Other methods to quantify T-cell proliferation include flow cytometric detection of thymidine analog BrdU (5-bromo-2′-deoxyuridine) following its incorporation into newly synthesized DNA [40], or by the expression of proliferation marker Ki-67 [41] in dividing cells.

2. *Peptide solubility and solvent issues:* The success of peptide proliferation assays is very much dependent on the purity and solubility of the peptides tested. Peptides with 90% purity are recommended for proliferation assays. It is advisable to test the solubility of peptides in aqueous solution in physiological pH prior to the assay. Peptide sequences that contain many hydrophobic residues tend to aggregate and are not generally soluble in aqueous solvents. Organic solvents such as dimethylsulfoxide (DMSO), acetonitrile, or dimethylformamide (DMF) are generally used to dissolve peptide sequences containing more than 50% hydrophobic residues. In general for in vitro cellular assays, DMSO is usually well tolerated up to 0.1% final concentration (v/v). Higher concentrations will affect proliferation and ultimately the quality of the data. DMSO concentrations above 1% (v/v) are toxic to cells. For peptides that require organic solvents, control assay conditions using appropriate dilution of solvent (without the peptide) must be incorporated.

3. Working stocks of peptides in 96-well plates can be prepared in advance and stored at −80 °C. Long-term storage of aqueous solution of peptides at 4 °C is not recommended.

4. The culture conditions need to be standardized and carefully monitored to prevent overgrowth. Excessive number of cells will deplete the nutrients in the medium, and lower pH (medium becomes yellow) resulting in cell death. Scintillation counts should not be taken in overgrown cells. Ideally, the cells should be in the log phase of proliferation to obtain reliable counts.

5. Sterile working stocks of tritiated thymidine can be prepared and stored at 4 °C by diluting in culture medium.

6. Cells supernatants for cytokine estimation (if needed) must be collected prior to addition of radioactive thymidine.
7. Adequate precautions must be taken for handling and disposal of radioactive substances following regulations of local laboratories and government agencies.

References

1. Saenz SA, Taylor BC, Artis D (2008) Welcome to the neighborhood: epithelial cell-derived cytokines license innate and adaptive immune responses at mucosal sites. Immunol Rev 226:172–190
2. Akdis CA (2012) Therapies for allergic inflammation: refining strategies to induce tolerance. Nat Med 18:736–749
3. Akdis CA, Agache I (2014) Global atlas of allergy. European Academy of Allergy and Clinical Immunology, Zurich
4. Scanlon ST, McKenzie AN (2012) Type 2 innate lymphoid cells: new players in asthma and allergy. Curr Opin Immunol 24:707–712
5. Wambre E, James EA, Kwok WW (2012) Characterization of CD4+ T cell subsets in allergy. Curr Opin Immunol 24:700–706
6. Woodfolk JA (2007) T-cell responses to allergens. J Allergy Clin Immunol 119:280–294 quiz 286–295
7. Akdis CA, Akdis M (2015) Mechanisms of allergen-specific immunotherapy and immune tolerance to allergens. World Allergy Organ J 8:17
8. Akdis M (2006) Healthy immune response to allergens: T regulatory cells and more. Curr Opin Immunol 18:738–744
9. Larche M, Akdis CA, Valenta R (2006) Immunological mechanisms of allergen-specific immunotherapy. Nat Rev Immunol 6:761–771
10. Muller U, Akdis CA, Fricker M, Akdis M, Blesken T et al (1998) Successful immunotherapy with T-cell epitope peptides of bee venom phospholipase A2 induces specific T-cell anergy in patients allergic to bee venom. J Allergy Clin Immunol 101:747–754
11. Couroux P, Patel D, Armstrong K, Larche M, Hafner RP (2015) Fel d 1-derived synthetic peptide immuno-regulatory epitopes show a long-term treatment effect in cat allergic subjects. Clin Exp Allergy 45:974–981
12. Patel D, Couroux P, Hickey P, Salapatek AM, Laidler P et al (2013) Fel d 1-derived peptide antigen desensitization shows a persistent treatment effect 1 year after the start of dosing: a randomized, placebo-controlled study. J Allergy Clin Immunol 131(103–109):e101–e107
13. Archila LD, Jeong D, Pascal M, Bartra J, Juan M et al (2015) Jug r 2-reactive CD4(+) T cells have a dominant immune role in walnut allergy. J Allergy Clin Immunol 136:983–992 e987
14. Ruiter B, Tregoat V, M'Rabet L, Garssen J, Bruijnzeel-Koomen CA et al (2006) Characterization of T cell epitopes in alphas1-casein in cow's milk allergic, atopic and non-atopic children. Clin Exp Allergy 36:303–310
15. Holen E, Elsayed S (1996) Specific T cell lines for ovalbumin, ovomucoid, lysozyme and two OA synthetic epitopes, generated from egg allergic patients' PBMC. Clin Exp Allergy 26:1080–1088
16. Bohle B, Radakovics A, Jahn-Schmid B, Hoffmann-Sommergruber K, Fischer GF et al (2003) Bet v 1, the major birch pollen allergen, initiates sensitization to Api g 1, the major allergen in celery: evidence at the T cell level. Eur J Immunol 33:3303–3310
17. de Jong EC, Spanhaak S, Martens BP, Kapsenberg ML, Penninks AH et al (1996) Food allergen (peanut)-specific TH2 clones generated from the peripheral blood of a patient with peanut allergy. J Allergy Clin Immunol 98:73–81
18. Pastorello EA, Monza M, Pravettoni V, Longhi R, Bonara P et al (2010) Characterization of the T-cell epitopes of the major peach allergen Pru p 3. Int Arch Allergy Immunol 153:1–12
19. Schulten V, Radakovics A, Hartz C, Mari A, Vazquez-Cortes S et al (2009) Characterization of the allergic T-cell response to Pru p 3, the nonspecific lipid transfer protein in peach. J Allergy Clin Immunol 124:100–107
20. Tordesillas L, Cuesta-Herranz J, Gonzalez-Munoz M, Pacios LF, Compes E et al (2009) T-cell epitopes of the major peach allergen, Pru p 3: identification and differential T-cell response of peach-allergic and non-allergic subjects. Mol Immunol 46:722–728
21. Tanabe S, Kobayashi Y, Takahata Y, Morimatsu F, Shibata R et al (2002) Some human B and T cell epitopes of bovine serum albumin, the major beef allergen. Biochem Biophys Res Commun 293:1348–1353
22. Ravkov EV, Pavlov IY, Martins TB, Gleich GJ, Wagner LA et al (2013) Identification and vali-

dation of shrimp-tropomyosin specific CD4 T cell epitopes. Hum Immunol 74:1542–1549
23. Jahn-Schmid B, Radakovics A, Luttkopf D, Scheurer S, Vieths S et al (2005) Bet v 1142-156 is the dominant T-cell epitope of the major birch pollen allergen and important for cross-reactivity with Bet v 1-related food allergens. J Allergy Clin Immunol 116:213–219
24. Bohle B, Radakovics A, Luttkopf D, Jahn-Schmid B, Vieths S et al (2005) Characterization of the T cell response to the major hazelnut allergen, Cor a 1.04: evidence for a relevant T cell epitope not cross-reactive with homologous pollen allergens. Clin Exp Allergy 35:1392–1399
25. Bohle B (2006) T-cell epitopes of food allergens. Clin Rev Allergy Immunol 30:97–108
26. Burks W, Sampson HA, Bannon GA (1998) Peanut allergens. Allergy 53:725–730
27. DeLong JH, Simpson KH, Wambre E, James EA, Robinson D et al (2011) Ara h 1-reactive T cells in individuals with peanut allergy. J Allergy Clin Immunol 127(1211–1218):e1213
28. Prickett SR, Voskamp AL, Phan T, Dacumos-Hill A, Mannering SI et al (2013) Ara h 1 CD4+ T cell epitope-based peptides: candidates for a peanut allergy therapeutic. Clin Exp Allergy 43:684–697
29. Van Hemelen D, Mahler V, Fischer G, Fae I, Reichl-Leb V et al (2015) HLA class II peptide tetramers vs allergen-induced proliferation for identification of allergen-specific CD4 T cells. Allergy 70:49–58
30. Nielsen M, Justesen S, Lund O, Lundegaard C, Buus S (2010) NetMHCIIpan-2.0-improved pan-specific HLA-DR predictions using a novel concurrent alignment and weight optimization training procedure. Immunome Res 6:-9
31. Nielsen M, Lund O (2009) NN-align. An artificial neural network-based alignment algorithm for MHC class II peptide binding prediction. BMC Bioinformatics 10:296
32. Pascal M, Konstantinou GN, Masilamani M, Lieberman J, Sampson HA (2013) In silico prediction of Ara h 2 T cell epitopes in peanut-allergic children. Clin Exp Allergy 43:116–127
33. Ramesh M, Yuenyongviwat A, Konstantinou GN, Lieberman J, Pascal M, et al. (2016) Peanut T-cell epitope discovery: Ara h 1. J Allergy Clin Immunol
34. Foster B, Foroughi S, Yin Y, Prussin C (2011) Effect of anti-IgE therapy on food allergen specific T cell responses in eosinophil associated gastrointestinal disorders. Clin Mol Allergy 9:7
35. Cesbron-Gautier A, Simon P, Achard L, Cury S, Follea G et al (2004) Luminex technology for HLA typing by PCR-SSO and identification of HLA antibody specificities. Ann Biol Clin (Paris) 62:93–98
36. Bui HH, Sidney J, Dinh K, Southwood S, Newman MJ et al (2006) Predicting population coverage of T-cell epitope-based diagnostics and vaccines. BMC Bioinformatics 7:153
37. Roederer M (2002) Multiparameter FACS analysis. Curr Protoc Immunol Chapter 5: Unit 5 8
38. Turcanu V, Maleki SJ, Lack G (2003) Characterization of lymphocyte responses to peanuts in normal children, peanut-allergic children, and allergic children who acquired tolerance to peanuts. J Clin Invest 111:1065–1072
39. Wallace PK, Tario JD Jr, Fisher JL, Wallace SS, Ernstoff MS et al (2008) Tracking antigen-driven responses by flow cytometry: monitoring proliferation by dye dilution. Cytometry A 73:1019–1034
40. Dolbeare F, Gratzner H, Pallavicini MG, Gray JW (1983) Flow cytometric measurement of total DNA content and incorporated bromodeoxyuridine. Proc Natl Acad Sci U S A 80:5573–5577
41. Soares A, Govender L, Hughes J, Mavakla W, de Kock M et al (2010) Novel application of Ki67 to quantify antigen-specific in vitro lymphoproliferation. J Immunol Methods 362:43–50

Chapter 16

Tetramer-Guided Epitope Mapping: A Rapid Approach to Identify HLA-Restricted T-Cell Epitopes from Composite Allergens

Luis L. Diego Archila and William W. Kwok

Abstract

Tetramer-guided epitope mapping (TGEM) is a technique in immunology that permits the rapid identification of allergenic epitopes through peptide screening procedures utilizing human lymphocyte antigen (HLA) class II tetramers as staining reagents for detection. The identification of allergenic epitopes is a prerequisite for the accurate characterization of allergen-specific $CD4^+$ T cells without in vitro stimulation. Additionally, these MHC-II/peptide complexes that interact with T-cell receptors (TCR) of pathogenic $CD4^+$ T cells are compatible with a different number of assays like Intracelullar Cytokine Staining (ICS), and Carboxyfluorescein succinimidyl ester (CFSE) making it a robust technology to study the functionality of allergen-specific $CD4^+$ T cells.

Key words Food allergy, Epitopes, MHC class II tetramers, T cells

1 Introduction

An epitope is part of a protein that is recognized by the immune system [1]. In the allergy context, allergens are considered to have antigenic properties if they bind specific IgE antibodies [2] and induce IgE-mediated reactions [3]. On the other hand, it is now firmly established that allergen-specific $CD4^+$ T cells play an important role in the cycle that perpetuates allergic inflammation [4, 5]. In this regard, linear epitopes within the allergen can trigger T-cell reactivity and their identification is essential to develop novel immunotherapies that could target these T cells directly. In addition, identification of epitopes will allow the tracking of allergen-specific CD4+ T cells in both allergic and non-allergic subjects. Several approaches have been utilized to identify T-cell epitopes, such as: ELISPOT, CD137 activation assay [6] and by intracellular cytokine staining [7]. Each of these approaches has its own advantages and disadvantages. Here, we describe another approach designated

Jing Lin and Marcos Alcocer (eds.), *Food Allergens: Methods and Protocols*, Methods in Molecular Biology, vol. 1592, DOI 10.1007/978-1-4939-6925-8_16, © Springer Science+Business Media LLC 2017

as Tetramer-Guided Epitope Mapping (TGEM). In TGEM, epitope identified will have known MHC restriction, and antigen-specific T-cell clones can be isolated in the process of epitope identification.

For the TGEM approach, soluble class II monomers with leucine zipper regions attached to the carboxyl terminals of the molecules loaded with specific peptides are assembled into "tetramer" complexes through fluorochrome-labeled streptavidin [8]. HLA/peptide complexes can engage αβTCR and permit the analysis of allergen-specific CD4+ T cells. The concept of using soluble HLA/peptide-labeled ligands to study these rare T-cell populations has been a successful strategy applied in numerous translational and clinical contexts [9]. As mentioned earlier, Class II tetramers can be used to identify novel T-cell epitopes. TGEM was first described to identify Herpes virus simplex virus VP16 [10] and has since been utilized to describe a variety of HLA-DR-restricted T-cell epitopes derived from multiple allergens, including seasonal allergens [11, 12], perennial allergens [13], and food allergens [14–17]. The protocol described below will focus on identifying of T-cell epitopes for allergens. Although tetramer assays are highly specific and sensitive, the HLA type of the subject and a library of overlapping peptides for a known antigen of interest is a prerequisite to apply TGEM.

The basis of this approach (Fig. 1) is to stimulate PBMC (Protocol can be carried out with either PBMC or isolated CD4+ T cells with antigen presenting cells. Both protocols will be described below.) from the subject with peptide mixtures. These mixtures are composed of multiple pools of peptides where each pool consists of 5 to 10 different overlapping peptides. Soluble class II molecules that match the HLA of the subject are loaded with each mixture of peptides, and matching tetramers are used to screen individual wells of stimulated PBMC usually at day 14 post-stimulation. The particular pooled peptide tetramer that provides a positive staining is identified. Next, individual peptides from the pool are then utilized to generate single peptide tetramers. Positive staining in a second round of FACS analysis with a particular tetramer will identify the peptide containing the allergenic epitope. Following up the identification of allergenic epitopes additional tetramer complimentary assays can be utilized for further analysis. Besides the fast identification of novel epitopes, tetramer assays offer important advantages over other methods by enabling the recovery of allergen-specific T cells through sorting of tetramer-positive T cells with flow cytometry. Epitope-specific T-cell clones can then be generated and permit further analysis. Additionally, the tetramer technology can be compatible with a number of assays such as intracellular cytokine assay that permit the accurate characterization of phenotype and functionality of CD4+ T cells [11]. Here, we will demonstrate how to efficiently use the TGEM approach to identify novel epitopes from food

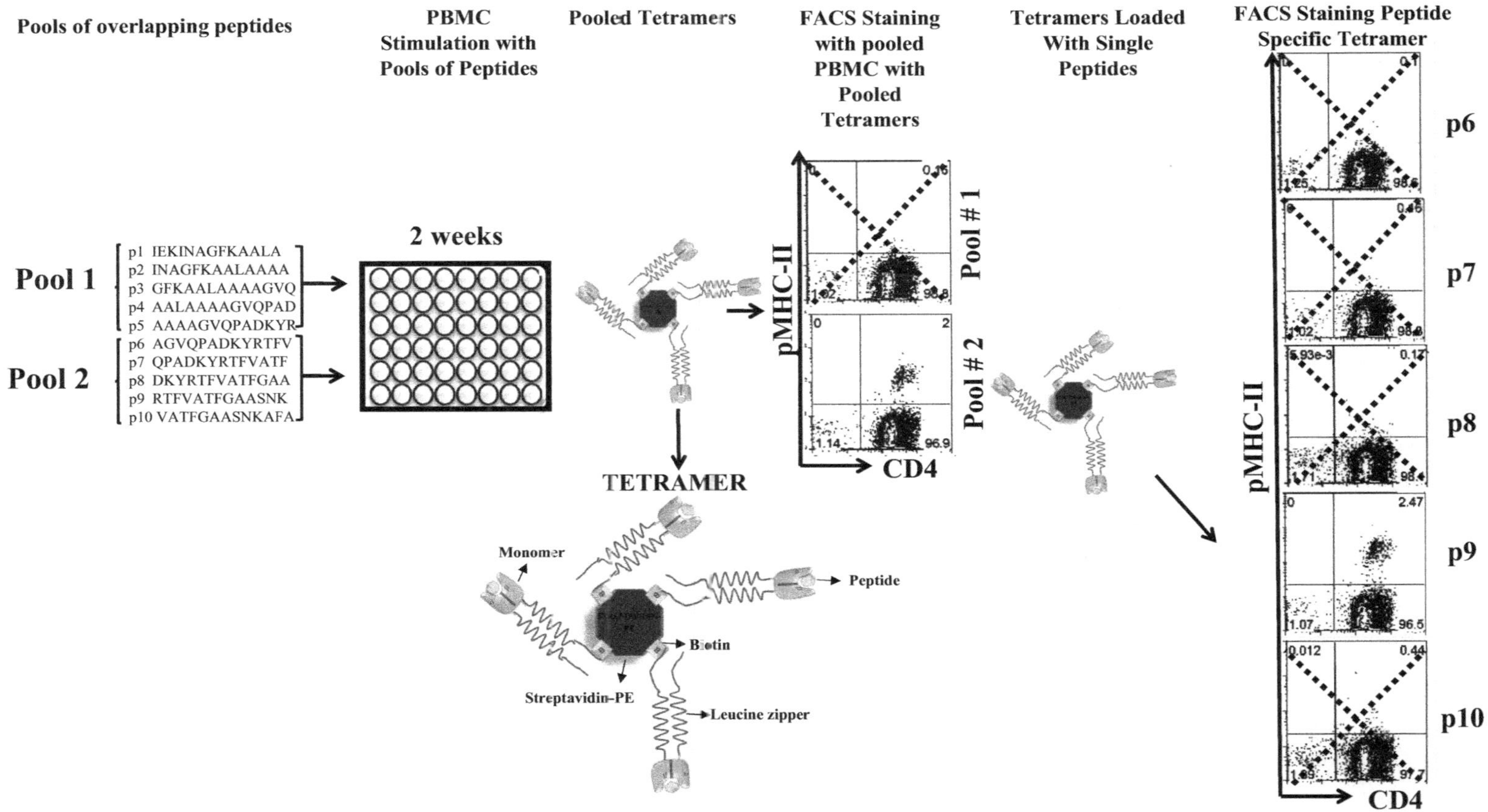

Fig. 1 Tetramer-guided epitope mapping. A panel of overlapping peptides that span the allergen of interest are divided into pools that consist of five peptides per pool. Each peptide pool is then utilized to stimulate individual wells plated with PBMC and cells will be cultured for 14 days. Peptide pools are also loaded onto soluble HLA class II molecules to generate pool peptide tetramers of the appropriate allergen. The pooled peptide tetramer that gives a positive staining is identified and peptides from that particular pool are utilized to generate tetramers loaded with individual peptides. Protocols for monomer production, assembly of pooled peptide tetramers, and single peptide loaded tetramers from monomers have been described elsewhere, and will not be described below. The particular tetramer that gives a positive staining is the allergenic HLA-restricted epitope

allergens in previously studied food allergens and will provide a step-by-step description of the methodological approach of using HLA class II tetramers in mapping T-cell epitopes.

2 Materials

2.1 Reagents

1. Class II tetramer at 0.5 mg/mL, BRI-A009.
2. RPMI 1640.
3. Penicillin-Streptomycin (P/S).
4. Pooled human serum.
5. IL-2 Stock (10,000 U), Roche.
6. Phytohaemagglutinin, Remel.
7. Running buffer: 2 mM EDTA, 0.5% BSA in 1× PBS.
8. Hemolytic buffer: 8.3 g NH_4Cl, 1.0 g $NaHCO_3$, 0.04 g disodium EDTA in 1 L of H_2O.
9. Ficoll-Paque, GE Healthcare.
10. Dulbecco's Phosphate Buffered Saline (1× PBS).
11. $CD4^+$ T-cell isolation kit human, Miltenyi Biotech.
12. *n*-Dodecyl-β-maltoside.
13. 1 mM Pefabloc SC.
14. R-PE streptavidin.

2.2 Equipment and Consumables

1. 50 mL polypropylene conical tubes.
2. 48 and 96-well culture cluster.
3. 37 °C, 5% CO_2, Incubator.
4. Centrifuge.
5. FACS tubes, Falcon.
6. FACS Calibur, BD Biosciences.
7. FACS ARIA II, BD Biosciences.
8. Cell irradiator.
9. Easysep™ Magnet, Stem cell technologies.

3 Methods

Carry out all procedures at room temperature and in a sterile Class II Biological Safety Cabinet unless otherwise specified.

3.1 PBMC Isolation

1. Cover work area in Class II Biological Safety Cabinet with an absorbing pad. Gather enough 50 mL conical tubes in a rack for each to contain 20 mL of whole blood per tube and dilute the blood to 40 mL with 1× PBS.

2. Underlay Ficoll utilizing a 10 mL pipette per conical tube. Draw up to 10 mL of Ficoll, insert into conical tube with tip placed on the bottom of tube and remove from pipet aid. Let the Ficoll gradually drain into the bottom.
3. Spin tubes at 448 rcf for 20 min with no brake at RT (above 26 °C). After spinning, the tubes should be layered top to bottom as follows: serum (yellow), PBMC (white), Ficoll (clear), and buffy coat/blood (red). Utilizing a transfer pipette carefully draw up the entire layer of PBMC. Get as many cells as possible and transfer equally to half as many conical tubes (e.g., if you start with eight conical tubes transfer cell suspension into four new conical tubes).
4. Dilute the cells to 50 mL with 1× PBS. Spin at 252 rcf for 15 min with low brake. Dispose of blood waste in a double bag filled with absorbent pellets during this spin.
5. Aspirate supernatant down to ~5 mL. Add 5 mL of pre-warmed hemolytic buffer to each tube. Resuspend by pipetting up and down with transfer pipette. Incubate at room temperature in the dark for 5 min. Dilute up to 50 mL with 1× PBS and spin at 112 rcf for 10 min.
6. Aspirate supernatant and resuspend pellet. Fill up to 50 mL with 1× PBS. Do cell counts. Spin at 112 rcf for 10 min.

3.2 In Vitro Stimulation of PBMC with Peptide

1. Aspirate supernatant and resuspend pellet with fresh medium up to desired cell concentration (2 or 2.5 million cells/mL) (*see* **Notes 1** and **2**). Add 1 mL of fresh medium containing PBMC to each individual well as necessary (*see* **Note 3**).
2. Add 1 μL (4 μg per mL final concentration for each individual peptide pool) of appropriate peptide pools to each well. Leave some wells without peptide as controls and incubate at 37 °C for 7 days. Next, carefully draw ½ of the media from each well and gently resuspend cells in remaining medium and transfer to a new well. Add 500 μL of culture medium and 50 μL/mL of IL-2 (10 U/mL). Every 2 days cells are fed with 500 μL of culture medium and 50 μL/mL of IL-2 and replate into additional wells when necessary.

3.3 Isolation of $CD4^+$ T Cells and In Vitro Stimulation of Cells with Peptide

1. Aspirate supernatant and resuspend pellet with running buffer up to desired cell concentration according to $CD4^+$ T-cell isolation kit human manufacturer's instructions (40 μL per every 10 million cells, e.g., if 100 million cells total: 40 μL × 10) (*see* **Note 1**).
2. Add $CD4^+$ T-cell Biotin-Antibody cocktail (10 μL per every 10 million cells). Resuspend cells by pipetting up and down with micropipette equivalent to total volume. Incubate at 4 °C for 10 min.

3. Add running buffer (30 μL per 10 million cells). Add $CD4^+$ T-cell microbead cocktail human (20 μL per 10 million cells) and gently mix with micropipette equivalent to total volume avoiding bubbles. Incubate at 4 °C for 10 min.
4. Get two sterile, capped polypropylene vials in EasySep™ magnet. Transfer about 50 million cells to each vial (100 million cells per vial maximum). Bring volume up to ~4 mL with running buffer. Incubate for 10 min at room temperature in Class II Biological Safety Cabinet in the dark.
5. Keeping polypropylene vials in magnets, quickly dump out unbound $CD4^+$ T cells into new 50 mL conical tube (This is a negative selection kit, non-$CD4^+$ T cells bind magnetic microbeads, $CD4^+$ T cells do not bind microbeads).
6. Add 1 mL of running buffer to polypropylene vial and resuspend non-$CD4^+$ T-cell fraction. Transfer to another 50 mL conical tube. Rinse out tube with 1 mL of running buffer and transfer to the 50 mL conical tube to recover cell fraction. Add 1× PBS to 50 mL in both $CD4^+$ T-cell fraction and non-$CD4^+$ T-cell fraction [Antigen presenting cells (APC)] conical tubes to do accurate cell counts. Next, spin both conical tubes at 112 rcf for 7 min. Resuspend non-$CD4^+$ T-cell fraction to 10 million cells/mL in T-cell media. Add 200 μL of non-$CD4^+$ T-cell fraction to each well of a 48-well TC treated flat-bottom dish to be used in culture.
7. Incubate for 1 h at 37 °C. During this incubation resuspend $CD4^+$ T-cell fraction in culture medium at the following concentration: 1.5 million cells/mL. Store this fraction at 4 °C.
8. After incubation thoroughly wash the plates with culture medium, especially around the edges of each well utilizing a transfer pipette. Remove all culture medium. Quickly check under the microscope to see that you have removed all of the floating cells from each well of the plate.
9. Add 1 mL of $CD4^+$ T-cell fraction to each well containing APC. Add 1 μL (4 μg per mL final concentration for each individual peptide) of appropriate peptide pools to each well. Leave some wells without peptide as controls and incubate at 37 °C for 7 days. Next, carefully draw ½ of the media from each well and gently resuspend cells in remaining medium and transfer to a new well. Add 500 μL of culture medium and 50 μL/mL of IL-2 (10 U/mL). Every 2 days cells are fed with 500 μL of culture medium and 50 μL/mL of IL-2 and replate into additional wells when necessary (*see* **Notes 4** and **5**).

3.4 Tetramer-Guided Epitope Mapping

1. For peptide loading into HLA-DR monomer, take the biotinylated monomer into a 1.5 mL Eppendorf tube and load with 0.2 mg/mL of peptide pools and incubate for 72 h at 37 °C in

the presence of 0.2 mg/mL *n*-Dodecyl-β-maltoside and 1 mM Pefabloc SC. Subsequently, add R-PE streptavidin at a molar ratio of 8:1 into the peptide-loaded monomers and gently resuspend.

2. After 14 days of in vitro expansion (*see* **Note 6**), aliquot at least 200 μL of cell suspension into 5 mL Falcon polystyrene tubes from each well. Add into each of the tubes 1 μL PE-labeled HLA-DR tetramer loaded with the same peptide pool as used in the specific stimulation (final concentration of 10 μg/mL). PE-labeled HLA-DR tetramer loaded with a control peptide can be used to monitor unspecific staining.
3. Stain T cells in the dark with HLA-DR tetramers for 2 h at 37 °C in a CO_2 incubator (*see* **Note 7**). Add 2 mL of running buffer and spin at 112 rcf for 5 min. Decant excess of running buffer and add 2 μL of antibodies specific for human CD4, CD3, and CD25 with fluorochromes other than PE (*see* **Note 8**). Stain cells for 10 min in the dark at room temperature. Wash each tube with 2 mL of running buffer.
4. Decant and add 200 μL running buffer, mix by tapping, and analyze in a flow cytometer. Perform tetramer analysis utilizing Flow Jo software to assess the tetramer positivity of each stimulated well by comparing positive versus negative tetramer staining. Tetramer staining should be at least one log above background.
5. After identifying the wells that are tetramer positive, generate PE-labeled HLA-DR tetramers loaded with same single peptides that belong to that particular pool and repeat **steps 2** and **3** (Fig. 2).

3.5 Isolation and Culture of Tetramer-Positive T-Cell Clones

Although it is not required, an additional procedure can also be utilized to confirm Tetramer positivity.

1. Repeat **steps 1** and **2** from Subheading 3.4.
2. Irradiate unmatched PBMC in 5 mL of culture medium in a 50 mL conical tube. Wash irradiated PBMC with 30 mL culture medium and spin at 112 rcf for 5 min. Aspirate supernatant and adjust cells at a concentration of 1×10^6 cells per 1 mL. Plate 100 μL of irradiated PBMC in culture medium per well.
3. Set up FACS Aria II for single cell sorting and sort tetramer-positive T cells into round-bottom 96-well containing 100 μL of culture medium per well.
4. Add an extra 100 μL of culture medium and expand sorted T cells by stimulation with 5 μg per 1 mL of phytohemagglutinin (PHA) and incubation in a CO_2 incubator at 37 °C. On the next day stimulate T cells by adding 10 U/mL of IL-2 and expand for 10 to 14 days.

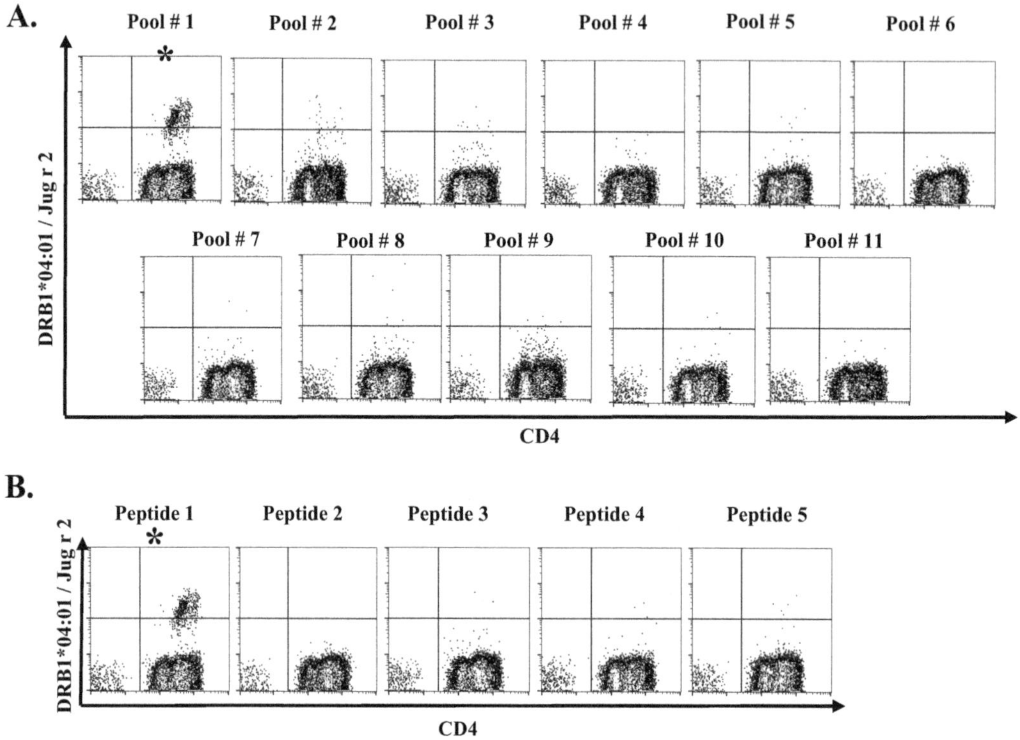

Fig. 2 TGEM studies of DRB1*04:01-restricted Jug r 2-reactive CD4+ T-cells. (**a**) PBMC from a DRB1*04:01 subject with walnut allergy were stimulated with 11 pools of Jug r 2 peptides for 2 weeks and subsequently stained with corresponding DRB1*04:01/Jug r 2 pooled peptide tetramers. (**b**) Cells that were stimulated with pool #1 were restained with individual peptides from the corresponding pool. The staining identified p1 (Jug r $2_{152\text{-}171}$) as DRB1*04:01 restricted Jug r 2 T-cell epitopes

5. On day 14 screen cells for growth and split confluent cells as needed by transferring half of the cells from each well into a new well and adding fresh culture medium and IL-2 as needed.
6. On day 20, screen cells by tetramer staining and repeat **steps 1** and **2** from Subheading 3.4. Tetramer-positive T-cell clone staining should be at least one log above negative population (Fig. 3).

4 Notes

1. To map a protein that is 300 amino acids long you will require approximately 28 wells for peptide pool stimulation, which is roughly equivalent to 70 million PBMC.
2. It is very critical to plate 2–2.5 million cells per well in a 48-well culture plate as antigen-specific T cells that are cultured in either too low or high cell confluency will not expand adequately.

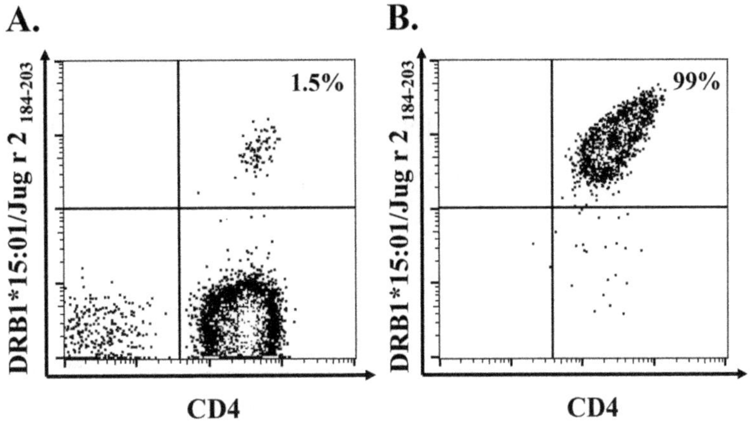

Fig. 3 Comparison of Tetramer staining in Tetramer-guided epitope mapping for walnut allergenic epitope Jug r 2 $_{184\text{-}203}$ and single cell sorted T-cell clones for the same allergenic epitope from a single walnut allergic subject. (**a**) Staining of cells with the DRB1*15:01/Jug r 2 $_{184\text{-}203}$ tetramer. (**b**) The tetramer-positive T cells were single cell sorted by flow cytometry, expanded with PHA and reexamined for positive tetramer staining

3. PBMC stimulation requires a more stringent every-day observation of your culture, as APC can also be expanded when adding fresh medium with IL-2. Thus, we find that transferring cells to a new well is advantageous the first 2 days after adding fresh medium with IL-2. Do not add new medium when transferring.
4. It is critical to split confluent cells as needed if there is high confluency. Do not split cells into a new well if confluency is too low. Adding fresh culture medium with IL-2 every 2 days is crucial for antigen-specific T-cell growth.
5. Avoid carrying APC plated from the original well of in vitro stimulation as these cells can outcompete antigen-specific T cells. If you encounter over carrying APC, gently pipette up and down and transfer into a new well.
6. TGEM should be performed within 10–16 days after in vitro stimulation, as apoptosis may prevent accurate detection of antigen-specific T cells.
7. Optimal time and temperature of different tetramer specificity can vary.
8. Tetramer-positive T cells express activation marker CD25, which is the α-chain of the IL-2 receptor (Fig. 4).

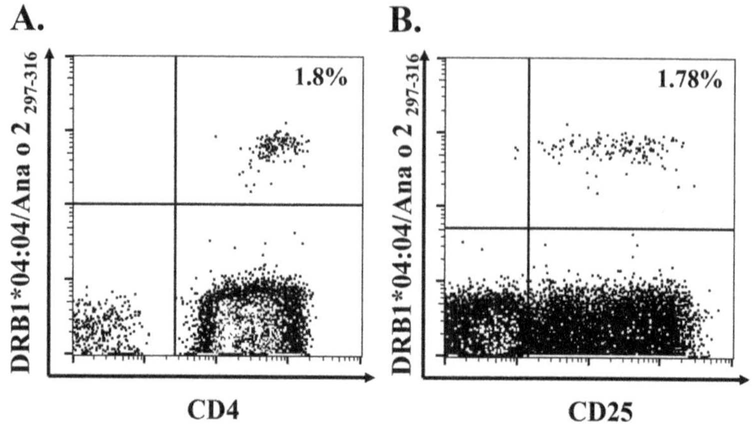

Fig. 4 Surface expression in tetramer-specific T cells. (**a**) In vitro expression of CD4 of DRB1*04:04/Ana o 2 $_{297-316}$ tetramer. (**b**) In vitro expression of CD25 of DRB1*04:04/Ana o 2 $_{297-316}$ tetramer

Acknowledgements

This work was supported by National Institutes of Health (NIH) contract HHSN272200700046C.

Disclosure of potential conflict of interest: L.D. Archila, W.W. Kwok has received research support from the US National Institutes of Health. The rest of the authors declare that they have no relevant conflict of interest.

References

1. Li PG, Ivaldi F, Moretti P, Manca F (2010) High throughput T epitope mapping and vaccine development. J Biomed Biotechnol 2010:325720
2. Andersson K, Lidholm J (2003) Characteristics and immunobiology of grass pollen allergens. Int Arch Allergy Immunol 130:87–107
3. Gieras A, Focke-Tejkl M, Ball T et al (2007) Molecular determinants of allergen-induced effector cell degranulation. J Allergy Clin Immunol 119:384–390
4. Woodfolk JA (2007) T-cell responses to allergens. J Allergy Clin Immunol 119:280–294
5. Wambre E, James EA, Kwok WW (2012) Characterization of CD4+ T cell subsets in allergy. Curr Opin Immunol 24:700–706
6. Wolfl M, Kuball J, Ho WY et al (2007) Activation-induced expression of CD137 permits detection, isolation, and expansion of the full repertoire of CD8+ T cells responding to antigen without requiring knowledge of epitope specificities. Blood 110:201–210
7. Archila LD, Delong JH, Wambre E, James EA, Robinson DM, Kwok WW (2014) Grass-specific CD4(+) T-cells exhibit varying degrees of cross-reactivity, implications for allergen-specific immunotherapy. Clin Exp Allergy 44:986–998
8. Reijonen H, Kwok WW (2003) Use of HLA class II tetramers in tracking antigen-specific T cells and mapping T-cell epitopes. Methods 29:282–288
9. Nepom GT (2012) MHC class II tetramers. J Immunol 188:2477–2482
10. Novak EJ, Liu AW, Gebe JA et al (2001) Tetramer-guided epitope mapping: rapid identification and characterization of immunodominant CD4+ T cell epitopes from complex antigens. J Immunol 166:6665–6670
11. Wambre E, Delong JH, James EA et al (2014) Specific immunotherapy modifies allergen-

specific CD4+ T cell responses in an epitope-dependent manner. J Allergy Clin Immunol 133(3):872–879

12. Wambre E, Delong JH, James EA, LaFond RE, Robinson D, Kwok WW (2012) Differentiation stage determines pathologic and protective allergen-specific CD4+ T-cell outcomes during specific immunotherapy. J Allergy Clin Immunol 129(544–51):551
13. Kwok WW, Roti M, Delong JH et al (2010) Direct ex vivo analysis of allergen-specific CD4+ T cells. J Allergy Clin Immunol 125:1407–1409
14. Delong JH, Simpson KH, Wambre E, James EA, Robinson D, Kwok WW (2011) Ara h 1-reactive T cells in individuals with peanut allergy. J Allergy Clin Immunol 127:1211–1218
15. Renand A, Newbrough S, Wambre E, Delong JH, Robinson D, Kwok WW (2014) Arginine kinase Pen m 2 as an important shrimp allergen recognized by T2 cells. J Allergy Clin Immunol 134:1456–1459
16. Archila LD, Chow IT, McGinty JW et al (2016) Ana o 1 and Ana o 2 cashew allergens share cross-reactive CD4(+) T cell epitopes with other tree nuts. Clin Exp Allergy 46:871–883
17. Archila LD, Jeong D, Pascal M et al (2015) Jug r 2-reactive CD4(+) T cells have a dominant immune role in walnut allergy. J Allergy Clin Immunol 136:983–992

Chapter 17

T-Cell Epitope Prediction

George N. Konstantinou

Abstract

An epitope is a part of an immunogenic protein that can be recognized by the immune system. The peptides that can be recognized by the T-cell receptors after a particular antigen has been intracellularly processed, bound to at least one MHC molecule and expressed on the surface of the antigen presenting cell as a MHC-peptide complex, are called a T-cell epitope. Individuals who have at least one MHC molecule able to most avidly bind to allergenic amino acid sequences from an allergen, and at the same time have the appropriate T-cell clone that can recognize this MHC-peptide complex, are expected to be genetically prone to allergic reactions against that allergen. This possibility can be examined in silico by utilizing modern computational techniques that are based on sophisticated mathematics and statistics. The design principles of these techniques are different and therefore variations in their predictions are expected. The available software programs that have been developed on this basis are able to combine the increasing amount and complexity of the available experimental data that have been organized in immunoinformatics databases to predict potential allergen T-cell epitopes. All relevant T-cell epitope prediction methods can be accessed online as a freeware.

Key words T-Cell epitope, Prediction, In silico, Bioinformatics, Peptide, Allergy, Allergen, Antigen, Processing

1 Introduction

1.1 Epitope Definition

All parts of an antigen that can be recognized and bind to either immune cells (e.g., T cells and B cells), free molecules (e.g., antibodies), or cell-surface proteins [e.g., major histocompatibility complex (MHC)] are characterized as epitopes. The epitopes are distinguished into two types according to the primary, secondary, or tertiary structure of the molecule they belong:

1. A continuous stretch of amino acid residues within a peptide is known as a *linear*, *sequential*, or *continuous* epitope.
2. Noncontinuous amino acid segments that are distantly separated within the same molecule but are brought into proximity by the folding of the molecule are called *conformational* or *discontinuous* epitopes.

Jing Lin and Marcos Alcocer (eds.), *Food Allergens: Methods and Protocols*, Methods in Molecular Biology, vol. 1592,
DOI 10.1007/978-1-4939-6925-8_17, © Springer Science+Business Media LLC 2017

B-cell epitopes can be either linear or conformational, but T-cell epitopes are always linear [1].

All antigens are displayed by antigen presenting cells (APC) after being internalized (most of the times by phagocytosis) and digested into smaller fragments/peptides. These peptides are presented in MHC molecules on APC surfaces. MHC molecules can bind only short peptides and consequently, all antigenic proteins have to be converted into peptides, a procedure that is known as *antigen processing*. There are two types of antigens that can be processed: intracellular or class I antigens and extracellular or class II antigens. The intracellular antigens are displayed on the MHC class I molecules that are found on the cell surface of all nucleated cells. The extracellular antigens are displayed on the MHC class II molecules found basically on dendritic cells that have phagocytosed exogenous pathogens (e.g., bacteria, parasites, toxins, allergens, etc.). In general, MHC class I molecules obtain peptides mainly from cytosolic proteins and MHC class II molecules from proteins in intracellular vesicles [2].

Each MHC molecule consists of an extracellular peptide-binding cleft or groove formed by appropriate folding of the amino termini of the MHC-encoded proteins. Each cleft has two walls and a floor that may vary on the amino acids composition among the different MHC alleles and is responsible for binding with the peptides that will be displayed to the antigen receptors of the T cells [2].

MHC molecules and peptides are bound with a noncovalent interaction mediated by amino acid residues on both the MHC clefts and the processed peptides. This interaction is class dependent. The association of a peptide with the MHC class I cleft depends mainly on the electrostatic interactions of the positively charged amino (N)-terminus and the negatively charged carboxyl (C)-terminus of the processed peptide to the MHC molecule. In most MHC class I molecules, the floor of the cleft contains hydrophobic pockets where hydrophobic amino acid residues of the C-terminal end of these peptides (e.g., valine, isoleucine, leucine, or methionine) can bind. Some MHC class I molecules have a preference for a basic amino acid residue at the C terminus (most of the times lysine or arginine). The hydrophobic bonds do not exclude complementary binding of other amino acid residues of a peptide (called anchor residues because they literally anchor the peptide in the cleft of the MHC molecule) with electrostatic, hydrogen, or van der Waals interactions that vary in strength according to avidity and affinity of this bond. In MHC class II molecules, such interactions may occur not only with the floor but also with the walls of the cleft contributing additionally to peptide binding and its strength [2].

The peptide-binding cleft of MHC class I molecules is large enough to accommodate peptides no larger than 8–11 amino acids long because the ends of their cleft are closed (Fig. 1). In contrast,

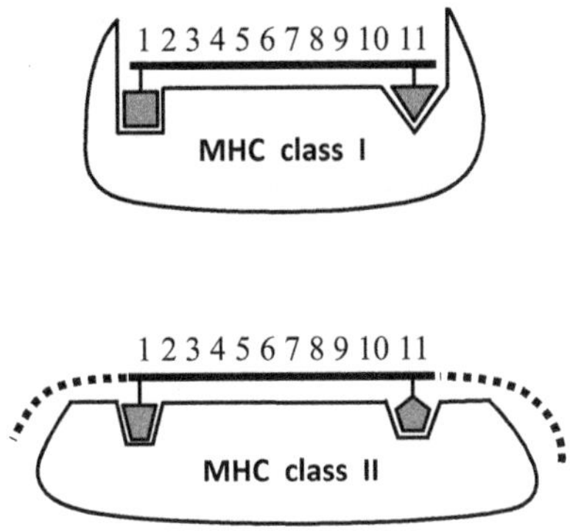

Fig. 1 Schematic representation of structure of MHC/peptide complexes

MHC class II molecules have open ends of the peptide-binding cleft so that they can bind peptides of 10–30 residues long or even longer, with the optimal length being 12–16 residues [2].

1.2 Antigen Processing T-Cell Epitope Dependence

The antigen processing procedure is dependent on the intracellular mechanisms of cleavage, transportation, and formation of the MHC binding.

In the MHC class I intracellular pathway, antigens in the cytosol are processed by the proteolytic activity of the proteasomes. Because MHC class I molecules are synthesized in the endoplasmic reticulum (ER), a mechanism is needed to deliver cytosolic cleavaged peptides into the ER. This delivery is mediated by the transporter associated with antigen processing (TAP). TAP exhibits a broad range of specificities and therefore it is expected to have higher transport affinity for some peptides over others. Its optimal activity, however, needs peptides 8–16 amino acids long that contain basic or hydrophobic carboxyl termini. The TAP-peptide dimer is transported to the ER, where they bind to class I MHC molecules. Once MHC class I molecules are loaded with the peptide, they exit the ER and are translocated to the cell surface.

The MHC Class II processing pathway involves the endocytosis of extracellular antigens into vesicles and their enzymatic degradation that takes place in these vesicles. MHC Class II molecules cannot bind with any peptides in the ER so that all ER-generated peptides are always associated with the MHC class I molecules as aforementioned. The MHC class II molecules are transported into exocytic vesicles toward the cell surface where they meet with the endocytic vesicles containing the processed antigens. The generated peptides are then associated with the appropriated MHC class II molecules in this fusion vesicle that is transported to the cell surface where the peptide-MHC class II complex is expressed [2].

1.3 MHC-Peptide Complex T-Cell Epitope Recognition

The antigen receptors of the T cells recognize the complex of the MHC molecule bound to a specific peptide. The fine specificity of antigen recognition is attributed to the peptide while the MHC residues are responsible for the MHC restriction of the T cells. Part of the bound peptide in the MHC cleft is exposed from the open top of the cleft, along with the adjacent amino acid residues of this MHC cleft. Only these exposed amino acid side chains can be recognized by a specific for this antigen complex T-cell receptor. It is self-explanatory that variations in either the peptide or the MHC cleft influence presentation and recognition of that peptide by the T cells (e.g., existence of a specific amino acid residue on either the MHC or the presenting peptide may enhance the immunogenicity of that peptide if this residue strengthens the binding between MHC-peptide complex and T-cell receptor). Thus, the structure of a processed peptide and the physicochemical properties of the component amino acids define the antigenic specificity of this epitope. Any change in the structure, including a single amino acid substitution or destruction, may influence antigenicity.

1.4 Immunogenicity of Protein Antigens

The immunogenicity of each antigen depends on the ability of the antigen-processing pathways to generate peptides that are able to bind with high avidity and affinity to the MHC molecules this organism has inherited. The MHC genes are the most highly polymorphic genes known. Because of this polymorphism a single MHC allele can present many different peptides to T cells and therefore the different MHC molecules are expected to present a great variety of different amino acid sequences and to cover all immunogenic amino acid sequences that exist in nature.

Each MHC molecule can accommodate only one peptide at a time. Therefore, only individuals that express MHC alleles that can bind this particular peptide may respond to that peptide. However, it has to be noted that a single T cell will be able to recognize only one of these huge amounts of MHC-peptide complexes. For instance, the individuals who have at least one MHC class II molecule able to most avidly bind to a peptide that is derived from grass pollen, and at the same time have the appropriate T-cell clone that can recognize this complex, are expected to be genetically prone to allergic reactions against that pollen.

2 Materials

Because of the MHC polymorphism, every single individual is expected to be unique. However, many of the different MHC molecules express similar peptide specificities because they have structural similarities according to which they are grouped into MHC supertypes [3]. A particular supertype is expected to bind to the same peptides. There are experimental data defining peptide sequences as epitopes able to bind with known MHC molecules and peptides that do not activate the MHC processing pathway (non-epitopes). These data are organized in immunoinformatics databases. To exploit the opportunities given by this huge amount of information, mathematical and statistical algorithms have been developed to analyze these peptide sequences so that T-cell epitope predictions can become an option. Based on the aforementioned antigen processing, this prediction cannot be simplified to directly utilizing peptide sequences and MHC or T-cell receptor structures. Proteosomal cleavage and TAP transportation should be taken into account since they are of equal importance, although unfortunately, there is scarcity of such experimental data.

There are online platforms that can combine the available information from databases that are constantly updated. This increasing amount and complexity of the available information complicates even more the prediction methods, highlighting the need to develop modern and sophisticated prediction algorithms based on statically learning theory. All these available tools, which can be accessed online and are available as freeware, will be presented in the following section.

The opportunity of in silico epitope prediction offers alternative options to minimize the cost of producing all the synthetic peptides needed to be experimentally tested and the enormous working time needed to perform all relevant experiments.

The accuracy of T-cell epitope predictions has been tested in Allergology, too. The potential of utilizing this analysis in Allergy field has implications not only in diagnostics but also for potential development of therapeutic options such as allergen immunotherapy. Utilizing the same online platforms and software, allergen T-cell epitope prediction has been proven to be of high precision when bioinformatics and experimental data are compared [4, 5]. This precision is very important for allergen epitope determination, for peptide-based allergen immunotherapy design, for allergenicity evaluation and modification, and for understanding immune tolerance mechanisms.

The constantly improved accuracy along with the cost and time minimization by following these approaches explain why in silico allergen T-cell epitope prediction is gaining ground in experimental settings.

3 Methods

There are three types of T-cell epitope prediction tools: MHC-binding prediction, Processing Prediction and Immunogenicity Prediction. The Immune Epitope Database (IEDB) and Analysis Resources platform incorporates all relevant available information of comparative studies having a state-of-the-art dynamic structure (*see* **Note 1**). At the same time, it follows continuous evaluation of new methods and datasets, and implements these data in a database that is constantly updated (*see* **Note 2**). Therefore, its platform is recommended as one of the best options to perform T-cell epitope predictions utilizing almost all available tools or, even better, a combination of them (*see* **Notes 3** and **4**). The following steps are based on the IEDB interface (*see* **Note 5**).

3.1 MHC-Binding Prediction

The peptide-binding strength is estimated by using two different types of thresholds to specify strong and weak binders: the binding affinity and a percentile rank.

The binding affinity is expressed in nanomolar of the half maximal inhibitory concentration (IC_{50}) values. The peptides are distinguished, according to the binding strength of the core peptides that are bound in the MHC cleft, into strong binders (predicted $IC_{50} < 50$ nM) or weak binders ($IC_{50} \leq 500$ nM). Nonsignificant peptides have $IC_{50} > 500$ nM but not above 5000 nM. MHC-binding prediction algorithms predict IC_{50} values for the specific peptide of interest that is supposed to bind a specific MHC molecule. Although, binding to MHC is necessary, it is not sufficient by itself for T-cell recognition.

The percentile rank is generated by comparing the peptide's IC_{50} against those of a set of random peptides derived, e.g., from Universal Protein Resource (UniProt) database. The smaller the numbered percentile rank is, the higher the expected affinity. In some algorithms the median percentile rank of the methods used is reported as the representative percentile rank.

There are tools that predict peptide binding to MHC class I or MHC class II molecules (*see* **Note 6**).

3.1.1 MHC-I-Binding Predictions

1. Specify sequences: Specify the sequences that will be scanned for binding peptides. Sequences can be entered either directly into the appropriate field or can be taken from appropriate protein databases like RCSB Protein Data Bank, NCBI protein database, or UniProt (*see* **Note 7**). The FASTA format is almost always the standard for inputting protein/peptide sequences.
2. Choose a prediction method: There are several different prediction methods that can be used to MHC class I binding:
   (a) Artificial neural network (ANN) [6].
   (b) Stabilized matrix method (SMM) [7].
   (c) SMM with a Peptide: MHC-Binding Energy Covariance matrix (SMMPMBEC) [8].
   (d) Scoring Matrices derived from Combinatorial Peptide Libraries (Comblib_Sidney2008) [9].
   (e) Consensus [10].
   (f) NetMHCpan [11].
   (g) NetMHCcons [12].
   (h) PickPocket [13].

The IEDB has a default prediction method for each MHC I allele which is based on availability of predictors and previously observed predictive performances. According to current (May 2016) performances the expected predictive performance of the aforementioned methods in decreasing order is Consensus, ANN, SMM, NetMHCpan, and CombLib.

3. Specify predictions details: Predictions are based on species-specific available data. The length and the type of the MHC molecule influence the predictions, too. Multiple allele/length pairs can be submitted at a time. For some allele/peptide length combinations, no prediction tools exist because there is too little experimental data available to generate them. Therefore, the selection of the allele/peptide length may influence the prediction outcome. Some platforms allow selection of distinct set of MHC alleles and peptide lengths according to existing data. If not a particular MHC allele of interest exist, there is an option to choose among frequently occurring alleles. Frequently occurring alleles are those that occur in at least 1% of the human population. A small set of such alleles can be compiled to cover most of the population of interest.
4. Specify the output: If the prediction will be based on IC_{50} there is an option to limit the outcomes displayed by defining an upper cutoff value. This option may influence the time needed for the calculations to be generated and the outcome to be displayed.
5. Submit the prediction: Click the submit button and wait for the result screen to appear.
6. Interpreting predicted affinities and percentile ranks: The predicted output can be given in units of IC_{50}nM. In that case, a lower number indicates higher affinity. Most known epitopes have high or intermediate affinity. Some epitopes have low affinity, but until now there is no known T-cell epitope with an IC_{50} value greater than 5000 nM. It has to be noted that although the predicted values seem to be quantitative, deviations are anticipated from the expected experimental IC_{50} values. This expected variability can be explained mainly by the mathematical/biostatistical way the prediction algorithms function and the differences in training and evaluation datasets that have been used in the developing process of these algorithms.

3.1.2 MHC-II-Binding Predictions

1. Specify sequences: Same as **step 1** in Subheading 3.1.1. MHC-I-binding predictions.
2. Choose a prediction method: The mostly recommended prediction methods for MHC class II binding are:
   (a) Consensus method [14].
   (b) Combinatorial library.

(c) NN-align (netMHCII-2.2) [15].
(d) SMM-align (netMHCII-1.1) [16].
(e) Sturniolo [17].
(f) NetMHCIIpan [18].

The IEDB has a default prediction method for each MHC class II molecule, which is based on availability of predictors and previously observed predictive performance that are based on large-scale evaluations of the performance of the different MHC class II binding algorithms [14, 19, 20].

3. Specify predictions details: Same as **step 3** in Subheading 3.1.1 MHC-I-binding predictions (specify species and select MHC alleles of interest). As in the MHC class I prediction method, the available predictions options are limited to alleles in which each of the prediction method has been trained and has available data.

Steps 4 and **5** same as **steps 4** and **5** in Subheading 3.1.1. MHC-I-binding predictions.

6. Interpreting predicted results: The predicted output can be given in units of IC_{50}nM for CombLib and SMM_align that are interpreted as mentioned in Subheading 3.1.1, **step 6**. The prediction result for Sturniolo is given as raw score in which higher score indicates higher affinity.

3.2 Processing Prediction

These tools predict epitope candidates based upon the processing of peptides in the cell.

3.2.1 MHC-I Processing Predictions

With this prediction method predictors of proteasomal processing, TAP transport, and MHC binding are combined to calculate an overall score for each antigen that is processing through the MHC class I antigen presentation pathway to become a potential MHC class I ligand.

1. Specify sequences: Same as **step 1** in Subheading 3.1.1MHC-I-binding predictions.
2. Choose a prediction method: Same as **step 2** in Subheading 3.1.1 MHC-I-binding predictions [according to current (May 2016) performances and comparisons the best prediction method seems to be the NetMHCpan because it supplies IC_{50} values and is available for all MHC alleles).
3. Specify predictions details: Same as **step 3** in Subheading 3.1.1 MHC-I-binding predictions (*see* **Note 8**).
4. Choose a proteasomal cleavage prediction type: There are two types of proteasomes: the constitutively expressed and the inducible immune-proteasomes regulated by IFN-γ secretion. Inducible proteasomes seem to enhance antigen presentation

and should be the preferable option to make a prediction when no more information is available.

5. Specify TAP prediction parameters: High affinity peptides exhibit high transport rates. The TAP score estimates an effective $-\log(IC_{50})$ values for the binding to TAP of a peptide or its N-terminal prolonged precursors.
6. Specify the output: Results can be sorted by proteasome, TAP, MHC, or processing score.
7. Submit the prediction: Click the submit button and wait for the result screen to appear.

3.2.2 Neural Network-Based Prediction of Proteasomal Cleavage Sites and T-Cell Epitopes

There are three methods to approach proteasomal processing and cleavage that are all based on neural network.

(a) NetChop predicts cleavage sites of the human proteasome.

(b) NetCTL predicts cytotoxic T-cell (CTL) epitopes in protein sequences.

(c) NetCTLpan (NetCTL update) allows for prediction of CTL epitope restricted to any MHC molecules of known protein sequence.

1. Choose a prediction method: Select either NetCHOP, NetCTL, or NetCTLpan method.
2. Specify sequences: Same as **step 1** in Subheading 3.1.1.
3. Method specific option: Depending on the selected method, enter the appropriate parameters or use the default options.
4. Submit the prediction: Click the submit button and wait for the result screen to appear.
5. Interpreting predicted results: A chart and a table outcome provides the prediction scores. NetCTL and NetCTLpan algorithms produce proteasome, TAP, MHC, or processing scores along with a global score for each peptide sequence.

3.2.3 Prediction of Peptides Naturally Processed by the MHC

This approach utilizes data obtained from MHC elution experiments with which the probability that a given peptide is naturally processed and binds to a given MHC molecule is assessed. The algorithm is named MHC-NP and is still unpublished, although it is one of the T-cell epitopes prediction option in IEDB. This method combines two predictors: one that has been trained to distinguish binding peptides from nonbinding peptides for a given allele, and one that has been trained to distinguish eluted peptides from other binding peptides. The generated score is based on the estimated probability that a processed peptide is eluted and a good binder. The greater the score, the more likely the peptide is naturally processed by the MHC allele.

Step 1 same as **step 1** in Subheading 3.1.1. MHC-I-binding predictions.

Step 2 same as **step 3** in Subheading 3.1.1 MHC-I-binding predictions (specify species and select MHC alleles of interest).

3. Specify the output: For each peptide, a score is predicted. This score is between 0 and 1 and the greater the value, the more likely a peptide is naturally processed by a specific allele.
4. Submit the prediction: click the submit button and wait for the result screen to appear.

3.3 Immunogenicity Prediction

This tool predicts the relative ability of a peptide/MHC class I complex to elicit an immune response and is based on the fact that some peptides are more immunogenic than others and therefore more likely to be T-cell epitopes [21]. This method has been validated for 9-mer peptides, but can produce prediction for any length.

Step 1 same as **step 1** in Subheading 3.1.1*MHC-I-binding predictions.*

2. Choose a masking option: The masked positions are dependent on the MHC class I molecule on which the peptide is presented. The first, second, and the C-terminal amino acid are masked by default, but additional amino acids may be masked depending on the expected anchor positions each MHC molecule exhibits.
3. Submit the prediction: Click the submit button and wait for the result screen to appear.

4 Notes

1. Although the IEDB Analysis Resource is a good option for performing T-cell epitope predictions, most of the previously described methods that are incorporated into IEDB website have their own websites for independent analysis.
2. The existing databases are updated almost weekly. Therefore, results from analyses performed different time points may differ. The same applies for the version of the same computational technique utilized.
3. The results among the different available online software may differ not only because of the mathematical approach but also because of the different datasets that have been used for the development and training of these algorithms.
4. The recommended method as the best performing at a certain time is usually based on comparative studies performed up to this time point. Since new techniques are developed and published, and new comparative studies are performed, the method of choice may change accordingly.

5. The software used for T-cell epitope prediction is available online as a freeware and in some cases they are available as standalone downloads.
6. For the allergen T-cell epitope prediction, the MHC Class II processing pathway is the one of interest. However, the autoallergy theory [22, 23] obliges the description of methods for MCH Class I processing, too.
7. Predictions can be made for molecules with unknown epitopes, provided that the datasets used to develop and train the computational technique do not include known data for this molecule of interest.
8. Select MHC alleles of interest and specify species although it must be highlighted that both the proteasome and TAP predictions have been developed from human experimental data that seem to be species-specific. Therefore, interpreting predictions for epitope processing in other species should be done with extra caution.

References

1. Barlow DJ, Edwards MS, Thornton JM (1986) Continuous and discontinuous protein antigenic determinants. Nature 322(6081):747–748. doi:10.1038/322747a0
2. Abbas AK, Lichtman AH, Pillai S (2015) Cellular and molecular immunology, 8th edn. Saunders/Elsevier, Philadelphia, PA
3. Reche PA, Reinherz EL (2007) Definition of MHC supertypes through clustering of MHC peptide-binding repertoires. Methods Mol Biol 409:163–173. doi:10.1007/978-1-60327-118-9_11
4. Pascal M, Konstantinou GN, Masilamani M, Lieberman J, Sampson HA (2013) In silico prediction of Ara h 2 T cell epitopes in peanut-allergic children. Clin Exp Allergy 43(1):116–127. doi:10.1111/cea.12014
5. Ramesh M, Yuenyongviwat A, Konstantinou GN, Lieberman J, Pascal M, Masilamani M, Sampson HA (2016) Peanut T-cell epitope discovery: Ara h 1. J Allergy Clin Immunol. doi:10.1016/j.jaci.2015.12.1327
6. Nielsen M, Lundegaard C, Worning P, Lauemoller SL, Lamberth K, Buus S, Brunak S, Lund O (2003) Reliable prediction of T-cell epitopes using neural networks with novel sequence representations. Protein Sci 12(5):1007–1017. doi:10.1110/ps.0239403
7. Peters B, Sette A (2005) Generating quantitative models describing the sequence specificity of biological processes with the stabilized matrix method. BMC Bioinformatics 6:132. doi:10.1186/1471-2105-6-132
8. Kim Y, Sidney J, Pinilla C, Sette A, Peters B (2009) Derivation of an amino acid similarity matrix for peptide: MHC binding and its application as a Bayesian prior. BMC Bioinformatics 10:394. doi:10.1186/1471-2105-10-394
9. Sidney J, Assarsson E, Moore C, Ngo S, Pinilla C, Sette A, Peters B (2008) Quantitative peptide binding motifs for 19 human and mouse MHC class I molecules derived using positional scanning combinatorial peptide libraries. Immunol Res 4:2. doi:10.1186/1745-7580-4-2
10. Moutaftsi M, Peters B, Pasquetto V, Tscharke DC, Sidney J, Bui HH, Grey H, Sette A (2006) A consensus epitope prediction approach identifies the breadth of murine T(CD8+)-cell responses to vaccinia virus. Nat Biotechnol 24(7):817–819. doi:10.1038/nbt1215
11. Hoof I, Peters B, Sidney J, Pedersen LE, Sette A, Lund O, Buus S, Nielsen M (2009) NetMHCpan, a method for MHC class I binding prediction beyond humans. Immunogenetics 61(1):1–13. doi:10.1007/s00251-008-0341-z
12. Karosiene E, Lundegaard C, Lund O, Nielsen M (2012) NetMHCcons: a consensus method for the major histocompatibility complex class I predictions. Immunogenetics 64(3):177–186. doi:10.1007/s00251-011-0579-8
13. Zhang H, Lund O, Nielsen M (2009) The PickPocket method for predicting binding specificities for receptors based on receptor pocket similarities: application to MHC-peptide binding. Bioinformatics 25(10):1293–1299. doi:10.1093/bioinformatics/btp137
14. Wang P, Sidney J, Dow C, Mothe B, Sette A, Peters B (2008) A systematic assessment of MHC class II peptide binding predictions and evaluation of a consensus approach. PLoS Comput Biol 4(4):e1000048. doi:10.1371/journal.pcbi.1000048

15. Nielsen M, Lund O (2009) NN-align An artificial neural network-based alignment algorithm for MHC class II peptide binding prediction. BMC bioinformatics 10:296. doi:10.1186/1471-2105-10-296
16. Nielsen M, Lundegaard C, Lund O (2007) Prediction of MHC class II binding affinity using SMM-align, a novel stabilization matrix alignment method. BMC Bioinformatics 8:238. doi:10.1186/1471-2105-8-238
17. Sturniolo T, Bono E, Ding J, Raddrizzani L, Tuereci O, Sahin U, Braxenthaler M, Gallazzi F, Protti MP, Sinigaglia F, Hammer J (1999) Generation of tissue-specific and promiscuous HLA ligand databases using DNA microarrays and virtual HLA class II matrices. Nat Biotechnol 17(6):555–561. doi:10.1038/9858
18. Nielsen M, Lundegaard C, Blicher T, Peters B, Sette A, Justesen S, Buus S, Lund O (2008) Quantitative predictions of peptide binding to any HLA-DR molecule of known sequence: NetMHCIIpan. PLoS Comput Biol 4(7): e1000107. doi:10.1371/journal.pcbi.1000107
19. Wang P, Sidney J, Kim Y, Sette A, Lund O, Nielsen M, Peters B (2010) Peptide binding predictions for HLA DR, DP and DQ molecules. BMC Bioinformatics 11:568. doi:10.1186/1471-2105-11-568
20. Zhang L, Udaka K, Mamitsuka H, Zhu S (2012) Toward more accurate pan-specific MHC-peptide binding prediction: a review of current methods and tools. Brief Bioinform 13(3):350–364. doi:10.1093/bib/bbr060
21. Calis JJ, Maybeno M, Greenbaum JA, Weiskopf D, De Silva AD, Sette A, Kesmir C, Peters B (2013) Properties of MHC class I presented peptides that enhance immunogenicity. PLoS Comput Biol 9(10):e1003266. doi:10.1371/journal.pcbi.1003266
22. Altrichter S, Peter HJ, Pisarevskaja D, Metz M, Martus P, Maurer M (2011) IgE mediated autoallergy against thyroid peroxidase--a novel pathomechanism of chronic spontaneous urticaria? PLoS One 6(4):e14794. doi:10.1371/journal.pone.0014794
23. Valenta R, Seiberler S, Natter S, Mahler V, Mossabeb R, Ring J, Stingl G (2000) Autoallergy: a pathogenetic factor in atopic dermatitis? J Allergy Clin Immunol 105(3):432–437. doi:10.1067/mai.2000.104783

Chapter 18

An Overview of Bioinformatics Tools and Resources in Allergy

Zhiyan Fu* and Jing Lin*

Abstract

The rapidly increasing number of characterized allergens has created huge demands for advanced information storage, retrieval, and analysis. Bioinformatics and machine learning approaches provide useful tools for the study of allergens and epitopes prediction, which greatly complement traditional laboratory techniques. The specific applications mainly include identification of B- and T-cell epitopes, and assessment of allergenicity and cross-reactivity. In order to facilitate the work of clinical and basic researchers who are not familiar with bioinformatics, we review in this chapter the most important databases, bioinformatic tools, and methods with relevance to the study of allergens.

Key words Food allergens, Allergy, Bioinformatics, Machine learning, Epitope prediction

1 Introduction

Allergy has become an emerging public health problem. It is an immunologically mediated adverse reaction, and the triggering agents are known as allergens that are otherwise not harmful. Allergic diseases are mainly mediated by immunoglobulin E (IgE) antibodies through the following mechanisms (Fig. 1): Exogeneous allergens are processed by endosomal proteases in antigen presenting cells (APCs) to peptides/epitopes, which are presented to T cells by major histocompatibility complex (MHC) class II molecules on cell surface. CD4+ T helper cells are activated upon recognition of these peptide-MHC complexes by T-cell receptor (TCR) molecules and start the production and secretion of cytokines (i.e., interleukin-4 (IL-4) and IL-13), which induce class switching and IgE production in stimulated B cells. Allergen-specific IgE (sIgE) antibodies play a central role in allergic reactions. Cross-linking of membrane-bound IgE antibodies by the specific allergens results in activation

*These authors contributed equally to this article.

Jing Lin and Marcos Alcocer (eds.), *Food Allergens: Methods and Protocols*, Methods in Molecular Biology, vol. 1592, DOI 10.1007/978-1-4939-6925-8_18, © Springer Science+Business Media LLC 2017

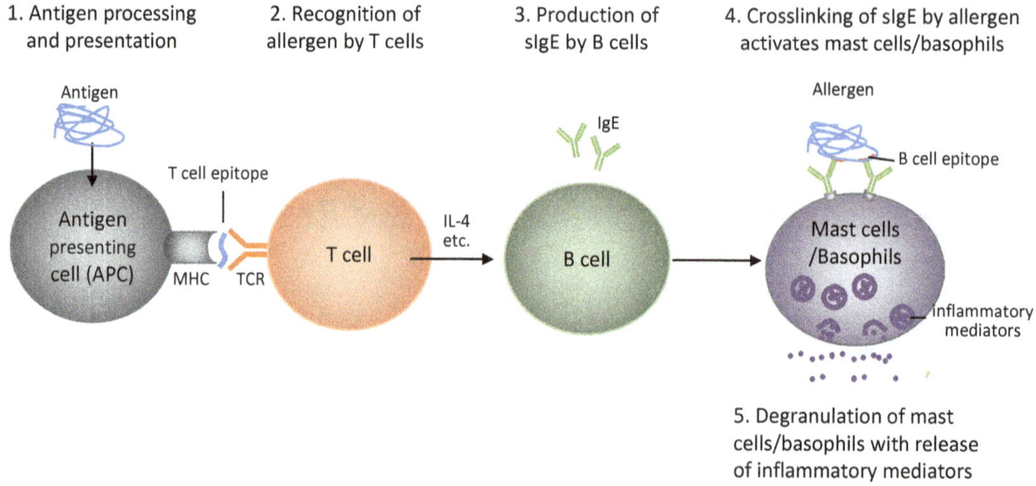

Fig. 1 A schematic diagram representing the IgE-mediated allergic reaction

and degranulation of effector cells (mast cells or basophils) with release of histamine and other inflammatory mediators, which together lead to the symptoms of allergic diseases [1]. In addition to IgE-mediated allergic diseases, other types of allergy also exist. For example, delayed allergic reactions to certain small therapeutic drugs (e.g., abacavir, nevirapine) are mediated by T cells and have been shown to be associated with specific MHC class I and/or II alleles [2].

Epitopes are the groups of amino acids within allergens that bind to antigen-specific receptors on lymphocytes or to secreted antibodies. There are two types of epitopes, continuous (or linear) and discontinuous (or conformational) in allergens. Continuous epitopes are short linear peptide fragments that are usually sequences of contiguous amino acids, while conformational epitopes are comprised of amino acids that line up because of the tertiary structure of an allergen. Studies of epitopes are important to both clinical and basic researchers in allergy or immunology in general as they hold huge potential for vaccine design, disease prevention, diagnosis, and treatment. For example, the current trends in allergy immunotherapy are to modify B-cell epitopes to prevent IgE binding, while preserving T-cell epitopes to retain the capacity for immunotherapy, or peptide-based immunotherapy containing major T-cell epitopes of the relevant allergen as an alternative strategy [3].

Epitopes can be categorized into B- and T-cell epitopes based on their respective receptors. B-cell epitopes are also known as IgE epitopes and can be either linear or conformational. The majority of T-cell epitopes are linear because antigens must be processed into peptide fragments or epitopes by proteasomes prior to MHC binding and presentation to Th cells.

Traditionally, studies of food allergens and allergenic epitopes depend exclusively on biochemical and immunological experiments, such as ELISA, protein/peptide microarray [4, 5], immunofluro-rescence, radioimmunoassay, Western blotting, immunohisto-chemistry, molecular cloning, NMR, and X-ray crystallography studies of antibody/antigen structure, most of which are expensive and time-consuming. In the post-genome era where massive amount of data of protein sequences and structures are available online, bioinformatics, which combine biomedical and computer science together, have progressed and developed vast varieties of methods and tools. These bioinformatics tools are now widely used for sequence analyses [6–8], protein structure modeling, and function annotation, reducing the time and effort spending on wet lab experiments [9].

In the last few years, machine learning technique, one of the computer science branches, advanced quickly and was widely applied in bioinformatics area [10]. For example, in addition to the traditional heuristic algorithms such as BLAST and FASTA used to detect sequence homology in large databases, better accuracy has been achieved using machine learning algorithms, such as support vector machine (SVM). An extensive number of customized kernels (functions that quantify the similarity between sequences) have been proposed and are more effective than general-purpose kernels (e.g., polynomial and radial basis function kernels) [11]. Classifiers developed to explicitly optimize the area under ROC curve (AUC) have been shown to be more useful than to optimize the classification error when the AUC is the performance metric of interest [12], and ensemble learning methods (e.g., boosting and bagging) have been shown effective in improving the performance of a single learning algorithm [13].

Now, with the aid of bioinformatics and machine learning, we are able to narrow protein of our interest, predict epitope using computation, increase allergy diagnostic accuracy, and drastically reduce the number of wet lab experiments. For example, we have applied bioinformatics tools in combination with peptide microarray experiment to identify epitope biomarkers that are capable of predicting clinical allergy with over 90% accuracy [14].

Currently, many bioinformatics resources with user-friendly web interface have been developed, which can facilitate the work of clinical and basic researchers who are not familiar with bioinformatics. However, the average researchers, who have no much background in computer science, can be easily overwhelmed by such a broad array of bioinformatics tools that are highly specific in use, not well understood or defined, and tested on limited data sets [15]. Our goal in writing this review is to introduce the essential updated bioinformatics resources in allergy field to clinicians and allergists and help them make informed selection among these tools.

2 Bioinformatic Prediction Methods

Current bioinformatics research in allergy field are primarily focused on assessment of protein allergenic potential, and prediction of B- and T-cell epitopes. Predicting the allergenic potential of a protein, particularly in novel foods, focuses on two main aspects: inherent protein allergenicity and cross-reactivity [16]. Inherent allergenicity refers to the potential of a protein to induce T-cell response and production of specific IgE antibodies, whereas cross-reactivity refers to the reactivity of a protein with pre-existing IgE antibodies that were previously induced by another allergen. The molecular basis of allergenicity of a protein can be studied through the analysis of its sequence, structure, and B- or T-cell epitopes. Online allergen databases are being used as reference for finding the sequence similarity for the purpose of allergenicity evaluation [17]. As allergen-specific IgE antibodies are the main effector molecules inducing allergic symptoms, prediction of allergen is closely related and often involves IgE epitope prediction. For example, in some of the allergen prediction methods, a protein is considered an allergen if it has a region or peptides identical to a known IgE epitope [18].

Allergen/epitope prediction dates back to 1981 when the first B-cell epitope prediction method was developed by Hopp and Woods [19]. Since then many methods have been developed or adapted from other computational tools. Despite the early start, however, prediction for B-cell epitopes is still in their infancy due to the difficulty in predicting discontinuous epitopes. For T-cell epitope prediction, MHC-I-binding predictions are now very strong by integration with predictions of proteasomal cleavage and TAP (transporter associated with antigen processing) binding sites. MHC-II-binding predictions are not as well developed as MHC I binding predictions, but are progressing at a fast pace. Based on the type of information being used, prediction methods can be categorized into sequence-based methods, structure-based methods, and hybrid methods.

2.1 Sequence-Based Prediction

Sequence-based method is based on the concept that protein sequence determines its structure and identical structures may lead to identical functions. Epitopes may have a common sequence pattern or motif, as well as MHC allele specificity determining patterns. BLAST and FASTA are common sequence–sequence comparison methods used to find sequence homologues and assign amino acid scores by multiple alignment of query protein sequence with template sequences in databases. However, experiments have shown that proteins with high sequence identity may possess differential functions due to folding, interactions among variable regions in different cellular compartmentization [20]. The methods using only sequence information are limited to the prediction of continuous epitopes.

Physico-chemical properties are also used to predict epitopes, such as charge, hydrophilicity, flexibility, number of proline residues, the distance/proximity to the N or C terminus, etc. Due to the enormous number of physico-chemical properties that may be associated with epitopes, simple quantitative descriptors of amino acid properties can be used for computation. The classical amino acid scale-based methods of identifying potential linear epitopes from sequences typically rely on the use of amino acid propensity scale that is to compute the scores of a residue i in a given protein sequence. The $i - (n - 1)/2$ neighboring residues on each side of the residue I are used to compute the score for residue i in a window size of n amino acids. The final score for residue i is the average of the scale values for n amino acids in the window. Pellequer [21] has compared several propensity scale methods using a dataset of 14 epitope-annotated proteins and found that the classical scores developed by Parker et al. [22], Chou and Fasman [23], Levitt [24], and Emini [25] provide better results than the other scores tested [26].

2.2 Structure-Based Prediction

Structure-based epitope prediction was first used by Kolaskaret al. in 1999 [27]. It is based on the 3D protein structural similarity between query protein and template proteins, and it also considers the related propensity scales, including geometric attributes and structure-based physico-chemical properties. With the development of various omics and bioinformatics, experimental data of conformational B-cell epitopes has been increasing rapidly in recent years. Current structure-based epitope identifying techniques mainly include mutagenesis, competition experiments, free energy scoring function, quantitative structure–activity relationship (QSAR) analysis [28], protein threading [29], rigid/flexible docking [30], and homology modeling [31]. Atomistic molecular dynamics simulations have also been applied but not broadly used as it is computational intensive.

The structure-based epitope prediction approaches generally give more accurate prediction due to their several advantages over the sequence-based one. For example, discontinuous epitopes can only be predicted based on structure. In addition, as protein functions can be predicted by its structure, the structure-based prediction can be used to predict epitopes for alleles/genes that have not been extensively studied, where sequence-based approaches have failed. However, the structure-based approach has been greatly restricted due to high computational cost, development complexity, and limited availability of protein 3D structures.

2.3 Hybrid Prediction: Combining Sequential with Structural Information

Due to the limitations of epitope predictors based only on either sequence or structure analysis, predictive methods taking advantage of both sequential and structural information have been developed. For example, a method that integrates 3D protein structure with properties of amino acids using Hidden Markov Model (HMM) improved the prediction precision to a significant degree [26].

In addition to the above three categories, prediction methods can also be categorized based on the techniques or algorithms, such as binding motifs [32], quantitative matrices (QM) [33], machine learning algorithms [34], linear programming [35], etc. They all have their relative advantages and disadvantages [36]. For example, in a comparative study, Yu et al. found that methods based on binding motifs gave the most accurate MHC-binding peptides predictions (potential T-cell epitopes) with a limited data-set, but as the data volume increased, machine learning predictions considering both structure and sequence information became more reliable [37]. Among machine learning methods, Bahsin and Ragahava have compared SVM (support vector machine) and ANN (artificial neural network) techniques, and found that SVM techniques performed better [38]. SVM is particularly attractive to biological analysis, due to its ability to filter noise, large input spaces, and good performance [10].

Ensemble methods (also known as consensus methods) combine the predictions of several predictors and often outperform individual predictors in many biomolecular sequence and structure classification studies. Several strategies for combining a set of predictors, *S*, into a single consensus or meta-predictor exist: (1) majority voting, (2) weighted linear combination, and (3) meta-learning [39]. A large number of nearest neighbor- and decision tree-based classifiers are trained using different sets of training data features for developing an ensemble of linear B-cell epitope classifiers [40].

2.4 Performance Evaluation of Prediction Methods

To evaluate and compare the performance of various prediction methods and software, ROC analysis is commonly used. An ROC analysis includes positive and negative predicative values (PPV, NPV), area under the curve (AUC), specificity, sensitivity, and accuracy. A ROC curve is obtained by plotting true positives on the *y*-axis against false positives on the *x*-axis. AUC that is the area under the rectangular hyperbola ROC curve represents the accuracy of prediction. AUC equals 0.5 (ROC plotted as a straight diagonal line) means the test is no better than random chance alone, while AUC equals 1.0 means the test has perfect accuracy. In order to make evaluation more accurate, cross-validation method is usually used [14]. Cross validation is a technique to evaluate predictive models by partitioning the original sample into a training set to train the model, and a test set to evaluate it. Usually, multiple rounds of cross-validation are performed using different partitions and the evaluation (i.e., AUC) obtained from cross validation is the average over rounds.

3 Allergen Prediction Tools and Resources

According to the guideline proposed by World Health Organization (WHO) and Food and Agriculture Organization (FAO) for evaluating protein allergenicity (FAO/WHO 2001) [41], a protein that has at least six to eight consecutive identical amino acids or >35% identity within any window of 80 amino acids when compared with any known allergens is considered an allergen. This guideline has been widely accepted for allergen prediction and implemented into some web tools, such as SDAP [42]. However, prediction methods based on the guideline are sequence-based and tend to produce results with high sensitivity but very low specificity. It has been reported that only 1 of 200 "positive matches" represents a true allergen when using the FAO/WHO guidelines [43].

Several allergenicity prediction methods have been developed which showed improvement over the FAO/WHO guideline. For example, Stadler developed a motif-based method to achieve higher specificity by generating a minimal set of motif sequences from a database of known allergens. A protein was classified as a potential allergen if it contained at least one of the motifs [43]. Bjorklund et al. compared the sequence of >570 allergens and 700 non-allergens and identified a dataset of allergen-representative peptides (ARP). Their data showed that the ARP-based allergen prediction method outperformed the methods based on the FAO/WHO guideline [44]. Epitope-based methods have also been reported which are based on similarity search against IgE epitope database [18]. ARP and epitope-based methods are restricted by the number of known epitopes and allergenic domains. More recently, Wang et al. [45] have tried to integrate the FAO/WHO guideline-based method with motif-based and SVM-based methods and achieve >90% accuracy in allergen prediction.

Online allergen sequence databases are essential for evaluating the allergenic potential of protein as they not only serve as reference for finding the sequence/structure similarity with known allergens, but also provide useful web tools for structural and physio-chemical property analysis. Here, we will briefly introduce a few important and currently online available allergen prediction databases and tools. These resources are summarized in Table 1.

The allergen nomenclature database (www.allergen.org) is the official site for the systematic allergen nomenclature that is approved by the World Health Organization and International Union of Immunological Societies (WHO/IUIS) Allergen Nomenclature Sub-committee and has been constantly updated [46].

The Allergome website (www.allergome.org) [47] has been designed to supply information on allergens. The primary data source

Table 1
Resources for allergen prediction

Names	URLs
Database of IUIS	http://www.allergen.org
Database of Allergome	http://www.allergome.org
SDAP	http://www.fermi.utmb.edu/SDAP/
AlgPred	http://www.imtech.res.in/raghava/algpred
proAP	http://gmobl.sjtu.edu.cn/proAP/main.html

for Allergome is the literature published since the early 1960s. It has a total of 2484 allergen sources and 33,097 uploaded bibliographic references (updated in March 2016). It contains allergens that are not in the IUIS list but these allergens are added after careful characterization under stringent criteria. The Allergome platform has developed several modules aiming to support specific purposes. For example, "Real Time Monitoring of IgE sensitization" (ReTiME) module allows uploading of raw data from both in vivo and in vitro experiments.

SDAP (Structural database of Allergenic Proteins) (http://fermi.utmb.edu/SDAP/) [42] is a web server that integrates a database of allergenic proteins with various computational tools that can assist structural biology studies related to allergens. In its latest update, it has 1526 allergens and isoallergens. SDAP provides links to retrieve related information from the most common databases of protein sequences and structures (e.g., SwissProt, PIR, NCBI, PDB), and tools to assess allergenic potential of proteins using the FAO/WHO guideline.

Two web tools, AlgPred [18] and proAP [45], allow allergen prediction using several different approaches, such as motif-based using MEME/MAST [43], ARP-based, or SVM-based methods, or a hybrid option to predict allergen using combined approach (SVMc + IgE epitope + ARPs BLAST + MAST).

One problem facing the development of allergenicity prediction methods is the lack of a standard dataset for training and testing, including a good negative dataset of non-allergens. Allergen-related data are currently scattered across various publicly accessible databases. The lack of a standard dataset has made comparison between the various methods difficult and is hindering progress.

4 Epitope Prediction Tools and Resources

4.1 B-Cell Epitopes

B-cell epitopes are either continuous/linear or discontinuous/conformational [26]. So far various kinds of B-cell epitope sequences and structures have been identified. However, experiments designed to identify B-cell epitopes are mostly based on linear epitopes [4, 5]. Because many of the B-cell epitopes are discontinuous, prediction of which requires 3D protein structure and notoriously difficult to predict, their predictive software and databases are generally with lower accuracy and based on a smaller scale of dataset. Currently, the top performing B-cell epitope prediction methods have average AUC values ranging between 0.6 and 0.7, depending on the evaluation dataset used [48–50]. Here, we will briefly introduce the most common software/tools and databases on B-cell epitopes (summarized in Table 2), all of which are currently available online.

4.1.1 Conformational B-Cell Epitope Prediction Software

As proteins can be recognized by B cells in their native forms, the input for conformational/discontinuous B-cell epitope prediction software is usually 3D protein structures and the output can be viewed graphically as 3D structures. Anderson et al. presented a method called DiscoTope [51], which used a combination of amino acid statistics, spatial information, and surface exposure, and could detect 15.5% of residues located in discontinuous epitopes with a specificity of 95%.

BEPro, formerly known as PEPITO, was initially developed as an alternative method to Discotope. Similar to Discotope, BEPro combines propensity scales with surface exposure information. BEPro utilizes the Discotope amino acid propensity scale in its algorithm, along with side-chain orientation and solvent accessibility data [48].

One of the most complete tools in this field is ElliPro [31], which is available on the IEDB analysis resource website. This tool predicts both linear and discontinuous epitopes based on protein's 3-D structure. ElliPro associates each predicted epitope with a structural related score, defined as a PI (Protrusion Index) value. In ElliPro, the input is protein sequence. Based on the structural template selected by the user, a 3-D structure will be predicted for the input protein sequence by homology modeling, and linear and discontinuous epitopes will be computed based on the predicted structure.

Three web servers SEPPA [52], Epitopia [49], and EPCES [53] were published in 2009. SEPPA employs two concepts, "unit patch of residue triangle" and "clustering coefficient" to describe the local spatial context and spatial compactness, and combines them to predict epitopes. Epitopia uses several structural and physiochemical features to represent the surface patch and applies machine-learning algorithm (Naive Bayes classifier) for epitope prediction. EPCES introduced a consensus scoring method for epitope prediction based on several structural and physicochemical features. In 2011, two server applications EPSVR and EPMeta were presented by the same author of EPCES [54]. EPSVR adopted the SVM regression method to integrate the scoring terms as EPCES, while EPMeta is a meta-server that combines EPSVR, EPCES, Epitopia, SEPPA, PEPITO, and Discotope1.2.

Table 2
List of B-cell epitope prediction servers

Method	Online service (program)	Predict discontinuous/ continuous epitopes	Brief notes (features used in prediction
DiscoTope	http://www.cbs.dtu.dk/services/DiscoTope/	Discontinuous	Amino acid statistics, spatial context, and surface accessibility
ElliPro	http://tools.iedb.org/ellipro/	Both	Prominent index
PEPITO/ BEPro	http://pepito.proteomics.ics.uci.edu/	Discontinuous	Half sphere exposure values
SEPPA	http://lifecenter.sgst.cn/seppa/index.php	Discontinuous	Unit patch of residue triangle
Epitopia	http://epitopia.tau.ac.il/	Both	Based on Naive Bayes classifier with physicochemical and structural geometrical properties
EPCES	http://sysbio.unl.edu/services/EPCES/	Discontinuous	Consensus score by six functions Shinji Soga Not stated Antibody-specific epitope propensity index
EPSVR &EPMeta	http://sysbio.unl.edu/services/	Discontinuous	Based on SVR and meta-analysis
MEPS	http://www.caspur.it/meps	Discontinuous	Surface mimicking peptides
MIMOX	http://immunet.cn/mimox	Discontinuous	The first free Mimotop-based web tool
Pepitope	http://pepitope.tau.ac.il	Both	The first method based on amino acid pairs
EpiSearch	http://curie.utmb.edu/episearch.html	Discontinuous	An automated sequence analysis based on sequence and 3D profiles
Pep-3D-Search	http://kyc.nenu.edu.cn/Pep3DSearch	Discontinuous	Ant colony optimization algorithm
MimoPro	http://informatics.nenu.edu.cn/MimoPro	Discontinuous	Based on both patch and graph searching
Bcepred	http://www.imtech.res.in/raghava/bcepred/	Continuous	Linear B-cell epitopes prediction by physico-chemical properties
BepiPred	http://www.cbs.dtu.dk/services/BepiPred/	Continuous	Linear B-cell epitope prediction
ABCPred	http://www.imtech.res.in/raghava/abcpred/	Continuous	Artificial neural network linear B-cell epitope predictor

The above B-cell epitopes prediction methods are based on the structure features of antigen. Most of them are available as web servers or can be downloaded as a standalone version (Table 2) with user-friendly interfaces. Researchers just need to enter the PDB ID (*see* Subheading 4.1.4) or upload the local file in PDB format, enter the Chain id for the protein chain of interest, and/or specify a threshold (may be changeable on the output view). Yao et al. [55] evaluated the performance of prediction methods available at that time and showed that overall the accuracy of EPMeta is the highest value by all conditions and methods.

4.1.2 Mimotope-Based Prediction Methods

One unique type of method to predict conformational B-cell epitope is Mimotope-based prediction, which is a combinatorial method that requires both a list of affinity-selected peptides and the protein 3D structure as input. To obtain the affinity-selected peptides, random peptides are generated and displayed on the surface of bacteriophages, and screened with immobilized antibodies (e.g., IgE from patients). The unbound phages are removed and the bound ones are then eluted, amplified, and used for further rounds of selection. After several rounds, phage clones displaying peptides with higher affinity binding to antibodies are highly enriched. These affinity-selected peptides are defined as mimotopes that have the similar functionality to and a high sequential similarity with the native epitope [56]. Mapping these mimotopes back to the source antigen can help in finding the native epitopes. Mimotope-based prediction methods are essential to map mimotopes back to the surface of a source antigen to locate the best alignment sequences and predict possible epitope regions. Currently available mimotope-based web servers (programs), algo rithms, and brief notes are listed in Table 2.

These include MIMOP [56], which predicts linear and conformational epitopes based on MimAlign and MimCons methods, MIMOX [57], Pepitope [58] which uses Pepsurf [59] and Mapitope [60] methods, Pep-3D-Search [61], and MimoPro [62] . These methods can be classified into two categories: sequence-sequence alignment category and sequence-structure alignment category [63]. MimAlign method of MIMOP belongs to the sequence-sequence alignment category that aligns mimotope sequences with the antigen sequence. The other methods belong to the sequence-structure alignment category that aligns mimotope sequences and the antigen 3D structure. In the sequence-structure alignment category, there are motif-based methods (i.e., MIMOX, MimCons method of MIMOP), pairs-based methods (i.e., Mapitope), patch-based methods (i.e., EpiSearch) [64], and graph-based methods (i.e., Pep-3D-Search and Pepsurf). To improve the performances of existing programs, hybrid methods such as MimoPro [62] and meta-servers such as Pepitope [58] were also developed.

4.1.3 Continuous B-Cell Epitope Prediction Software

Continuous B-cell epitopes are easier to predict than discontinuous ones, and share many common characteristics with T-cell epitopes that are mostly continuous. The input format for continuous B-cell epitope prediction software can be either sequence or structure. Methods for predicting continuous B-cell epitopes are generally sequence-based methods, amino acid propensity scale-based methods, or machine-learning methods. Common predictive software on continuous B-cell epitope includes ABCpred, BcePred, BepiPred, and the prediction tool provided on IEDB.

ABCpred is based on standard feed-forward (FNN) and recurrent neural network (RNN) for predicting B-cell epitopes in an antigenic sequence with an estimated accuracy of 65.9% [65].

BcePred server predicts linear B-cell epitopes with 53–58% accuracy [66] based on the physico-chemical properties (i.e., hydrophilicity, flexibility/mobility, accessibility, polarity, exposed surface, and turns) or combination of properties. It was developed based on a dataset of 1029 B-cell epitopes obtained from Bcipep database and an equal number of non-epitopes obtained randomly from Swiss-Prot database.

Bepipred [67] predicts linear B-cell epitopes using a combination of machine learning technique-hidden Markov model (HMM), and one of the two propensity scale methods, Parker [22] and Levitt [24]. When tested on the validation data set constructed from three datasets of linear B-cell epitopes: annotated proteins from literature, AntiJendatabase [68], and Los Alamos HIV database (http://www.hiv.lanl.gov), it achieves ~60–66% of accuracy for continuous epitope prediction.

4.1.4 B-Cell Epitope Databases

Experimental data plays an essential role in B-cell epitope prediction. The 3D structure of allergens or antigen-antibody complexes can be found in the Protein Data Bank (PDB) database [69], which is a database for the 3D structural data of proteins and nucleic acids. Its data are typically obtained by X-ray crystallography, NMR spectroscopy, or cryo-electron microscopy. One can search structure according to the PDB-id at the home page and then view or download the structure in several formats.

Bcipep [70] provides comprehensive information about experimentally verified B-cell epitopes and tools for mapping these epitopes on an antigen sequence.

IEDB database (immune epitope databases and analysis resources) [71] is the most commonly used and most authoritative database containing a large number of epitopes (237,460 peptidic epitopes as in May 2016), and displays relatively complete information about each epitope as well as cross linked to other databases. IEDB covers a wide range of epitopes, including both B- and T-cell epitopes, and for a spectrum of host organisms, including human. It can be browsed and searched by different categories, such as epitope type (linear, discontinuous, etc.), source (organism or antigen name), or diseases (allergic, infectious, autoimmune, etc.). It predicts continuous B-cell epitopes with the option of various methods, including six amino acid property-based methods, Bepipred Linear Epitope Prediction, etc. For prediction of discontinuous B-cell epitopes, it also provides methods based on antigen structure, such as ElliPro and DiscoTope, which have been mentioned in earlier sections.

Conformational epitope database (CED) [72] provides a collection of conformational epitopes and related information (e.g., location, immunological property, corresponding antibody) of the epitope. All epitopes in the database have been manually curated from the published literature. Most epitopes in CED can also be viewed interactively in the context of their 3D structures. In addition, the entries are also hyperlinked to other databases such as Swiss-Prot, PDB, KEGG, and PubMed, providing wide background information.

For mimotope-based methods, it needs both the antigen structure and the sequence data of mimotopes. Since the 3D structure can be obtained from PDB or by computational homology modeling, the small number of mimotope sequences derived from phage display becomes a limitation for the development of mimotope-based conformational B-cell epitope prediction. In recent years, several databases have been released, which integrated the structure data, the mimotopes data, and other associated information. One such example is ASPD, a curated database that incorporated data on peptides and proteins mainly from phage display experiments [73]. The current version released in 2001 has 195 entries. ASPD has a user-friendly interface, and researchers can search the needed information by means of simple search system or SRS (Sequence Retrieval System).

PepBank is a database of peptides based on sequential text mining and public peptide data sources and it has incorporated the short peptide sequences of the ASPD database [74]. This database only stores peptides with available sequences and 20 amino acids or shorter in length. PepBank has a web-based user interface with a simple, Google-like search function, advanced text search, and BLAST and Smith-Waterman search capabilities.

BDB (Biopanning Data Bank, formerly known as MimoDB) is an information portal to biopanning results of random libraries [75]. It is the latest and largest database for mimotopes. In its latest release (April 2016), it has >25,000 peptides grouped into ~3000 sets and collected from >1300 papers. For each entry, the target, template, library, and structure information are provided. In addition, BDB provides tools for simple and advanced search, structure visualization, BLAST, and alignment view on the fly.

These databases are listed in Table 3. They are important resources for B-cell epitope prediction, and provide a basis for computational biologists to derive benchmark and customize

Table 3
Databases for B-cell epitopes

Databases	Websites
PDB	http://www.rcsb.org/pdb/home/home.do
BCIPEP	http://www.imtech.res.in/raghava/bcipep
CED	http://immunet.cn/ced/
IEDB	http://www.iedb.org/
ASPD	http://wwwmgs.bionet.nsc.ru/mgs/gnw/aspd
PEPBANK	http://pepbank.mgh.harvard.edu
BDB	http://immunet.cn/bdb

datasets for tool evaluation and new algorithm development. However, limitations exist due to limited number/types of epitope entries in databases, limited number of discontinuous epitope databases, incomplete epitope information, and rare integration of databases and epitope prediction software.

4.2 T-Cell Epitopes

A functional T-cell response requires binding of antigenic peptides with MHC class I or class II molecules (also known as HLA, human leukocyte antigen) and a proper interaction of the peptide-MHC complex with TCR on T cells. Therefore, currently T-cell epitopes are largely predicted indirectly by predicting peptide binding to MHC molecules.

MHC-binding prediction consists of MHC-I and II-binding prediction, which are distinct from each other. This is because the peptide-binding groove of MHC class I molecules is closed, while the corresponding groove on class II is open at both ends that can accommodate peptides of variable length, typically 13–25 amino acids long [76]. As a result, MHC-II-binding prediction has much lower accuracy rate than that of MHC I. T-cell epitope prediction methods and algorithms can be roughly grouped into five distinct types: quantitative matrix, machine learning techniques (ANN, SVM, etc.), MHC peptide threading, 3DQSAR (three-dimensional quantitative structure and activity relations), and molecular modeling [77]. Their performance in predicting T-cell epitopes is compared in Table 4. The number of MHC-binding predictive software is expanding rapidly and achieved impressive prediction accuracies of 70–99% sensitivity but only 40–80% specificity with limited range of MHC allele coverage and for peptide with fixed length [78]. A few commonly used T-cell epitope predictive software with publicly available web interfaces are listed in Table 5. Most of these software and databases are user friendly with straightforward output, providing online tutorials for those who are not familiar in this field to select the suitable tools.

Table 4
Comparison of T-cell epitope prediction methods

Method	Training dataset	Prediction dataset	Accuracy	AUC	Correlation coefficient
3D QSAR	A*0201	A*0201			0.679
EpiDock	A*0201	A*0201, B*2705	75–85%		
Threading	10 alleles		71%		−0.61 to 0.07
HMM-SMM	DRB1*0101	DRB1*0101		0.89	
ANN + QM	30 alleles		93.6%		
SVM	30 alleles	30 alleles	86–99%		

However, T-cell epitope prediction based only on MHC-binding prediction has its limitations. Binding to MHC is necessary but not sufficient for recognition by T cells. Many factors are involved in epitope recognition and not every peptide with high affinity to MHC proteins are epitopes. Therefore, combining the prediction results of multiple well-selected tools can achieve more accurate prediction than any single tool. For example, to predict T-cell epitopes from an antigenic protein sequence, an integrated prediction of proteasomal cleavage, TAP transport efficiency, and MHC class I binding affinity will yield better results than a single-prediction software [79]. A study by Trost et al. has shown that a consensus method combining the predictions of 16 MHC-I-binding peptide prediction servers performed better than any individual server [80].

4.2.1 Software for MHC-I-Binding Prediction

Although MHC class I molecules are not directly associated with antigen presentation to T helper cells and B-cell stimulation, bindings of certain drugs with specific MHC class I molecules have been shown to associate with drug allergy and prediction of these bindings can help with drug allergy prediction.

MHC I epitope prediction is quite reliable and currently provided in most software. Software exclusively focused on MHC I epitopes includes BIMAS, CTLpred, ProPred-1, various tools provided on IEDB, etc. BIMAS allows users to locate and rank potential 8- to 10-mer peptides based on a predicted half-time of dissociation to MHC class I molecules. The analysis is based on coefficient tables deduced from the paper published by Parker et al. [81]. BIMAS and SYFPEITHI [82] used to be two of the most commonly used T-cell epitope prediction tools.

MMBPred [83] server predicts mutated promiscuous and high-affinity MHC class I-binding peptide from protein sequence. It uses the matrix data in a linear prediction model, in which peptide conformation is ignored.

NetMHC server [84] uses artificial neural network (ANN) and weight matrices. It has been trained on data from 55 MHC peptides (43 human and 12 nonhuman) and position-specific scoring matrices (PSSMs) for additional 67 HLA alleles.

Similar to NetMHC, NetMHCpan [85] is also based on neural-network method. It generates a quantitative prediction of the affinity of any peptide-MHC class I interaction, covering HLA-A and HLA-B for humans as well as chimpanzee, macaque, gorilla, cow, pig, and mouse, which very few databases can achieve. Both NetMHC (ANN) and NetMHCpan tools are currently provided by the IEDB Analysis Resource website for T-cell epitope prediction.

In addition to MHC I binder prediction, the web server EpiJen [77] has tried to model the entire process of the MHC I degradation pathway, and includes proteasome cleavage and TAP binding into its prediction algorithm. It is a multi-step algorithm for T-cell epitope prediction, which belongs to the next generation of in silico T-cell epitope identification methods. Similar to EpiJen, NetCTL [86], and WAPP (Whole Antigen Processing Pathway) [87] web servers, based on ANN and SVM, respectively, also integrate predictions of proteasomal cleavage, TAP transport efficiency, and MHC class I binding affinity for T-cell epitope prediction. NetCTLpan [79], a pan-specific MHC class I epitope predictor, is an improved and extended version of NetCTL.

4.2.2 Software for MHC-II-binding prediction

As mentioned earlier, MHC-II-binding peptides and epitopes are more difficult to predict than MHC I epitopes, owning to the inherent physical and chemical properties of MHC II molecules. A few web-based tools (listed in Table 5), built specifically for MHC-II-binding prediction, are currently available, such as ProPred, MHC2Pred, and MHC-II-binding tools provided by IEDB.

Propred [33] is a graphical web tool for predicting MHC class II binding regions in antigenic protein sequences, using quantitative matrices derived from the published literature by Sturniolo et al. [88]. MHC2Pred is a SVM-based method for the prediction of promiscuous MHC class II binder. The average accuracy of the SVM-based method for 42 alleles is 80%. The performance of the method was lower for some alleles due to a smaller size of dataset [33].

The MHC-II-binding prediction server on IEDB provides various tools for predicting MHC II binders. The input format can be space separated sequences, one continuous sequence, or in FASTA format. When choosing the prediction method, by default the consensus method that combines several other tools is selected, as it has the highest overall performance ranking than any single tool.

4.2.3 Software for MHC-I and II-Binding Prediction

Software that can be used to predict both MHC I and II binders are usually hybrid method, or have combined several methods. SVMHC [34] is a software based on SVM for both MHC I and II epitope prediction. The server can be used to find the most likely binders in a protein sequence and to investigate the effects

Table 5
List of T-cell epitope prediction servers

Server name	Link	Predictive server for	Predictive method
BIMAS	http://www-bimas.cit.nih.gov/molbio/hla_bind/	MHC I	Published coefficient tables
ProPred I	http://www.imtech.res.in/raghava/propred1/	MHC I	QM
MMBPred	http://www.imtech.res.in/raghava/mmbpred/	MHC I	QM
NetMHC	http://www.cbs.dtu.dk/services/NetMHC/	MHC I	ANN
NetMHCpan	http://www.cbs.dtu.dk/services/NetMHCpan-3.0/	MHC I	ANN
IEDB binding	http://tools.immuneepitope.org/analyze/html/mhc_processing.html	MHC I	SVM + ANN
EpiJen	http://www.ddg-pharmfac.net/epijen/EpiJen/EpiJen.htm	MHC I	Multi-step algorithm
NetCTL	http://www.cbs.dtu.dk/services/NetCTL	MHC I &TAP	ANN-regression
NetCTLpan	http://www.cbs.dtu.dk/services/NetCTLpan/	MHC I &TAP	ANN-regression
MHCPred	http://www.ddg-pharmfac.net/mhcpred/MHCPred/	MHC I &II	Additive method
SYFPEITHI	http://www.syfpeithi.de/bin/MHCServer.dll/EpitopePrediction.htm	MHC I &II	Published motifs
RANKPEP	http://bio.dfci.harvard.edu/RANKPEP/	MHC I &II	PSSM
SVMHC	http://abi.inf.uni-tuebingen.de/Services/SVMHC	MHC I &II	SVM
ProPred	http://www.imtech.res.in/raghava/propred/	MHC II	QM
MHC2Pred	http://www.imtech.res.in/raghava/mhc2pred/	MHC II	SVM
CTLPred	http://www.imtech.res.in/raghava/ctlpred/	MHC I &CTL	SVM + ANN
TAP Pred	http://www.imtech.res.in/raghava/tappred/	TAP	SVM
WAPP	http://abi.inf.uni-tuebingen.de/Services/WAPP/information	TAP	SVM
PAProC	http://www.paproc.de	Proteasomal cleavages	
FRAGPREDICT	http://www.mpiib-berlin.mpg.de/MAPPP/cleavage.html	Proteasomal cleavages	
NetChop	http://www.cbs.dtu.dk/services/NetChop	Proteasomal cleavages	ANN
Pcleavage	http://www.imtech.res.in/raghava/pcleavage	Proteasomal cleavages	SVM

QM quantitative matrix, *SVM* support vector machine, *ANN* artificial neural network, *PSSM* position-specific scoring matrices

of SNPs (single nucleotide polymorphisms) in terms of MHC-peptide binding.

RANKPEP predicts peptide binders to MHC I and MHC II molecules from protein sequences or sequence alignments using Position Specific Scoring Matrices (PSSMs), which derived from a set of aligned peptides known to bind to a given MHC molecule. The binding potential of any peptide sequence (query) to the MHC molecule is determined by comparing the query to the PSSM. In addition, it also determines whether the C-terminus of the predicted MHC I peptide binders are the result of proteasomal cleavage [89].

MHCPred [90] uses the additive method to predict the binding affinity to MHC I and II molecules and also to the TAP. It is composed of a number of allele-specific Quantitative Structure Activity Relationship (QSAR) models created using PLS, a robust multivariate statistical method.

4.2.4 Software for Proteasomal Cleavage Sites Prediction

Predictions of proteasomal cleavage sites provide an alternative way for T-cell epitope prediction, although their prediction sensitivity is not very high. This is expected because proteasomal cleavage is only the first stage in antigen degradation and MHC presentation process, and the majority of peptides may not bind to MHC molecules during later stages. However, they may complement predictive software based on other mechanisms. A few commonly used software with publicly available web interfaces for proteasomal cleavage site prediction, including PAProC, NetChop, FRAGPREDICT, and Pcleavage, are listed in Table 5.

PAProC [91] is a prediction tool that predicts cleavages by human and yeast 20S proteasomes, based on experimental cleavage data. Pcleavage [92] is a SVM-based software for the prediction of constitutive and immunoproteasome cleavage sites in antigenic sequences. It uses SVM, Parallel Exemplarbased Learning (PEBLS), and Waikato Environment for Knowledge Analysis (Weka). Pcleavage and NetChop [93] that are based on neural network prediction are considered to be the best methods for proteasomal cleavage site prediction.

4.2.5 Software for TAP-Binding Prediction

The transporter associated with antigen processing (TAP) delivers the peptide fragments of the proteolyzed antigen to the endoplasmic reticulum, where they bind to MHC class I molecules. Therefore, prediction of TAP-binding peptides is helpful in identifying the MHC class I-restricted T-cell epitopes and has been implemented into several T-cell epitope prediction software (i.e., EpiJen, NetCTL, and WAPP). But as TAP binding alone is not very informative, there are only very few software exclusively for TAP-binding prediction. For example, TAPPred [94] is an online tool to predict binding affinity of peptides toward the TAP transporter. The server allows the user to predict TAP binders using a simple SVM model or cascade SVM model, and to customize the display/output.

Table 6
T-cell epitope related databases

Database	URL	Description
IEDB	http://epitope2.immuneepitope.org/home.do	Biothreat pathogen T-cell epitope database
IMGT/TR	http://imgt.cines.fr/textes/IMGTrepertoire	Aligned and annotated T-cell receptor sequences
IPD-IMGT/HLA	http://www.ebi.ac.uk/ipd/imgt/hla/	Aligned and annotated HLA sequences by WHO nomenclature
SYFPEITHI	http://www.syfpeithi.de	MHC binders, MHC-specific anchor and auxiliary motifs

4.2.6 T-Cell Epitope Databases

There are more databases containing larger amount of data (usually tens of thousands of epitopes) of T-cell epitopes than B-cell epitope databases as discontinuous epitopes are more difficult to analyze. A few commonly used T-cell epitope databases are listed in Table 6. These databases usually provide user-friendly search interface to search or browse for epitopes. Among these databases, IEDB, which has been mentioned earlier in B-cell epitope databases, is one of the several complete databases containing a large number of epitopes, including both T- and B-cell epitopes. When searching for epitopes, it allows specifying MHC restriction to limit the search by one or more MHC classes or specific alleles.

Syfpeithi [32] is a database comprising more than 7000 peptide sequences known to be MHC class I and II ligands and peptide motifs of humans and other species, such as apes, cattle, and mouse. The database is based on previous publications on T-cell epitopes and MHC ligands. Syfpeithi also allows prediction of T-cell epitopes based on published motifs by calculating a score based on amino acids in the anchor, auxiliary anchor positions, and other frequent amino acids. However, the Syfpethi website has not been updated since August 2012.

IMGT® [95] (the international ImMunoGeneTics information system®) has a wide collection of immunoglobulins, T-cell receptors, MHC, and related proteins of the immune system of human and other vertebrates. It consists of sequence databases (IMGT/LIGM-DB, IMGT/MHC-DB, IMGT/PRIMER-DB, etc.), genome database (IMGT/GENE-DB), structure database (IMGT/3Dstructure-DB), monoclonal antibodies database (IMGT/mAb-DB), Web resources (IMGT Repertoire, etc.), and interactive tools (IMGT/V-QUEST, IMGT/JunctionAnalysis, IMGT/StructuralQuery, etc.).

As part of the IMGT, the IPD-IMGT/HLA Database [96] provides a specialist database for sequences of the human MHC (currently containing 14,473 allele sequences) and includes the official sequences named by the WHO Nomenclature Committee for Factors of the HLA System.

5 Conclusions

Bioinformatics methods, software, and databases related to the studies of allergens and allergenic epitopes are developing and expanding quickly. This review is intended to provide an introduction and overview of the publicly accessible bioinformatics tools and databases related to allergy field. We hope to assist researchers in locating and leveraging on these tools and to provide insights into future development in this field. Although current prediction methods and tools are not perfect, especially for allergen and B-cell discontinuous epitopes discovery, a good selection and combination of the proper methods can still save researchers a considerable amount of work and effort. As this field progresses, more data sources and improvements on the methods are expected to make prediction more reliable and discovery even less expensive and time consuming.

References

1. Larche M, Akdis CA, Valenta R (2006) Immunological mechanisms of allergen-specific immunotherapy. Nat Rev Immunol 6(10): 761–771
2. Bharadwaj M, Illing P, Theodossis A et al (2012) Drug hypersensitivity and human leukocyte antigens of the major histocompatibility complex. Annu Rev Pharmacol Toxicol 52:401–401
3. Tanabe S (2007) Epitope peptides and immunotherapy. Curr Protein Pept Sci 8(1):109–118
4. Lin J, Bardina L, Shreffler WG et al (2009) Development of a novel peptide microarray for large-scale epitope mapping of food allergens. J Allergy Clin Immunol 124(2):315–322 322 e311–313
5. Ayuso R, Sanchez-Garcia S, Pascal M et al (2012) Is epitope recognition of shrimp allergens useful to predict clinical reactivity? Clin Exp Allergy 42(2):293–304
6. Mou C, Zhang S, Lin J et al (2002) EST analysis of mRNAs expressed in neurula of Chinese amphioxus. Biochem Biophys Res Commun 299(1):74–84
7. Fu Z, Lu Y, Ye L et al (2002) Construction and application of a large scale cDNA sequences analysis system based on Unix. Acta Sci Nat Univ Sunyatseni 41(5):60–63
8. Liu Z, Lin J, Fu Z et al (2001) A sequence-based typing method for HLA-DPB1 genotyping. Acta Sci Nat Univ Sunyatseni 40(5): 83–87
9. Fu Z (2008) Post-structural genomics: correlate protein sequence, structure, and function. ProQuest, Ann Arbor, MI
10. Fu Z, Lin J (2015) Applying supervised machine learning in bioinformatics analysis. In: Clary TS (ed) Horizons in computer science research, vol 12. Nova, New York, NY
11. Saigo H, Vert JP, Ueda N et al (2004) Protein homology detection using string alignment kernels. Bioinformatics 20(11):1682–1689
12. Hakenberg J, Bickel S, Plake C et al (2005) Systematic feature evaluation for gene name recognition. BMC Bioinformatics 6(Suppl 1):S9
13. El-manzalawy YM (2008) Machine leearning approaches for epitope prediction. Graduate theses and dissertations, Iowa State University
14. Lin J, Bruni FM, Fu Z et al (2012) A bioinformatics approach to identify patients with symptomatic peanut allergy using peptide microarray immunoassay. J Allergy Clin Immunol 129(5):1321–1328 e1325
15. De Groot AS (2006) Immunomics: discovering new targets for vaccines and therapeutics. Drug Discov Today 11(5–6):203–209

16. Aalberse RC (2000) Structural biology of allergens. J Allergy Clin Immunol 106(2):228–238
17. Brusic V, Petrovsky N, Gendel SM et al (2003) Computational tools for the study of allergens. Allergy 58(11):1083–1092
18. Saha S, Raghava GP (2006) AlgPred: prediction of allergenic proteins and mapping of IgE epitopes. Nucleic Acids Res 34((Web Server issue)):W202–W209
19. Hopp TP, Woods KR (1981) Prediction of protein antigenic determinants from amino-acid-sequences. Proc Natl Acad Sci U S Am Biol Sci 78(6):3824–3828
20. Rosenberg HF, Dyer KD (1995) Eosinophil cationic protein and eosinophil-derived neurotoxin. Evolution of novel function in a primate ribonuclease gene family. J Biol Chem 270(50):30234
21. Pellequer JL, Westhof E, Van Regenmortel MH (1991) Predicting location of continuous epitopes in proteins from their primary structures. Methods Enzymol 203:176–201
22. Parker JM, Guo D, Hodges RS (1986) New hydrophilicity scale derived from high-performance liquid chromatography peptide retention data: correlation of predicted surface residues with antigenicity and X-ray-derived accessible sites. Biochemistry 25(19): 5425–5432
23. Chou PY, Fasman GD (1978) Prediction of the secondary structure of proteins from their amino acid sequence. Adv Enzymol Relat Areas Mol Biol 47:45–148
24. Levitt M (1978) Conformational preferences of amino acids in globular proteins. Biochemistry 17(20):4277–4285
25. Emini EA, Hughes JV, Perlow DS et al (1985) Induction of hepatitis A virus-neutralizing antibody by a virus-specific synthetic peptide. J Virol 55(3):836–839
26. Greenbaum JA, Andersen PH, Blythe M et al (2007) Towards a consensus on datasets and evaluation metrics for developing B-cell epitope prediction tools. J Mol Recognit 20(2):75–82
27. Kolaskar AS, Kulkarni-Kale U (1999) Prediction of three-dimensional structure and mapping of conformational epitopes of envelope glycoprotein of Japanese encephalitis virus. Virology 261(1):31–42
28. Doytchinova IA, Flower DR (2001) Toward the quantitative prediction of T-cell epitopes: coMFA and coMSIA studies of peptides with affinity for the class I MHC molecule HLA-A*0201. J Med Chem 44(22):3572–3581
29. Schueler-Furman O, Altuvia Y, Sette A et al (2000) Structure-based prediction of binding peptides to MHC class I molecules: application to a broad range of MHC alleles. Protein Sci 9(9):1838–1846
30. Logean A, Rognan D (2002) Recovery of known T-cell epitopes by computational scanning of a viral genome. J Comput Aided Mol Des 16(4):229–243
31. Ponomarenko J, Bui HH, Li W et al (2008) ElliPro: a new structure-based tool for the prediction of antibody epitopes. BMC Bioinformatics 9:514
32. Rammensee H, Bachmann J, Emmerich NP et al (1999) SYFPEITHI: database for MHC ligands and peptide motifs. Immunogenetics 50(3–4):213–219
33. Singh H, Raghava GP (2001) ProPred: prediction of HLA-DR binding sites. Bioinformatics 17(12):1236–1237
34. Donnes P, Kohlbacher O (2006) SVMHC: a server for prediction of MHC-binding peptides. Nucleic Acids Res 34(Web Server issue):W194–W197.
35. Murugan N, Dai Y (2005) Prediction of MHC class II binding peptides based on an iterative learning model. Immunol Res 1:6
36. Doytchinova IA, Taylor P, Flower DR (2003) Proteomics in vaccinology and immunobiology: an informatics perspective of the immunone. J Biomed Biotechnol 2003(5):267–290
37. Yu K, Petrovsky N, Schonbach C et al (2002) Methods for prediction of peptide binding to MHC molecules: a comparative study. Mol Med 8(3):137–148
38. Bhasin M, Raghava GP (2004) Prediction of CTL epitopes using QM, SVM and ANN techniques. Vaccine 22(23–24):3195–3204
39. El-Manzalawy Y, Honavar V (2010) Recent advances in B-cell epitope prediction methods. Immunol Res 6(Suppl 2):S2
40. Sollner J (2006) Selection and combination of machine learning classifiers for prediction of linear B-cell epitopes on proteins. J Mol Recognit 19(3):209–214
41. FAO/WHO (2001) Allergenicity of genetically modified foods. Report of a joint FAO/WHO expert consultation on allergenicity of foods derived from biotechnology. FAO/WHO, Rome
42. Ivanciuc O, Schein CH, Braun W (2003) SDAP: database and computational tools for allergenic proteins. Nucleic Acids Res 31(1):359–362
43. Stadler MB, Stadler BM (2003) Allergenicity prediction by protein sequence. FASEB J 17(9):1141–1143
44. Bjorklund AK, Soeria-Atmadja D, Zorzet A et al (2005) Supervised identification of allergen-representative peptides for in silico

detection of potentially allergenic proteins. Bioinformatics 21(1):39–50

45. Wang J, Yu Y, Zhao Y et al (2013) Evaluation and integration of existing methods for computational prediction of allergens. BMC Bioinformatics 14(Suppl 4):S1
46. Radauer C, Nandy A, Ferreira F et al (2014) Update of the WHO/IUIS allergen nomenclature database based on analysis of allergen sequences. Allergy 69(4):413–419
47. Mari A, Scala E, Palazzo P et al (2006) Bioinformatics applied to allergy: allergen databases, from collecting sequence information to data integration. The Allergome platform as a model. Cell Immunol 244(2):97–100
48. Sweredoski MJ, Baldi P (2008) PEPITO: improved discontinuous B-cell epitope prediction using multiple distance thresholds and half sphere exposure. Bioinformatics 24(12):1459–1460
49. Rubinstein ND, Mayrose I, Martz E et al (2009) Epitopia: a web-server for predicting B-cell epitopes. BMC Bioinformatics 10:287
50. Kringelum JV, Lundegaard C, Lund O et al (2012) Reliable B cell epitope predictions: impacts of method development and improved benchmarking. PLoS Comput Biol 8(12):e1002829
51. Haste Andersen P, Nielsen M, Lund O (2006) Prediction of residues in discontinuous B-cell epitopes using protein 3D structures. Protein Sci 15(11):2558–2567
52. Qi T, Qiu T, Zhang Q et al (2014) SEPPA 2.0—more refined server to predict spatial epitope considering species of immune host and subcellular localization of protein antigen. Nucleic Acids Res 42((Web Server issue)):59–63
53. Liang S, Zheng D, Zhang C et al (2009) Prediction of antigenic epitopes on protein surfaces by consensus scoring. BMC Bioinformatics 10:302
54. Liang S, Zheng D, Standley DM et al (2010) EPSVR and EPMeta: prediction of antigenic epitopes using support vector regression and multiple server results. BMC Bioinformatics 11:381
55. Yao B, Zheng D, Liang S et al (2013) Conformational B-cell epitope prediction on antigen protein structures: a review of current algorithms and comparison with common binding site prediction methods. PLoS One 8(4):e62249
56. Moreau V, Granier C, Villard S et al (2006) Discontinuous epitope prediction based on mimotope analysis. Bioinformatics 22(9): 1088–1095
57. Huang J, Gutteridge A, Honda W et al (2006) MIMOX: a web tool for phage display based epitope mapping. BMC Bioinformatics 7:451
58. Mayrose I, Penn O, Erez E et al (2007) Pepitope: epitope mapping from affinity-selected peptides. Bioinformatics 23(23):3244–3246
59. Mayrose I, Shlomi T, Rubinstein ND et al (2007) Epitope mapping using combinatorial phage-display libraries: a graph-based algorithm. Nucleic Acids Res 35(1):69–78
60. Bublil EM, Freund NT, Mayrose I et al (2007) Stepwise prediction of conformational discontinuous B-cell epitopes using the Mapitope algorithm. Proteins 68(1):294–304
61. Huang YX, Bao YL, Guo SY et al (2008) Pep-3D-Search: a method for B-cell epitope prediction based on mimotope analysis. BMC Bioinformatics 9:538
62. Chen WH, Sun PP, Lu Y et al (2011) MimoPro: a more efficient Web-based tool for epitope prediction using phage display libraries. BMC Bioinformatics 12:199
63. Huang J, Ru B, Dai P (2011) Bioinformatics resources and tools for phage display. Molecules 16(1):694–709
64. Negi SS, Braun W (2009) Automated detection of conformational epitopes using phage display Peptide sequences. Bioinf Biol Insights 3:71–81
65. Sun P, Ju H, Liu Z et al (2013) Bioinformatics resources and tools for conformational B-cell epitope prediction. Comput Math Methods Med 2013:943636
66. Saha S, Raghava GP (2006) Prediction of continuous B-cell epitopes in an antigen using recurrent neural network. Proteins 65(1):40–48
67. Larsen JE, Lund O, Nielsen M (2006) Improved method for predicting linear B-cell epitopes. Immunol Res 2:2
68. Toseland CP, Clayton DJ, McSparron H et al (2005) AntiJen: a quantitative immunology database integrating functional, thermodynamic, kinetic, biophysical, and cellular data. Immunol Res 1(1):4
69. Berman HM, Westbrook J, Feng Z et al (2000) The protein data bank. Nucleic Acids Res 28(1):235–242
70. Saha S, Bhasin M, Raghava GPS (2005) Bcipep: a database of B-cell epitopes. BMC Genomics 6:79–79
71. Vita R, Overton JA, Greenbaum JA et al (2015) The immune epitope database (IEDB) 3.0. Nucleic Acids Res 43((Database issue)):D405–D412
72. Kulkarni-Kale U, Bhosle S, Kolaskar AS (2005) CEP: a conformational epitope prediction server. Nucleic Acids Res 33((Web Server issue)):W168–W171
73. Valuev VP, Afonnikov DA, Ponomarenko MP et al (2002) ASPD (Artificially selected proteins/

peptides database): a database of proteins and peptides evolved in vitro. Nucleic Acids Res 30(1):200–202

74. Shtatland T, Guettler D, Kossodo M et al (2007) PepBank—a database of peptides based on sequence text mining and public peptide data sources. BMC Bioinformatics 8:280
75. Huang J, Ru B, Zhu P et al (2012) MimoDB 2.0: a mimotope database and beyond. Nucleic Acids Res 40((Database issue)):D271–D277
76. Meydan C, Otu HH, Sezerman OU (2013) Prediction of peptides binding to MHC class I and II alleles by temporal motif mining. BMC Genomics 14((Suppl. 2)):S13
77. Doytchinova IA, Guan P, Flower DR (2006) EpiJen: a server for multistep T cell epitope prediction. BMC Bioinformatics 7:131
78. Cui J, Han LY, Lin HH et al (2007) Prediction of MHC-binding peptides of flexible lengths from sequence-derived structural and physicochemical properties. Mol Immunol 44(5):866–877
79. Stranzl T, Larsen MV, Lundegaard C et al (2010) NetCTLpan: pan-specific MHC class I pathway epitope predictions. Immunogenetics 62(6):357–368
80. Trost B, Bickis M, Kusalik A (2007) Strength in numbers: achieving greater accuracy in MHC-I binding prediction by combining the results from multiple prediction tools. Immunol Res 3:5–5
81. Parker KC, Bednarek MA, Coligan JE (1994) Scheme for ranking potential HLA-A2 binding peptides based on independent binding of individual peptide side-chains. J Immunol 152(1):163–175
82. Schuler MM, Nastke MD, Stevanovikc S (2007) SYFPEITHI: database for searching and T-cell epitope prediction. Methods Mol Biol 409:75–93
83. Bhasin M, Raghava GP (2003) Prediction of promiscuous and high-affinity mutated MHC binders. Hybrid Hybridomics 22(4):229–234
84. Lundegaard C, Lamberth K, Harndahl M et al (2008) NetMHC-3.0: accurate web accessible predictions of human, mouse and monkey MHC class I affinities for peptides of length 8–11. Nucleic Acids Res 36((Web Server issue)):W509–W512
85. Hoof I, Peters B, Sidney J et al (2009) NetMHCpan, a method for MHC class I binding prediction beyond humans. Immunogenetics 61(1):1–13
86. Larsen MV, Lundegaard C, Lamberth K et al (2007) Large-scale validation of methods for cytotoxic T-lymphocyte epitope prediction. BMC Bioinformatics 8:424
87. Donnes P, Kohlbacher O (2005) Integrated modeling of the major events in the MHC class I antigen processing pathway. Protein Sci 14(8):2132–2140
88. Sturniolo T, Bono E, Ding J et al (1999) Generation of tissue-specific and promiscuous HLA ligand databases using DNA microarrays and virtual HLA class II matrices. Nat Biotechnol 17(6):555–561
89. Reche PA, Reinherz EL (2007) Prediction of peptide-MHC binding using profiles. Methods Mol Biol 409:185–200
90. Guan P, Hattotuwagama CK, Doytchinova IA et al (2006) MHCPred 2.0: an updated quantitative T-cell epitope prediction server. Appl Bioinformatics 5(1):55–61
91. Nussbaum AK, Kuttler C, Hadeler KP et al (2001) PAProC: a prediction algorithm for proteasomal cleavages available on the WWW. Immunogenetics 53(2):87–94
92. Bhasin M, Raghava GP (2005) Pcleavage: an SVM based method for prediction of constitutive proteasome and immunoproteasome cleavage sites in antigenic sequences. Nucleic Acids Res 33(Web Server issue):W202–W207.
93. Nielsen M, Lundegaard C, Lund O et al (2005) The role of the proteasome in generating cytotoxic T-cell epitopes: insights obtained from improved predictions of proteasomal cleavage. Immunogenetics 57(1–2):33–41
94. Bhasin M, Lata S, Raghava GP (2007) TAPPred prediction of TAP-binding peptides in antigens. Methods Mol Biol 409:381–386
95. Lefranc MP, Giudicelli V, Ginestoux C et al (2009) IMGT, the international ImMunoGeneTics information system. Nucleic Acids Res 37((Database issue)): D1006–D1012
96. Robinson J, Waller MJ, Fail SC et al (2009) The IMGT/HLA database. Nucleic Acids Res 37((Database issue)):1013–1017

Part IV

Methods Currently Being Developed and Future Development

Chapter 19

The Use of a Semi-Automated System to Measure Mouse Natural Killer T (NKT) Cell Activation by Lipid-Loaded Dendritic Cells

Ashfaq Ghumra and Marcos Alcocer

Abstract

Cell-based assays are widely used in all aspects of research ranging from understanding basic biological function to identifying compounds for disease intervention. Immortalized cell lines have been ideal components of these assays due to the low cost of growth, easy maintenance, and the ability to obtain homogenous cell populations. Like other molecular assays, cell-based systems have been automated to reduce experimental error. Complex lipids are now recognized as important components of the allergic response, the study of the interaction between NKTs and lipid-activated DCs opens a new perspective into the intrinsic allergenicity of proteins. Here, we describe a semi-automated method to measure IL-2 release upon activation of mouse NKT cells (DN32.D3) by various lipids in a 384-well plate using the Biomek® 3000 laboratory automated workstation (Beckman Coulter).

Key words Cell-based assays, Natural Killer T (NKT) cells, Robotics, ELISA, Biomek® 3000

1 Introduction

The exact role of lipids in the intrinsic allergenicity of proteins is still poorly characterized. Accumulating evidence demonstrated that large numbers of protein allergens possess a lipid-binding site or lipid transfer functions. The presence of the hydrophobic site and the observation that other components copresented with proteins can influence the initial stages of allergic sensitization, are therefore of growing interest. It is now well described that immune response can be modulated by lipids presented by Antigen Presenting Cells (APCs) and subsequently recognized by NKT cells in a Toll receptor independent system. Once activated, NKT cells can rapidly secrete large amounts of Th1 and Th2 cytokines which leads to the activation of various immune cells playing a central role bridging innate and adaptive immune responses [1]. The majority of NKT cells express highly restricted TCRs with an invariant α-chain

Jing Lin and Marcos Alcocer (eds.), *Food Allergens: Methods and Protocols*, Methods in Molecular Biology, vol. 1592,
DOI 10.1007/978-1-4939-6925-8_19, © Springer Science+Business Media LLC 2017

(Vα24-Jα18 (TRAV10-TRAJ18) in humans and Vα14-Jα18 in mice) and limited β-chains. These are referred to as Type I or invariant NKT (iNKT cells) [2]. Type II cells form the remaining NKT cells and express noninvariant TCRs. Most NKTs recognize lipid antigens presented by a CD1 molecule, a major histocompatibility complex (MHC) class I-like antigen presenting molecule expressed in APCs, which consists of a binding pocket adapted for glycolipid antigens. CD1d are constitutively expressed on APCs such as dendritic cells, B cells, and macrophages [3]. Natural ligands for CD1 include a wide range of both self and non-self-glycolipids with the α-galactosylceramide isolated from marine sponge being one of the most potent CD1 ligands known. Some pollen lipids and fractions from Brazil nut have shown to be recognized by this pathway [4]. In addition to activating NKT cells, lipids have also been shown to have an immune-stimulatory and regulatory effect; however, the underlying mechanisms underpinning these effects are not fully understood [5]. Here, we have established an assay that can be used to identify lipids that activate NKT cells.

Automation of cell-based assays has become less specialized and user-friendly workstations are slowly replacing time-consuming tissue culture techniques by providing a controlled environment for the study of biological interactions. The Biomek 3000® workstation (Beckman Coulter) is one platform that has provided reliable results in highly demanding scientific areas such as forensic genetic DNA typing [6]. In this study, we investigate the interaction between the NKT receptor expressed on the surface of the mouse DN32.D3 cells and lipid-loaded CD1d that is expressed on the surface of mouse JAWS II dendritic cells. This interaction has been shown to result in the release of IL-2 cytokine that can be measured by Enzyme-Linked-Immunosorbent Assays (ELISAs) [7]. In this study, we corroborated this finding and furthermore we miniaturized the experiment to reduce cost and adapt the assay so that it can be used in a semi-automated system to reduce manual work and human error.

2 Materials

Prepare all solutions using ultrapure water (18 MΩ at 25 °C) and analytical grade reagents. Follow all waste disposal regulations when disposing waste materials (*see* **Note 1**).

2.1 In-Vitro Culturing of Mouse Cell Lines

1. Mouse NKT cell line DN32.32 was kindly donated by Prof A. Bendelac (University of Chicago, USA).
2. Immature dendritic mouse cell line: JAWS II (ATCC® CRL-11904™).
3. DN32 Medium: Rosewell Park Memorial Institute (RPMI) 1640 medium supplemented with 10% Fetal Bovine Serum

(FBS), 1% penicillin-streptomycin (10,000 U/mL) and 2 mM l-Glutamine.

4. JAWS II medium: Alpha minimum essential medium (MEM) with ribonucleosides and deoxyribonucleosides supplemented with 20% FBS, 4 mM l-Glutamine, 1 mM Sodium Pyruvate, and 5 ng/mL Granulocyte Macrophage-Colony Stimulating Factor (GM-CSF).
5. Cell dissociation reagent: Trypsin-EDTA (0.25%).
6. Cell counting: Luna-II™ Automated Cell Counter (Logos Biosystems) requires Luna™ Cell Counting Slides and 0.4% Trypan Blue.

2.2 Co-culturing of Lipid-Loaded JAWS II with DN32.D3 Cells

1. Corning sterile 384-well plates (Sigma).
2. RPMI DMSO: for a 50 mL solution add 2.5 mL of Dimethyl Sulfoxide (DMSO) to 47.5 mL of supplemented RPMI (DN32 medium) to a final concentration of 5% DMSO.
3. Lipids used in this study were obtained from various sources. Alpha-galactosylceramide (Funakoshi-KRN 7000), Glucocerebrosides (bovine/buttermilk), Cerebrosides, *N*-hexadecanoyl-ceramide tri-hexoside, Lactosylceramides (porcine RBC), Sulfatides (bovine, Na^+ salt), and Lyso-sulfatide (NH_4^+ salt) (Matreya LLC). Other lipids used were Phosphatidylinositol, digalactosyldiacylglycerol, Beta-sitosterol, Oleoyl-l-alpha-lysophosphatidic acid, Lecithin soybean, Sodium lauryl sulfate, NaCl dodecylbenzenesulfonate, and Lysophosphatidylethanolamine.
4. Sonication water bath.
5. Automated workstation: Biomek® 3000 laboratory automated workstation (Beckman Coulter) enclosed in a sterile environment and preferably in Class II Biological Safety Cabinet.
6. Biomek® AP96 P50 sterile tips and half modular reservoirs for Biomek® workstation.
7. Autoclaved tub is required to empty the contents of the plates.
8. Cut 100 mm × 150 mm pieces of autoclaved 3 mm Whatman paper.
9. Bench Centrifuge.

2.3 IL-2 Enzyme-Linked Immunosorbent Assay (ELISA)

1. Nunc® MaxiSorp™ 384-well ELISA plates.
2. Mouse IL-2 ELISA Ready-SET-Go!® (eBioscience) contains all the reagents for the ELISA to detect mouse IL-2.
3. Phosphate-Buffered Saline (PBS): add five ready-made tablets (Sigma-Aldrich) in 1 L of deionized water.
4. Phosphate-Buffered Saline Tween (PBST): Add 0.5 mL of Tween-20 to the I L solution of PBS to a final Tween-20 concentration of 0.05% (PBST).

5. Plate washer: BioTek ELx50 or similar.
6. The Biomek® 3000 laboratory automated workstation is used for all the steps in the ELISA (*see* Subheading 3).
7. 2 M sulfuric acid: add 11.1 mL of concentrated sulfuric acid to 89.9 mL of deionized water.

3 Methods

3.1 In-Vitro Culturing of Mouse Cell Line DN32.D3

All procedures are to be carried out under sterile conditions and at room temperature unless otherwise specified.

1. Remove a cryovial containing DN32.D3 cells and place immediately in a water bath that has been pre-warmed to 37 °C.
2. After 5 min and when the contents of the vial are thawed, remove the vial from the water bath and transfer it into a Class II Biological Safety Cabinet. From this point onward, tubes containing cells are always to be opened in the Class II cabinet that has a HEPA-filtered vertical unidirectional airflow providing a sterile environment for tissue culture.
3. Transfer the contents of the cryovial into a 15 mL Falcon™ conical centrifuge tube (Fisher scientific) and add 10 mL of DN32 media described in Subheading 2.1, **item 3**.
4. Centrifuge the tube for 5 min at 1000 × *g*.
5. Aspirate the supernatant and resuspend the cell pellet in 10 mL of DN32 media and transfer the contents into a 25 cm^2 T-25 culture flask and place into a 37 °C incubator with a supply of 5% CO_2.
6. After 2 days, use a cell scraper to remove all the cells that have been adhered to the bottom of the flask and resuspend into the media. After mixing the cell culture suspension, take a 10 μL aliquot and place into a 1.5 mL eppedorf tube. Add 10 μL of 0.4% Trypan Blue solution to the cell culture aliquot, mix by pipetting up and down, and load into one of the wells of the cell-counting slide. Place the slide into the Luna-II™ and start the count.
7. Maintain DN32.D3 cells at a density of 1×10^6 cells/mL and therefore dilute by adding more DN32 media accordingly. **Step 6** should be repeated every 2 days to monitor the growth of these cells and to maintain the number at 1×10^6 cells/mL.

3.2 In-Vitro Culturing of Mouse Cell Line JAWS II

1. Carry out the same steps as described for DN32.D3 in Subheading 3.1 except to use JAWS II media instead of DN32 media. Also note that the JAWS II cells grow at a slower rate compared to DN32.D3 and therefore routine counting and maintenance can be carried out every 5 days instead of 2.

3.3 Co-culturing of Lipid-Loaded JAWS II and DN32.D3 Cells

1. Make top concentration of all 15 lipids in RPMI-DMSO and place into wells A1 to O1 of a 384-well plate. All lipid stocks were dissolved in DMSO to get a concentration of 1 mg/mL and placed in a sonication bath for 15 min. After the lipids had been dissolved, a concentration of 10 μg/mL was prepared by adding 1 μL of lipid stock to 99 μL of RPMI-DMSO. All 100 μL were pipetted into wells A1 to O1. The P1 well can be used as a control that may contain RPMI-DMSO.
2. Take the flask containing JAWS II cells and remove the media. Add 5 mL of sterile PBS to rinse the internal sides of the flask that contain adherent cells. Discard the PBS and add 5 mL of Trypsin-EDTA. Place the flask into the 37 °C incubator for 5 min and observe whether the cells have been detached under a light microscope. Tap the side of flask to aid the detachment of cells.
3. Add 5 mL of JAWS II media to trypsin cell suspension and transfer the mixture to a 15 mL falcon tube and centrifuge at $1000 \times g$ for 5 min.
4. Remove the supernatant and resuspend the cell pellet in 10 mL of JAWS II media and perform a cell count using the Luna-II automated system, as described in Subheading 3.1, **step 6**.
5. Calculate the total number of JAWS II cells required for the co-culture experiment. Each well of a 384-well plate should hold 1.25×10^4 cells in 30 μL for this assay. A total of 4.8×10^6 cells in 11.53 mL are required to test 15 lipids in a 384-well plate. To allow for pipetting error, an excess solution of cells is required and therefore it is advisable to prepare 5.4×10^6 in 13 mL. Take an appropriate volume of JAWS II cells (5.4×10^6), centrifuge at $1000 \times g$ for 5 min, and resuspend the cell pellet in 13 mL of RPMI-DMSO.
6. Take the 384-well plate containing the lipids, JAWS II cells in RPMI-DMSO, and 20 mL of RPMI-DMSO media to the Biomek 3000® workstation. Make sure that the working area around the workstation is decontaminated using disinfectant (Distel) and 70% ethanol, start the Biological Safety Cabinet, and maintain a sterile environment for the next steps.
7. Using the Biomek software (Beckman Coulter) to develop a protocol to carry out 1:10 serial dilutions of the lipids (*see* **Note 2**). Place the RPMI-DMSO in the right chamber of an autoclaved two-chamber reservoir and start the programme to carry out a 1:10 dilution of the lipid from well A1–P1 to well A8-P8.
8. Continue following the instructions prompted by the programme (*see* **Note 3**). Add JAWS II cells to the left chamber of the autoclaved reservoir and place a new 384-well plate adjacent to the plate in which the lipid is diluted. The programme will dispense 30 μL of JAWS II cells to each well.

9. Continue with the programme and turn the lipid plate 180° in a clockwise direction. The programme will dispense 20 μL of each lipid dilution into the wells of a plate containing JAWS II cells (*see* **Note 4**). This will be done in triplicates (A1–P1 to A8–P8, A9–P9 to A16–P16 and A17–P17 to A24–P24) so that each row of a 384-well plate will correspond to one lipid.
10. Seal the plate containing JAWS II cells and lipids with parafilm and incubate in a 37 °C/CO_2 incubator for 4 h.
11. After 4 h, count the number of DN32.D3 cells as described in Subheading 3.1, **step 6**. This step requires 1.25×10^5 DN32.2 cells per well (in 45 μL). All 384 wells of the plate are to be used in this assay where the effects of 15 lipids are to be investigated and would require 5.5×10^7 in 20 mL of DN32 media. Calculate the volume of cell suspension required to obtain 5.5×10^7 cells, take the required amount, and spin down for 5 min at 1000 ×*g*. Discard the supernatant and resuspend the cell pellet in 20 mL of DN32 media.
12. Spin down the JAWS II plate containing lipids at 1000 × g for 5 min.
13. Take the plate into the safety cabinet containing the Biomek® workstation and flick out the contents into an autoclaved tub. Make sure to dab the empty plate onto autoclaved Whatman blotting paper to remove any excess supernatant.
14. Load the programme on the Biomek software that is configured to wash the plate with DN32 media (*see* **Note 5**). Follow the instructions, placing the 384-well plate into the correct position. Add DN32 media to the right chamber of an autoclaved two-chamber reservoir and start the programme. This step would lead to dispensing of the media into the plate. Follow the instructions and centrifuge the plate as **step 12**.
15. After the centrifugation, repeat **step 13** in Subheading 3.3 and place the 384-well plate in the correct position within the Biomek® workstation. Add the DN32.D3 cells prepared from **step 11** in Subheading 3.3 to the left side chamber of an autoclaved 2-chamber reservoir and continue with the programme. The dispensing unit will pipette 45 μL of DN32.D3 cells into each well of a 384-well plate.
16. After dispensing the DN32 cells. Seal the plate using parafilm and place overnight in a 37 °C/CO_2 incubator.

3.4 ELISA to Detect IL-2 in DN32.D3/JAWS II Co-culture Supernatants (See Note 6)

1. Coat Nunc® MaxiSorp™ plates with the purified anti-mouse IL-2 capture antibody. Prepare 12.5 mL 1× coating buffer by 1.25 mL of 10× coating buffer to 11.25 mL of deionized water. Add 50 μL of 250× anti-mouse IL-2 capture antibody to 12.5 mL of 1× coating buffer. Use the Biomek® workstation and software to develop a programme to pipette 30 μL of capture antibody solution (placed in the reservoir) in each well of a 384-well plate

(Plate 1). An extra 24 wells are coated on a separate plate (Plate 2) which will be used for internal standard controls.

2. Seal the plate with parafilm and place at 4 °C overnight.
3. On the following day, prepare 1 L of PBST as described in Subheading 2.3, **item 3**.
4. Rinse the BioTek plate washer with deionized water and prime the instrument with prepared PBST.
5. Remove the ELISA plates, take off the parafilm, and wash each well with 100 μL of PBST using the plate washer. Carry out three washes with 10 s of shaking in between. Invert the plates and tap them onto tissue paper to remove the excess buffer from the wells.
6. Prepare "blocking buffer" by adding 10 mL of 5× Assay Diluent to 40 mL of deionized water.
7. Add 60 μL of blocking buffer to each well of washed plates 1 and 2 using the Biomek® workstation and software. Leave the plates at room temperature for 1 h.
8. Repeat Subheading 3.4, **step 5**.
9. Using a programme developed by the Biomek® software, apply 15 μL to DN32 media to each well of 384-well ELISA plate (Plate 1), which will require 6.5 mL of DN32 media to be added to the reservoir chamber. Remove the 384-well plate containing the DN32.D3-JAWS II co-culture and centrifuge for 5 min at 1000 × *g*. Place the co-culture plate next to the ELISA plate that contains DN32 media and continue the programme. The programme will transfer 15 μL of supernatant from the co-culture plates to the ELISA plate for each of the 384 wells (*see* **Note** 7). Seal plate 1 with parafilm and leave at room temperature for 2 h.
10. Plate 2 has 24 coated and blocked wells that will be used for IL-2 standards. Prepare the IL-2 standard by adding 0.8 mL of deionized water to one vial of lyopholized IL-2. Allow to sit for 15 min prior to dilution. The concentration of the reconstituted standard is 15 ng/mL. Add 100 μL of standard to 7.4 mL of blocking buffer to prepare the top standard concentration (200 pg/mL). Carry out 8× Twofold serial dilution of the IL-2 standard starting with the top concentration at 200–1.25 pg/mL. Transfer 30 μL of each concentration in three wells (triplicates) in plate 2, seal the plate with parafilm and leave at room temperature for 2 h.
11. Repeat **step 5** in Subheading 3.4.
12. Prepare 13 mL of biotin-conjugated anti-mouse IL-2 by adding 52 μL of 250× biotin-conjugated anti-mouse IL-2 to 12.95 mL of blocking buffer prepared in **step 6** in Subheading 3.4. Use the Biomek® apparatus to apply 30 μL to each well of plate 1 and the 24 wells of plate 2. Leave the plates at room temperature for 1 h.

13. Repeat **step 5** in Subheading 3.4 followed by **step 12** in Subheading 3.4 except to use 250× Avidin-HRP instead of the 250× biotin-conjugated anti-mouse IL-2.
14. Repeat **step 5** in Subheading 3.4 followed by **step 12** in Subheading 3.4 except to use 60 μL of 1× TMB solution to each well and incubate the plates at room temperature for 15 min as you observe the appearance of a blue-colored product. Stop the reaction by using the Biomek® apparatus to apply 30 μL of 2 M sulfuric acid.
15. Read the plate by taking an absorbance value at 450 nm wavelength using a spectrophotometer (Fluostar Optima, BMG Biotech).

3.5 Results

As shown in Fig. 1, more than 500 pg/mL of IL-2 was detected in supernatants from alpha-galactosylceramide presentation by JAWS II cells to DN32.D3.

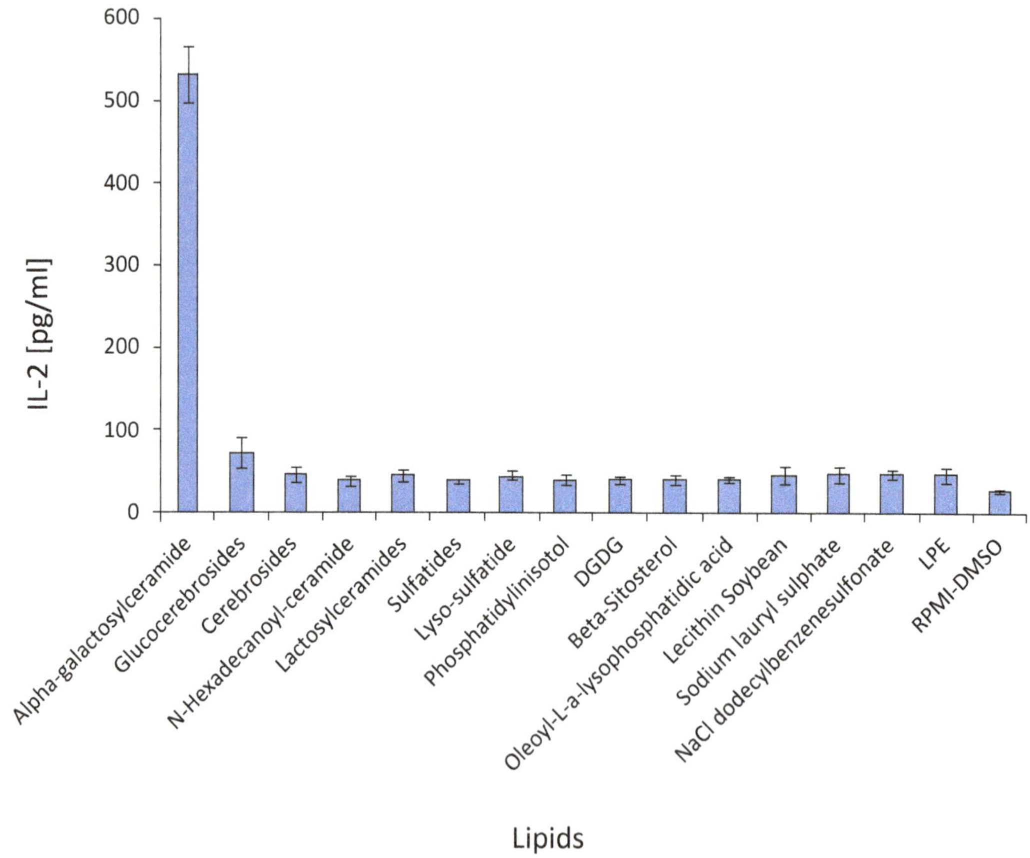

Fig. 1 IL-2 ELISA results. Graph shows ELISA results representative of three experiments. Each lipid was tested in triplicate co-cultures and triplicate supernatants were tested by ELISA. More than 500 pg/mL of IL-2 was detected in supernatants from alpha-galactosylceramide presentation by JAWS II cells to DN32.D3 cells. All other lipids lacked the ability to induce IL-2 release when presented in the same manner. *DGDG* digalactosyl diacyl glycerol, *LPE* lysophosphatidylethanolamine

4 Notes

1. Thawing and maintaining cell viable cell cultures require good sterile technique using all other relevant materials such as 15 and 50 mL sterile tubes, pipette dispensers, pipettes, 25 cm^2 and 75 cm^2 tissue culture flasks, water bath, Class II Biological Safety Cabinet, centrifuge, and a 37 °C incubator that can provide 5% CO_2.
2. Figure 2 shows the programing steps used in the Biomek software to carry out lipid dilution.
3. Figure 3 shows the programing steps used in the Biomek software for the addition of JAWS II cells.

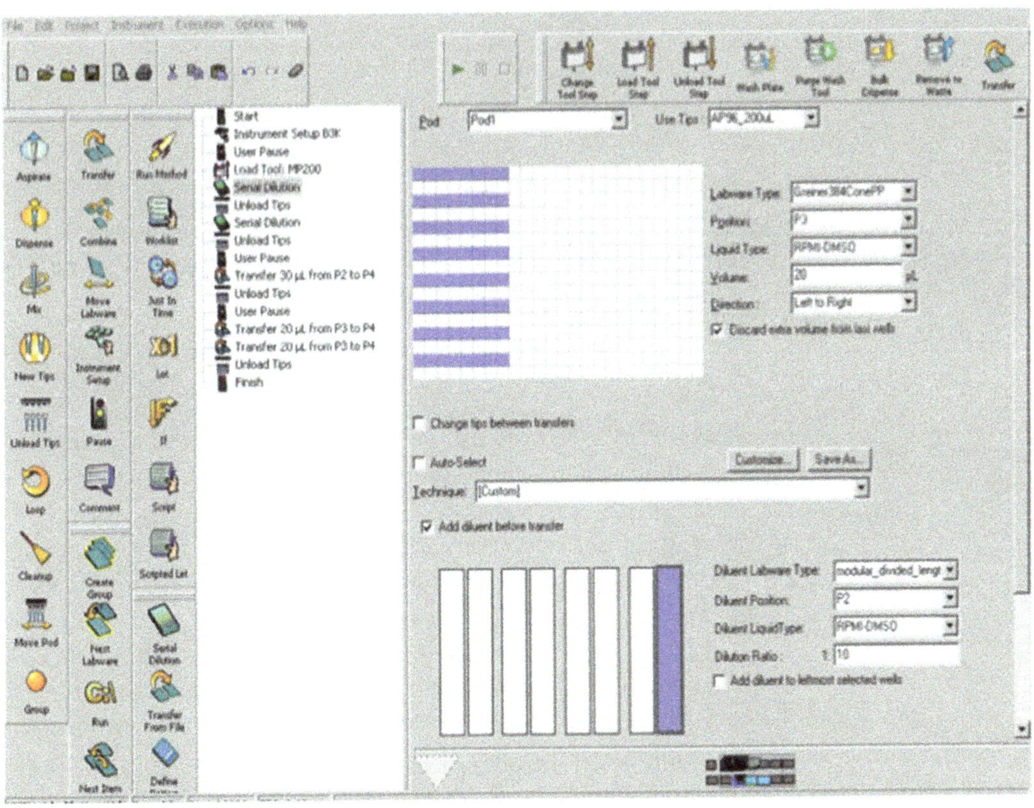

Fig. 2 Use of Biomek® software to carry out lipid dilution. Column 1 contains top concentration of lipids previously diluted and pipette manually (Subheading 3.3, *step 1*). The programme is devised such that serial dilution of lipids is done in two steps. RPMI-DMSO is placed on the right-hand side of the half modular reservoir. The first step will carry out a dilution of the lipids from column 1 to column 6 for *rows A, C, E, G, I, K, M,* and *O*. The second step will carry out a dilution of the lipids from column 1 to column 6 for rows *B, D, F, H, J, L,* and *N*

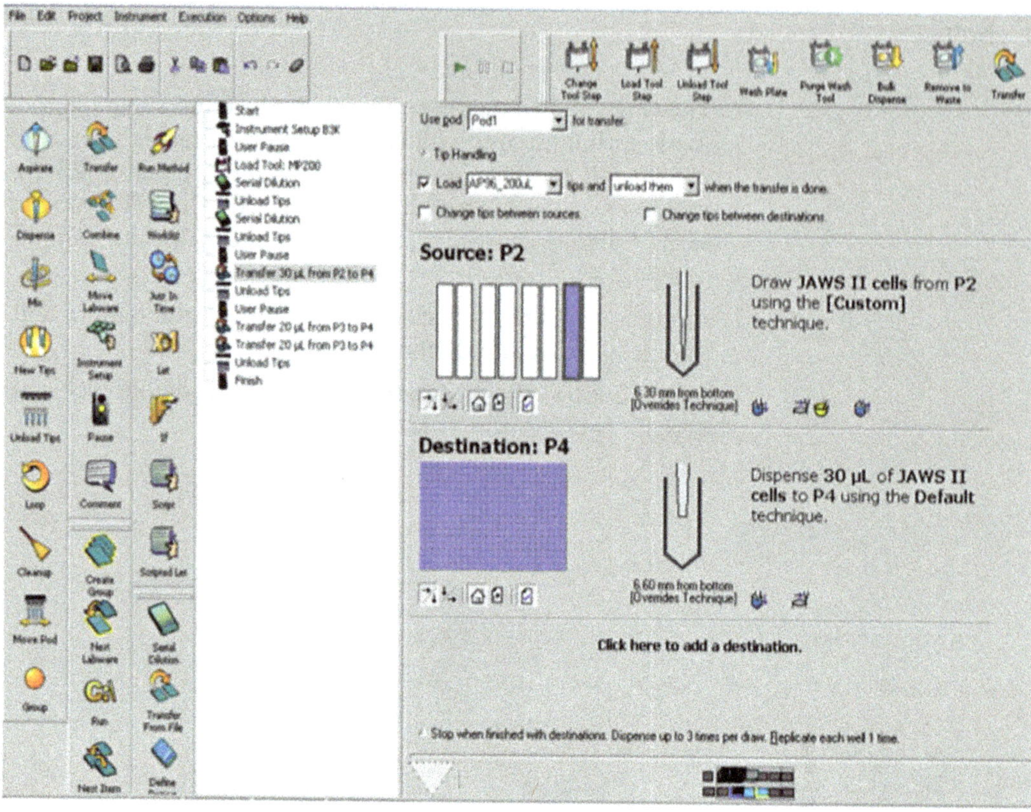

Fig. 3 Addition of JAWS II cells to 384-well plates. The left-hand side chamber of the half module reservoir containing JAWS II cells is used as shown in Source P2. A new 384-well plate is used and 30 μL of cells is placed in each well

4. Figure 4 shows the programing steps used in the Biomek software for transferring diluted lipids into plates containing JAWS II cells.
5. Figure 5 shows the programing steps used in the Biomek software for the removal of the excess lipids and washing the wells.
6. All procedures are to be carried out using the Mouse IL-2 ELISA Ready-SET-Go! Kit from eBioscience. The following protocol is described in the manufacturer's guidelines but has been adapted in this procedure for a 384-well plate to be used.
7. Figure 6 shows the programing steps used in the Biomek software for the final addition of DN32.D3 cells.

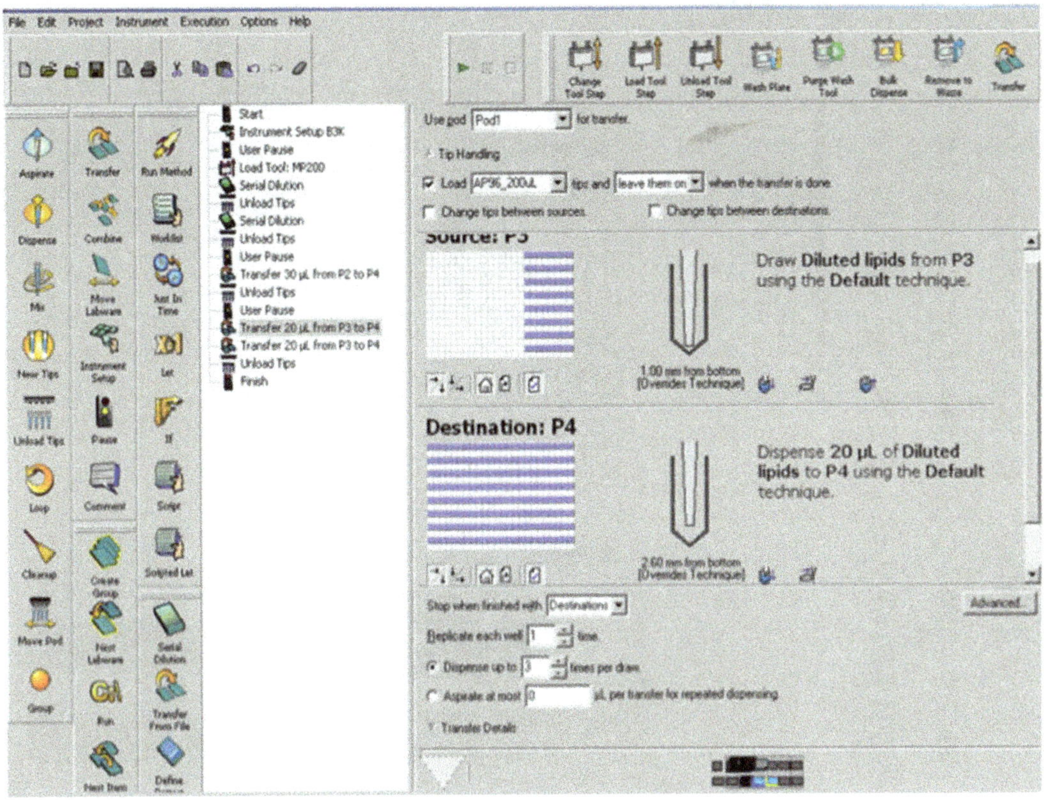

Fig. 4 Transferring diluted lipids into plates containing JAWS II cells. Source P3 contains the 384-well plate containing the serially diluted lipids. The plate has been inverted to allow minimal distance movement of tips from one plate to another to avoid contamination. The first step will carry out transfer of lipids from rows *A*, *C*, *E*, *G*, *I*, *K*, *M*, and *O*. The second step will carry out transfer of lipids from rows *B*, *D*, *F*, *H*, *J*, *L*, and *N*. Destination 4 is the 384-well plate containing JAWS II cells into which lipids are dispensed. Each row in destination 4 will have triplicates of all eight lipid dilutions from source P3

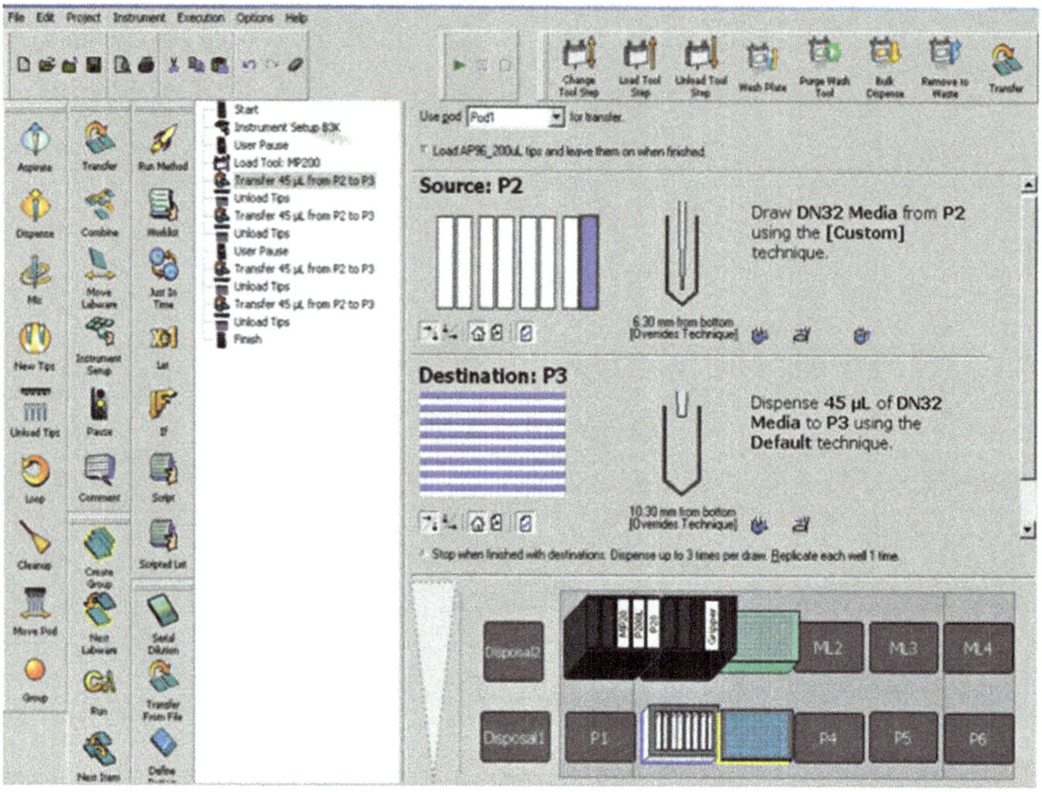

Fig. 5 Remove excess lipids and wash the wells. This step shows the actions of the Biomek® 3000 workstation after centrifugation and removal of the excess unbound lipid. The dispenser takes 45 μL of DN32 media from the right chamber of the half module reservoir (Source P2) and places it into each well of a 384-well plate (Destination P3). Washing is carried out in two steps. The first step adds media to rows *A*, *C*, *E*, *G*, *I*, *K*, *M*, and *O*. The second step will carry out transfer of lipids from rows *B*, *D*, *F*, *H*, *J*, *L*, and *N*

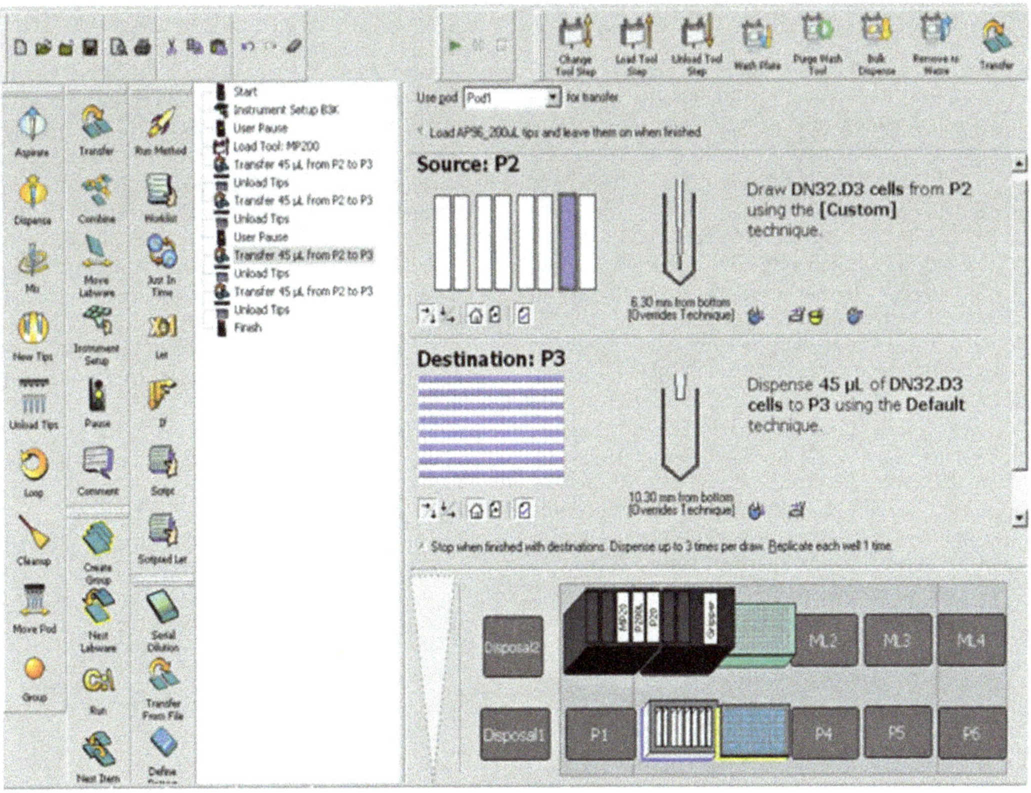

Fig. 6 Addition of DN32.D3 cells. DN32.D3 cells were placed in the left chamber of the half module reservoir (Source P2) and 45 µL dispensed in each well of a 384-well plate (Destination P3). This dispensing of cells is also carried out in two steps. The first step adds media to rows *A*, *C*, *E*, *G*, *I*, *K*, *M*, and *O*. The second step will carry out transfer of lipids from rows *B*, *D*, *F*, *H*, *J*, *L*, and *N*

References

1. Amprey JL, Im JS, Turco SJ, Murray HW, Illarionov PA, Besra GS, Porcelli SA, Späth GF (2004) A subset of liver NK T cells is activated during Leishmania donovani infection by CD1d-bound lipophosphoglycan. J Exp Med 200(7):895–904
2. Rhost S, Löfbom L, Rynmark BM, Pei B, Månsson JE, Teneberg S, Blomqvist M, Cardell SL (2012) Identification of novel glycolipid ligands activating a sulfatide-reactive, CD1d-restricted, type II natural killer T lymphocyte. Eur J Immunol 42(11):2851–2860
3. O'Konek JJ, Illarionov P, Khursigara DS, Ambrosino E, Izhak L, Castillo BF 2nd, Raju R, Khalili M, Kim HY, Howell AR, Besra GS, Porcelli SA, Berzofsky JA, Terabe M (2011) Mouse and human iNKT cell agonist β-mannosylceramide reveals a distinct mechanism of tumor immunity. J Clin Invest 121(2):683–694
4. Mirotti L, Florsheim E, Rundqvist L, Larsson G, Spinozzi F, Leite-de-Moraes M, Russo M, Alcocer M (2013) Lipids are required for the development of Brazil nut allergy: the role of mouse and human iNKT cells. Allergy 68(1):74–83
5. Bashir ME, Lui JH, Palnivelu R, Naclerio RM, Preuss D (2013) Pollen lipidomics: lipid profiling exposes a notable diversity in 22 allergenic pollen and potential biomarkers of the allergic immune response. PLoS One 8(2):e57566
6. Stangegaard M, Meijer PJ, Børsting C, Hansen AJ, Morling N (2012) Biomek 3000: the workhorse in an automated accredited forensic genetic laboratory. J Lab Autom 17(5):378–386
7. Jacques P, Venken K, Van Beneden K, Hammad H, Seeuws S, Drennan MB, Deforce D, Verbruggen G, Apostolaki M, Kollias G, Lambrecht BN, De Vos M, Elewaut D (2010) Invariant natural killer T cells are natural regulators of murine spondylarthritis. Arthritis Rheum 62(4):988–999

Chapter 20

Recent Advances in the Detection of Allergens in Foods

Silvia de la Cruz, Inés López-Calleja, Rosario Martín, Isabel González, Marcos Alcocer, and Teresa García

Abstract

Food allergy is a public health issue that has significantly increased worldwide in the past decade affecting consumers' quality of life and making increasing demands on health service resources. Despite recent advances in many areas of diagnosis and treatment, our general knowledge of the basic mechanisms of the disease remained limited, i.e., not at pace with the exponential number of new cases and the explosion of the new technologies. For sensitized individuals, the only effective way to prevent allergic reactions is the strict avoidance of the offending food. For this reason, a number of regulatory bodies in several countries have recognized the importance of providing information about the presence of food allergens by enacting laws, regulations, or standards for food labeling of "priority allergens." This has resulted in the need for the development of analytical methods for protection of food-allergic consumers that should be among others highly specific, sensitive, and not influenced by the presence of the food matrix components. Several analytical approaches target either the allergen itself or a corresponding allergen marker such as peptide fragment or gene segment and have been used in the detection and quantification of allergens in food products. In this short review, some of the conventional and new methods for the detection of allergens in food are listed and briefly discussed.

Key words Food allergy, Allergens, Sensitization, Analytical methods, ELISA, Mass spectrometry

1 Introduction

Food allergy is a public health issue that has significantly increased worldwide in the past decade, affecting consumers' quality of life and making increasing demands on health service resources [1–3]. The statistics vary but according to the EAACI 2015 report approximately 17 million people in Europe are suffering from food-related allergies and critical hospital admission for children has increased by sevenfolds within the past 10 years. Food allergy affects around 2–4% of the population peaking at 6–8% at 1 year of age and declining gradually to 2–4% in older children and adults [4–6].

This decline reflects the fact that many infants grow out of their food allergies as they age. The rate and probability of resolution varies significantly among specific foods. Frequently,

Jing Lin and Marcos Alcocer (eds.), Food Allergens: Methods and Protocols, Methods in Molecular Biology, vol. 1592, DOI 10.1007/978-1-4939-6925-8_20, © Springer Science+Business Media LLC 2017

egg, milk, wheat, and soy allergies resolve relatively early in life, whereas allergies to peanuts, tree nuts, sesame seeds, fish, crustacean shellfish, and buckwheat are likely to persist. Truthfully, to this day, it remains unclear why some children or adults achieve natural tolerance and others do not. The estimated rates of resolution also vary among studies for any specific food and only contributing resolution factors such as sensitization to multiple food allergens, high allergen-specific IgE antibody levels, a history of anaphylaxis, atopic dermatitis, and particular IgE-binding patterns for food allergies.

The degree and type of childhood food allergy, in particular, is an evolving public health problem that appears to have risen rapidly in industrialized countries. However, although it is estimated that 10–15% of children report symptoms of food allergy, the actual prevalence of IgE-mediated food allergies (i.e., symptoms of food allergy in the context of a positive skin prick test) is reported to be much lower at approximately 6–8% in children less than 3 years old [4, 5]. By contrast, not much is known about the prevalence of non-IgE-mediated food allergies, although both eosinophilic esophagitis and celiac disease have been documented to be increasing. Despite the increasing number of studies mounted to investigate the rise of both allergic diseases in general and food allergy in particular, the causes behind the putative epidemic of food allergy remain elusive. In general terms it is estimated that about a quarter of the population will have an adverse reaction to food (of which food allergy is just one type) during their lifetime, most of which will occur during infancy and early childhood.

Regarding the type of food involved and despite the geographical variations attributed to differences in environmental or individual factors, it is observed that 75% of allergic reactions among children are linked to a limited number of foods, which include egg, peanut, cow's milk, fish, and various nuts. Conversely in adults, fruits of the latex group (e.g., kiwi, banana), fruits of the Rosaceae family (e.g., apples, pears, prunes), vegetables of the Apiaceae family (e.g., carrot, celery), and various nuts and peanuts are responsible for 50% of allergic reactions [7–9].

1.1 Clinical Symptoms

IgE-mediated allergic reactions to food are represented by well-defined clinical features. These allergic reactions may manifest as a variety of signs and symptoms that can involve the digestive, respiratory, cardiovascular, or cutaneous organ systems [10]. Reaction severity varies from mild (skin rashes, itchy nose and eyes, sneezing, wheezing, coughing, itchy lips and mouth, nausea, cramp, bloating, vomiting, and diarrhea) to severe (such as systemic shock). Reactions involving multiple organ systems are generally called anaphylaxis. Fortunately, most allergic reactions to food are relatively mild but in very rare cases allergic reactions can be fatal. Reaction severity depends on the age, sensitivity of the individual, the level of exposure (amount of food consumed), and modifying factors such as the presence of other conditions (e.g., uncontrolled asthma) or the use of medications such as steroids or antihistamines. Clinical studies have shown that the range of sensitivity in the allergic population can encompass many orders of magnitude [11, 12]. This means that the same exposure might result in a mild reaction in one individual, a severe reaction in another, and death in a third.

1.2 What Defines an Allergen?

In general terms, food allergy can be defined as an immune-mediated sensitivity to food proteins [10]. It is essentially "immunity gone wrong" where normally harmless substances (food allergens) are perceived as a threat and acted upon by the body's immunological defenses. In a type I hypersensitivity reaction the adaptive immune system responds by producing IgE antibodies against the allergens. It is a two-step process where the capacity to respond through an allergic reaction when exposed to the particular allergen must be first established. This induces the immune system to generate specific IgE antibodies against the allergen in a so-called induction phase, or sensitization. Once sensitized to a particular allergen, the individual may develop a symptomatic allergic reaction when exposed again to the allergen in question in a provocation or later triggering phase [13].

Interestingly what defines a major allergen is still largely unknown. More importantly, the intrinsic factors that differentiate a common everyday food protein from a fatal allergen to a particular group of patients remain largely unknown. Despite attempts by a large number of groups to define the basic intrinsic characteristics of an allergenic protein, only two mechanisms, both described in the *Dermatophagoides pteronyssinus* (house dust mite), are currently known: a protease-dependent (Der p 1) and a protease-independent one (Der p 2). In the former, Der p 1 protease activity has been shown to cleave CD23, CD25, and CD40, inhibiting IL-12 secretion with the possible activation of the PAR family of G coupled proteins in the process [14]. In the latter mechanism, it has been elegantly shown that Der p 2 structurally mimics MD2, a component of the TLR4 complex that can coopt other signaling components to activate its target cells [15]. Hence, the involvement of complex lipids and Toll receptors has been clearly demonstrated. However, as most of the well-characterized allergens are not proteases and it is unlikely that MD2 homology could be a general mechanism for allergenicity these suggest that other mechanisms certainly exist [16].

This means that current understanding of the molecular mechanisms underlying the development of IgE responses is incomplete and as a result any risk assessment regarding allergenicity has to rely on historic evidences. Factors such as the age when the initial sensitization occurred, genetic susceptibility, environmental factors including geographic distribution, exposure route, type of food,

food matrixes, adjuvants among many others should be considered. As a consequence of this complexity decision-tree approaches have been proposed to facilitate the allergenicity assessment (ILSI and its revised version proposed by a joint FAO/WHO committee) [17]. The criticism and limitations of the different approaches currently used in the assessment of allergenicity are beyond the scope of this article; however, it should be noted that even the now ethically challenging and expensive animal experiments have shown not to mimic the ability of humans to become sensitized, hence alternative methodologies are sought.

1.3 Processing and Threshold

Cooking and food processing as a whole can affect the ability of the food components to trigger a reaction in an unpredictable manner. Nevertheless, information on minimal eliciting doses for various food allergens has emerged in recent years. The minimum allergen concentration to trigger an allergic reaction or threshold for hazelnut, for example, is about 30 μg of the nut [18] with values of 0.07 μg for milk, 0.003 μg for egg, 0.5 μg for peanut, and 0.3 mg for soybean [19]. However, due to the large differences in threshold values between individuals, a universal figure for the maximum concentration of an allergen within a food has yet not been determined since trace amounts of allergens can induce severe and even fatal reactions in sensitive patients. While there is interest by several stakeholder groups (i.e., food industry, regulatory agencies, allergic consumers, and clinicians) on threshold information, many countries' regulatory agencies have not yet got them implemented [12]. As there is so much uncertainty regarding each individual, any exposure to protein from a food allergen is considered to be of public health significance; hence, the food industry is tasked with essentially a zero threshold level of allergenic residue. This is operationally impossible given the complexity of manufacturing facilities and the numerous routes of allergen contamination and cross contact that can occur throughout the supply chain.

1.4 Legislation

The availability of information about the presence of allergenic food ingredients that are intentionally used in a food product has improved significantly in the last 15 years. Initially, a list of priority allergens was developed by the Codex Alimentarius 1999 [20] and used as a starting point by the European Commission and other regulatory bodies [21]. Although more than 180 allergenic food proteins have been described to date, in practical terms and based on prevalence, severity, and potency, a relatively limited number of food components have been identified as allergens [21, 22]. The European Regulation (EU) 1169/2011/EC (OJEU, 2011) provides a list of 14 groups of allergenic food components that manufacturers are required to declare on their labels if the ingredients are present regardless of their quantity. The list includes gluten-containing cereals, crustaceans, eggs, fish, peanuts, soybeans, milk, nuts (almond, hazelnut, walnut, cashew, pecan nut, Brazil nut, pistachio nut and macadamia nut), celery, mustard, sesame seeds, lupine, and molluscs, and products thereof. In addition, sulfur dioxide/sulfites are also required to be labeled at levels >10 ppm as they can trigger asthma attacks in those who are sensitive to this ingredient, and have also been associated with anaphylaxis [23].

While declaration of ingredients derived from allergenic sources used as direct ingredients or processing aids has helped to provide allergic consumers with more transparent allergen information, labeling laws do not address the potential risk involved with undeclared or hidden allergens. Hidden allergens may be present in the food products as a result of their unintentional or undeclared presence in the raw materials used, and also due to cross-contamination produced in shared equipment (e.g., use of common equipment, improper production scheduling, or improper use of rework material), to the mixture of ingredients at the supply chain level, or to a fraudulent adulteration. Cross-contact can occasionally occur despite the food manufacturer's best efforts to remove the allergenic residue [24].

2 Introduction to Techniques

Several analytical approaches have been developed for the detection and quantification of allergens in food products. These techniques target either the protein allergen itself or a corresponding allergen marker (peptide fragment or gene segment). Due to the diverse nature of food allergens and the complexity of the respective food matrices, the choice of detection methods can be challenging at times. With the recent advances in molecular biology, biochip technology, mathematical modeling among others and access to large volume of information on genomics, genomic-associated studies, cell culture, cell engineering, microbiome, and many of the new omics, the whole diagnostic, therapeutic, and basic immunology area of food allergy is undergoing a large transformation. At the protein level allergens are mainly determined by antibody-based enzyme-linked immunosorbent assays (ELISA), protein biosensors, and mass spectrometry (MS) methods [25–27]. However, due to their thermo/mechanical and chemical instability protein-based methods are only applicable to raw or slightly processed food components [28]. In contrast, the higher stability of nucleic acids makes it possible to apply DNA-based methods to both raw and highly processed food. Most DNA-based methods involve amplification of the target sequence by PCR or real-time PCR [29, 30]. Analytical methods used for the detection of residues of allergenic foods must not only be highly specific, sensitive, and rugged enough to be applicable in food matrices but also reliable. Moreover, the testing methods should detect levels of contaminants at concentrations in low parts per million range (ppm). Within this context in the next paragraphs a brief description of the common techniques applied in the detection of allergens in food products is listed and discussed.

2.1 Protein-Based Techniques

2.1.1 Immunoassays

Immunoassays are a collection of techniques that utilize specific antibodies raised against a specific antigen. The antibodies normally employed in immunoassays are mainly of two categories: polyclonal, when antiserum comprises immunoglobulins secreted by different B cell clones that recognize different epitopes, or monoclonal, if the immunoglobulins are secreted by clones of a single hybridized B cell and therefore react against a single epitope. Polyclonal and monoclonal antibodies are principally raised in animals, and mainly fall into the IgG antibody class, although when produced in egg yolk they are designated IgY [11, 31, 32]. A different strategy aimed to overcome the downsides of traditional antibodies (variations among different batches, use of live animals, etc.) entails their replacement by recombinant antibodies, such as scFv and Fab as described in Chap. 9 in this volume. Recombinant antibody technology makes it possible to create libraries of antibody fragments derived from immune cells or synthetic libraries and to employ phage display technology for panning antibody fragments with the desirable affinity [33]. Antibodies can also be replaced by oligonucleotide aptamers, ligands selected from combinatorial libraries or peptide molecules that bind their targets with high affinity [34, 35]. Due to their high sensitivity and specificity, immunoassays are frequently used analytical methods for the detection of food allergens, providing an accurate analysis of the test sample. Among immunoassay methods, enzyme-linked immunosorbent assay (ELISA) and lateral-flow devices (LFD) are the most commonly used formats.

ELISA

The enzyme-linked immunosorbent assay (ELISA) is the most widespread technique employed in industries and official food control agencies for the detection of allergenic ingredients in food products. It is reasonably quick, reliable, user-friendly and does not require special equipment allowing the simultaneous analysis of several samples [32, 36–38]. Several companies have developed commercial test kits that have become very popular for the food industry (Table 1). As described in Chap. 8 one of the main issues with ELISAs relates to the efficiency of the extraction methods. It has been demonstrated that certain food matrix components can inhibit the extraction of proteins or interfere on the detection of the analytes. To optimize the extractability of allergens, the use of extraction additives such as fish gelatin, skim milk powder, bovine serum albumin, is advisable [39]. ELISA methods employed in food industry are usually presented in a sandwich format. In this design, a capture antibody aimed to retain the antigens present in

Table 1
Commercial ELISA kits for detection of food allergens

	Company name									
ELISA	**ELISA Technologies**	**BioCheck**	**Crystal Chem**	**BioFront**	**ELISA Systems**	**Morinagra**	**Neogen**	**R-biofarm**	**Romer Labs**	**Elution technologies**
Targets	Gluten Lupin	b-Lactoglobulin Almond Casein Cashew Crustacean Egg Fish Hazelnut Lupin Milk Mustard Peanut Pistachio Sesame Soya Walnut	β-Lactoglobulin Buckwheat Casein Gliadin/gluten Egg Peanut	Almond Cashew Hazelnut Peanut Pecan Pistachio	Almond β-Lactoglobulin Buckwheat Casein Crustacean Hazelnut Mustard Peanut Sesame Soy Gliadin Lupin	β-Lactoglobulin Buckwheat Casein Peanut Ovalbumin	Almond β-Lactoglobulin Casein Crustacea Egg Gliadin/gluten Hazelnut Lupine Milk Mustard Peanut Sesame Soy Walnut	Almond β-Lactoglogulin Casein Crustaceans Egg Gliadin/gluten Hazelnut Lysozyme Lupine Macadamia Milk Mustard Peanut Sesame Soy	Almond β-Lactoglobulin Casein Cashew Crustaceans Egg white Fish Gluten Hazelnut Lupin Lysozyme Milk Mustard Ovalbumin Peanut Pistachio Sesame Soy Walnut	Almond Brazil nut Casein Cashew Coconut Crustaceans Egg Fish Macadamia Milk Mollusk Mustard Peanut Pecan Pine nut Sesame Soy Walnut

the sample is coating the plate surface. Captured antigens are later detected by a secondary antibody, which can be conjugated to an enzyme converting the substrate in a detectable product. However, when detecting small-size proteins, the preferred format is the competitive ELISA assay format where antigen is coated to a plate surface and the antibody is incubated with a diluted sample extract (inhibitor) before being added to the plate [31, 40]. ELISA results can be affected by cross-reactivity problems; thus positive ELISA results might require a confirmatory analysis by a non-immunological technique to corroborate data and to improve detection specificity [41].

Lateral Flow Devices (LFD)

LFD are fast and easy-to-use immunoassays test employed routinely in food industries (Table 2). They consist of a membrane strip with a sample pad on which a liquid sample containing antibodies or antigens is applied. Their major advantage is that they do not require specific instrumentation, but they solely determine the presence or absence of the target, not being suited to quantification of the amount of analyte present in the sample [31, 42]. Similar to ELISA lateral LFD are presented in two different formats: sandwich and competitive. Sandwich LFD is the most widespread design in food allergen testing where the sample is loaded into a membrane strip containing the specific antibodies against the target that remain unbound to the membrane. The detection

Table 2
Commercial ELISA kits for detection of food allergens

	Company name			
LFD	**Crystal Chem**	**R-biofarm**	**Romer Labs**	**Elution technologies**
Targets	Casein Gliadin/gluten Egg	Almond Brazil nut Cashew Coconut Crustaceans Egg Lysozyme Gliadin/gluten Hazelnut Macadamia nut Milk Mustard Peanut Pistachio Sesame Walnut	Almond β-lactoglobulin Brazil nut Casein Cashew/pistachio Coconut Crustaceans Egg Hazelnut Lupin Macadamia Mustard Peanut Sesame Soy Milk Walnut	Almond Cashew Coconut Egg Fish Gluten Milk Peanut Pecan Pistachio Soy Walnut

antibodies are labeled with colored particles (latex or gold nanoparticles), enzymes, or fluorescent molecules. In competitive LFD format, the analyte is attached to an antibody or protein that is labeled with latex or a colloidal metal (detection reagent). After loading the sample, the detection reagent and the sample containing the target molecule will wick onto the membrane; they will reach the test line region containing the capture antibodies (immobilized antibodies against the target analyte), which will capture some of the analytes and some of the detection reagents. The more analyte present in the sample (that is unlabeled), the more will compete with the limited amount of labeled particles comprising the detection reagent. The test line will appear as a colored band in samples not containing target molecules. The control line will appear as a band as the labeled antibody is captured by an antibody that is specific for the labeled antibody.

2.1.2 Protein Biosensors

Biosensors provide a novel approach for the detection of allergenic ingredients in food products [43]. They can be small portable real-time devices that may be used for on-site analyses. By the immobilization of a sensor onto a chip surface, whether it is an antibody recognizing the allergenic protein, a specific DNA fragment encoding for an allergen recognizing a complimentary strand or an aptamer selected to bind the specific allergen, the binding interaction between the two can be measured quantitatively. Biosensors consist of a sensing component of biological origin for selective detection of target, and a receptor-transducer analytical device that transforms the interaction into a measurable chemical-physical signal proportional to the target concentration [44]. According to the physical change accompanying the reaction, biosensors can be classified into optical and electrochemical types.

Optical biosensors detect changes in light absorption when the analyte is recognized by the receptor, or differences in light output as a result of a luminescent process. Many optical biosensors are based on surface-plasmon resonance (SPR), which exploits the changes in the refractive index close to a sensor surface. SPR biosensors have been applied in several food allergen detection methods. Pollet et al. [26] reported a fiber optic SPR biosensor that employed paramagnetic nanoparticles coupled to Ara h1 antibodies that allowed amplifying SPR signals when detecting Ara h1 peanut allergen. Billakanti and coworkers [45] presented a SPR technology for the simultaneous quantitative determination of five whey proteins employing antibodies immobilized on a GLC biosensor chip (Bio-Rad Laboratories). The instrument employed was a ProteOn XPR36 protein interaction array system (Bio-Rad Laboratories, CA, USA). Rebe Raz et al. [46] employed an angle scanning imaging SPR in combination with antibody array to rapidly quantify 13 major food allergens in foodstuffs. Studies that employ optical biosensors different to SPR are also described in the literature. Yman et al. [47] developed an optical biosensor for both direct and sandwich immunoassays detection of proteins from milk, egg, hazelnut, peanut, shellfish, and sesame in food samples. Godoy-Navajas and coworkers [48] developed a long-wavelength fluoroimmunoassay to determine the presence of soy proteins in food samples employing nile blue-doped silica nanoparticles. Furthermore, an assay for the simultaneous identification of eight food allergens (soybean, wheat, peanut, cashew, shrimp, fish, beef, and chicken) by employing silicon-based optical thin-film biosensor chip was reported by Wang et al. [49]. As the method allowed appreciating the change in color by the naked eye, there was not need of sophisticated equipment.

Electrochemical biosensors provide analytical information using a biological-recognition element (biochemical receptor), which is retained in direct spatial contact with an electrochemical transduction element. Electrochemical biosensors can be classified into potentiometric, amperometric, voltammetric, and impedance types, according to the mode of physico-chemical signal transduction. Cao et al. [50] determined the presence of casein through differential pulse voltammetry employing an immunosensor based on anti-casein antibody immobilized on a composite film based on gold nanoparticles and poly (l-Arginine)/multi-walled carbon nanotubes. Eissa and coworkers [51] developed a label-free voltammetric immunosensor to detect β-lactoglobulin employing graphene-modified screen-printed electrodes. Yang and coworkers [52] reported a concanavalin A-based electrochemical biosensor for the detection of chicken ovomucoid based on self-assembled ZnO quantum dots. Jiang and coworkers [53] developed a cell-based electrochemical biosensor to quantify Pen a1 shrimp allergen. To that end, mast cells were immobilized on l-cysteine/gold nanoparticle-modified gold electrodes. Immobilizing a monoclonal antibody on a gold electrode, Huang and coworkers [54] developed an impedance biosensor aimed to detect peanut allergenic protein Ara h1. They also described an electrochemical biosensor in which gold electrode is replaced by a degenerate Si electrode [55]. Singh and coworkers [56] reported a nanopore biosensor to detect peanut protein Ara h1, which is constructed by immobilizing an antibody within gold-coated pores of commercial nanoporous polycarbonate membranes. As the pores are obscured by the antibody-antigen complexes, electrolyte conductivity within the membrane decreases.

Electromechanical biosensors or quartz crystal microbalance (QCM) biosensors, the biological-recognition event generates a mass change of the sensing layer, giving rise to a change in the resonant frequency of the microbalance. The application commonly requires the immobilization of antibodies or DNA fragments on the transducer surface. Xiulan et al. [57] developed a QCM-based immunosensor aimed to determine the presence of shrimp allergen in food. Antibodies against shrimp were attached onto the crystal surface via a nanogold-modified composite film. The presence of the antigen bound to the antibody will induce a change in the frequency proportional to the concentration of the binding antigen. Chu and coworkers [58] described a QCM biosensor for the detection of gliadin in foods. The incorporation of gold nanoparticles increased by 48% the shift in the frequency of the biosensor in the detection of 2 ppm gliadin.

2.1.3 LC-Mass Spectrometry Techniques

Mass spectrometry (MS) is an analytical technique employed in food allergy research to obtain structural and functional information about food allergens, and it also serves as a non-immunological method to detect the presence of allergens in foodstuff. MS serves as a non-immunological method for fast, accurate, and sensitive analysis of traces of food allergens. The term "allergenomics" has been coined to define the application of proteomic technologies to the analysis of food allergens [59, 60]. The most widely employed soft-ionization techniques in use are matrix-assisted laser desorption ionization (MALDI) and electrospray ionization (ESI). MS is usually coupled with separation techniques as 2D PAGE, or liquid chromatography (LC), which enables the analysis of proteins or its peptides with high sensitivity and specificity. 2D PAGE allows the simultaneous separation of a large number of proteins according to their isoelectric point and their molecular weight. Protein spots are excised from the gel, digested with trypsin, and identified by MS or tandem mass spectrometry (MS/MS). MS identifies the protein by peptide mass fingerprint, providing evidence for the most probable identity of the protein, whereas MS/MS analysis offers structural information of the molecule (amino acid sequence of detected peptides), making the search highly specific and discriminating [32, 61, 62]. This methodology is known as the bottom-up approach. An alternative strategy, known as top-down proteomics implies the introduction of the intact protein into the mass spectrometer to measure the intact and fragment ions masses. This approach allows the full characterization of proteoforms (highly related protein molecules arising from all combinatorial sources of variation giving rise to products arising from a single gene). The latter approach is nowadays possible due to the high mass accuracy of new high-resolution mass spectrometers [63–65]. On the other hand, shotgun proteomics employs liquid chromatography (LC) coupled to MS analysis as an alternative to electrophoretic methods to separate proteins. In such an approach, the entire protein extract is digested by trypsin before being separated by LC (usually reverse-phase chromatography (RP))-ESI (electrospray ionization)-MS/MS. Liquid-phase separation method has higher analytical dynamic range, thus allowing the detection of low-abundance components—which becomes very useful when detecting traces of food allergens—but its resolution is limited compared to 2D–PAGE [66–68].

Therefore, to separate highly complex peptide mixtures, multidimensional identification (MultiID) technology is the preferred option, as it offers good resolution and peak capacity. The most common combination is strong cation-exchange resin coupled with reverse-phase LC (RPLC), but other formats employed included size-exclusion chromatography (SEC) with RPLC, and RPLC with capillary electrophoresis (CE). Recent advances in MultiID include peptide separation by ultra-high pressure LC (UHPLC) and anion-and-cation mixed-bed ion-exchange techniques [69, 70].

Capillary-liquid chromatography (CLC) and nano-LC are miniaturized techniques with great potential in the analytical field. Nano-LC employs capillaries with an internal diameter (ID) lesser than 100 μm and flow rates of 50–800 nL/min, whereas in CLC capillaries with an I.D. of 100–320 μm and flow rates of 1–100 μL/min are used. The reduction of column ID translates in shorter times of analysis, lower consumption of mobile phase, and easier coupling with MS because of the lower flow rates when comparing it with conventional LC. It also increases mass sensitivity due to the reduction of the mobile-phase flow responsible for the decrease in sample dilution. However, low I.D capillaries require a reduction in extra-column effects that can affect the efficiency of the technique. Considering the injected volumes, the sensitivity of the technique can be questionable for practical purposes. To solve this problem, it has been proposed the use of more sensitive detectors and/or applying sample pre-concentration (off-and on-column) [71].

When working with MS techniques, it must be taken into account that the quality of the protein identification will depend upon the quality of the mass spectrometry data, the accuracy of the database, and the power of the search algorithms and software used. Some examples of MS application in food allergen detection are stated below: Weber and coworkers [72] employed a CLC-Q-TOF MS/MS to detect αS1-casein in spiked foods, employing as a marker the casein peptide *m/z* 634.3. Monaci and coworkers [69] developed a CLC-ESI-MS/MS method for the detection of α and β-casein derived peptides in fined white wine, in which four specific peptide ions (*m/z* 742.2, 729.2, 634.2, and 692.6) could be identified by CLC-ESI-MS/MS analysis followed by bioinformatics search. They described a LOD 50 μg/mL for caseinate added to wine, when the *m/z* 742.2 ion is used as a caseinate marker. In Monaci et al. [73], they described the detection of milk protein and caseinates in two commodities (cookies and white wine) using a RP-LC separation coupled to an ion-trap mass spectrophotometer. Heick and coworkers [74] developed a LC-MS/MS method for the simultaneous detection of seven allergenic foods (milk, egg, soy, peanut, hazelnut, walnut, and almond) in processed and unprocessed samples. The influence of the baking process was assessed, and the results were compared to those obtained with commercially available ELISA kits. The MS method showed superior detection capability for the processed samples when comparing its results to those obtained with commercially available ELISA kits, with the advantage of its capability of multiplexing.

In order to identify peptide markers of the allergenic proteins of peanut taking their thermal stability into account, Chassaigne and coworkers [75] described a CLC method combined with Q-TOF MS/MS. They defined two specific markers for the allergenic protein Ara h 1 (VLEENAGGEQEER (*m/z* 786.88, charge 2+)) and DLAFPGSGEQVEK (*m/z* 688.85, charge 2+), one for the Ara h 2 ((RQQWELQGDR (*m/z* 439.23, charge 3+)) and two for the Ara h 3 (peptides, SPDIYNPQAGSLK (*m/z* 695.35, charge 2+) and SQSENFEYVAFK (*m/z* 724.84, charge 2+). Pedreschi et al. [67] employed shotgun proteomics to detect the presence of the proteotypic Ara h 3/4 marker peptides AHVQVVDSNGNR (*m/z* 432.5, 3+) and SPDIYNPQAGSLK (*m/z* 695.4, 2+) in baked cookies, employing as the representative food allergen source the standard IRMM-481 f. Mattarozzi et al. [66] described a sensitive and selective LC-ESI-MS/MS method to detect and quantify lupine's allergens (conglutins) in pasta and biscuits.

Undoubtedly, MS methods are a powerful tool to be employed in food allergen detection, overcoming the problems encountered with immunological techniques due to lack of detection of allergens after food-processing treatments that cause structural changes of proteins. However, their application requires the use of expensive equipment with high maintenance costs, and it needs to be operated by highly trained personnel. Therefore, at the present, MS methods cannot be employed as a routine analysis to trace the presence of food allergens, but can used as an auxiliary method to confirm the results obtained with less expensive assays platforms routinely employed in food industry.

2.2 DNA-based techniques

Methodologies based on genetics and molecular biology have become an interesting approach for tracking down the presence of trace amounts of allergens at any stage along the food supply chain [76, 77]. DNA-based technology is a relatively new approach for the detection of food allergens, a field traditionally dominated by immunoassays. DNA assays have been used for food authentication, including speciation, and for the detection of products of agricultural biotechnology to ensure label accuracy and compliance with regulations. DNA methods are indirect methods to detect food allergens as they do not detect the allergenic protein itself, but the DNA sequences in the allergenic food. Usually, DNA methods are based on the amplification of specific DNA fragments either by means of end point PCR, which offers a qualitative result (i.e., it detects the presence of a specific DNA sequence), or by real-time PCR, which gives a quantitative account. In this sense, the polymerase chain reaction (PCR), together with real-time PCR, can be a valuable tool to indicate the presence or absence of a particular allergen in food (below a concentration of 10 ppm). These DNA-based analytical methods are rapid, sensitive, and provide specific detection of the targeted DNA. The targeted DNA sequences are not necessarily located in the genes encoding for the allergenic protein, and thus the analysis detects genomic DNA of the offending ingredient, but does not necessarily indicate the presence of the protein that is responsible for the allergic response [78].

Advantages of DNA-based methods over protein-based methodologies rely in that the target DNA is efficiently extracted from raw and cooked products and is not affected by the heating process, because DNA typically remains intact after being exposed to the cooking temperatures of most foods. Although some components from food matrix may interfere with the PCR or real-time PCR assay, and therefore lower the amplification efficiency, PCR inhibitors can be removed during DNA extraction and purification steps with the help of suitable DNA clean-up procedures [79]. Quantification of allergens, either by immunological or by DNA-based methods, is a challenging problem, mainly due to the unavailability of certified reference materials (CRMs). Certified reference materials (CRMs) are materials or substances whose property values are sufficiently homogenous and well established to be used for method development and validation, or for proof of method performance, and possess certificate and traceable assigned values (to an international system, method or artifact). The use of these CRMs has in general contributed to facilitate compliance with food labeling laws and to improve the accuracy of analytical methods.

However, there is a current lack of reference materials for the development of allergen detection methods, which has prompted the scientific community to proactively working at this regard. Up to date, only a CRM has been developed for the detection of food allergens, and only for peanuts (Reference samples supplied by the Institute for Reference Materials and Measurements of the European Commission's Joint Research Centre, Belgium). Several research networks are currently involved in the production of food allergen reference materials, like egg powder and skimmed milk powder provided by NIST [28]. Even though reference materials are commercially available for the most important food allergens, the results obtained may not be comparable as these are not certified.

2.2.1 PCR and Real-Time PCR

A high number of PCR assays have been published for the detection of allergen residues in raw ingredients, and processed products (Table 3). PCR-based methods to detect DNA from an allergenic source in a food product consist of three steps:

1. DNA extraction and purification.
2. Amplification of specific DNA sequence(s).
3. Detection of the amplified DNA.

Table 3
Published DNA-based methods for detection of food allergens [RT-PCR (real-time PCR) NR (not reported)]

Allergen	Method	Target gene	LOD	Food matrices tested	Reference
Peanut	PCR	*trnL (chloroplast tRNA)*	NR	Peanut	[117]
		Peanut agglutinin precursor	10 ppm peanut DNA in wheat DNA samples	Tree nuts, soybean, potato, corn, rice, wheat, meats, fish, commercial foods	[118]
	RT-PCR	*Arah2*	2 ppm peanut in biscuit	Tree nuts, meat, fish, seeds, biscuits, chocolate, cake, pastry, sausage	[119]
		Arah2	<10 ppm peanut	Cereal bars, chocolates, cookies, pudding	[120]
		Arah3	<2.5 pg peanut DNA or 10 ppm peanut in food	Cereals, legumes (soy, lupine), tree nuts, meat, seeds, cookies	[121]
		Arah2 (1) *ITS (2)*	10 ppm (1)/0.1 ppm (2)	Tree nuts, seeds, meat, plants, commercial food products	[89]
Almond	RT-PCR	*Pru1*	NR	Cookies	[91]
		ITS1	0.1 ppm	Commercial food products	[122]
Hazelnut	PCR-ELISA	*Cor a 1.0401*	<10 ppm hazelnut	Food and food ingredients	[123]
	PCR-HPLC	*Cora1*	5 pg hazelnut DNA	Breakfast cereals, chocolate, biscuits, snacks	[124]
	PCR	*Cora1*	10 ppm	Chocolates, snacks, muesli	[125]
		Nad1	10 ppm in chocolate	Chocolate	[126]
	RT-PCR	*Cor a 1.04*	0.1 ng DNA	Seed, fruits, chocolate, hazelnut creams, biscuits, cornflakes, snacks	[127]
		Hsp1	13 pg DNA, 100 ppm hazelnut in model pastry	Confectionery and bakery products	[128]
		Cora8	10 ppm	Commercial food products and bakery products	[129]
		ITS1	0.1 ppm	Tree nuts, seeds, meat, plants, commercial food products	[90]

(continued)

Table 3
(continued)

Allergen	Method	Target gene	LOD	Food matrices tested	Reference
Cashew nut	RT-PCR	*2S albumin*	5 pg cashew DNA, 100 ppm cashew in chocolate cookies	Chocolate chip cookies, fruit and nut bars, cereal, crackers, chocolate, granola	[81]
		2S albumin	25 pg cashew DNA, 100 ppm cashew in model pastry	Tree nuts, cereal flours, cocoa and milk powder, chocolate, breakfast cereals, snacks, biscuits, nougate	[130]
		Ana o3	2 ppm	Pesto	[98]
Pecan	RT-PCR	*Vicilin-gene*	1 pg pecan DNA, 100 ppm pecan in model pastry	Pecan, walnut, cereals, flours, potato starch, biscuits, chocolate, praline	[82]
Walnut	PCR-RFLP	*MatK*	10 ppm walnut	Walnut-containing food products	[131]
	RT-PCR	*Jur r 2*	0.24 ng walnut DNA, 100 ppm walnut in pastry samples	Bakery, confectionary	[85]
Walnut	RT-PCR	*Vicilin-gene*	10 ppm of walnut	Commercial food products	[132]
		Vicilim.gene	NR	Confectionery and bakery products	[133]
		Vicilin-gene	NR	Confectionery and bakery products	[134]
Walnut/ Pecan	RT-PCR	*ITS1*	0.1 ppm	Tree nuts, seeds, meat, plants, commercial food products	[88]
Pistachio	PCR	*Rbcl*	<100 mg/kg	Mortadella	[135]
	RT-PCR	*ITS*	4 ppm	Pastry	[136]
		ITS	0.1 ppm	Tree nuts, seeds, meat, plants, commercial food products	[87]
Macadamia	RT-PCR	*Vicilin-gene*	200 ppm	Confectionery and bakery products	[86]
Brazil nut	RT-PCR	*11S Globulin*	1000 ppm	Commercial food products	[84]
		2S albumin	5 ppm	Processed food products	[137]
		2S albumin *(Bere1)*	2.5 ppm	Commercial food products	[100]

Sesame	RT-PCR	*2S albumin*	5 pg DNA, 50 mg/kg	Breakfast cereals, crackers, chocolate, cookies, fruit bars	[138]
		Ses i 1	50 pg DNA sesame, 500 ppm sesame in bread	Chocolate, sesame oil, tahini, snacks, bread	[139]
		2S albumin	50 ppm (w/w) in spice and flour	Spice, flour	[140]
Soy	PCR + nested PCR	*le1 (lectin gene)*	10,000 ppm protein concentrate	Processed meat products	[141]
		trnL (chloroplast tRNA)	NR	Soybeans	[117]
		Gly m Bd 30K	100 ppm soy flour	Legumes, cakes, hamburgers, sausage	[142]
		SIRE-1	10 ppm soy flour	Fish, bread, soymilk, tofu, lecithin, soy sauce, seasoning, biscuits	[143]
		le1	2000 ppm soy flour, 10000 ppm soy protein isolate	Bread, flour	[144]
	RT-PCR	*Lecitin*	100 ppm	Meat products	[145]
Soy/ Hazelnut	RT-PCR	*Gly m Bd 28K/Cora1*	5–15 genome copies	Plant and tree nuts	[92]
Lupine	RT-PCR	*ITS1*	0.1 ppm	Legumes, seeds, nuts, spices, fruit, meat	[97]
Celery	PCR	*Manitol dehydrogenase gene*	490–1530 pg DNA, 1000 ppm celery in pat_e model	Meat pâte, seasoning, bouillon	[146]
	RT-PCR	*api g 1*	60 pg DNA (root), 30 pg (seed), 250 pg (powder)	Rinse solution after cleaning	[147]
		Manitol dehydrogenase gene	One DNA copy, 5–10 mg/kg celery seed	Sausage, seasoning, sauces, bouillon	[94]
		Manitol dehydrogenase gene	100–10 ppm celery powder	Meat, spice, flour, swab test	[140]

(continued)

Table 3
(continued)

Allergen	Method	Target gene	LOD	Food matrices tested	Reference
Mustard	RT-PCR	*sin a 1*	50 ppm in spice and flour	Spice, flour	[140]
	RT-PCR	*MADS D protein*	5 ppm	Meat products	[148]
Wheat	PCR +Nested PCR	*Triticin precursor*	500 ppm	Grains and processed food products	[149]
		Wheat gliadin	10–1000 ppm or 0.04–0.4 mg	Oat flake and kernels	[117]
		Triticin precursor	NR	Commercial processed foods	[150]
Wheat	RT-PCR	*Triticin precursor*	20 pg DNA/1.5 ppm	Commercial processed foods	[95]
Wheat and barley	RT-PCR	*w-Gliadin w-Secalin Hordein Avenin*	For four cereals, LOD; between 5 and 50 pg DNA or 0.1–100 ppm	Cereals, flours, bran, crunch, cookies, ice cream, pankcakes	[151]
Wheat, barley, rice, sunflower	RT-PCR	*Acetyl-CoA carboxylase RALyase g -Hordein*	Wheat and barley: LOD 1 genome copy, LOQ 10 genome copies	Cereal flours and cereal-based food products	[152]
Wheat, barley and rye	RT-PCR	*TrnL (chloroplast rRNA)*	20 pg DNA (wheat), 2 pg DNA (barley, rye)	Cereals, bread, baby food	[153]
Buckwheat	RT-PCR	*ITS1 5.8S rRNA region*	1 ppm buckwheat (w/w) <10 ppm buckwheat flour	Buckwheat, wheat	[96]
Fish: Three mackerel species	PCR	*5S rDNA NTS*	NR	No food matrix; raw fish	[154]
Mackerel	PCR	*Parvalbumin*	5 ng mackerel DNA	Surimi, fish paste	[155]
Crustaceans: shrimp, lobster, crab, crawfish	PCR-RFLP	*16S rRNA gene*	15–20 ng DNA, <1000 ppm shrimp in raw pork meat	Raw pork, shrimp cake	[156]

Multiplex					
Wheat, buckwheat	Duplex PCR	Tricitin precursor, Allergenic storage protein	NR	Japanese food products	[102]
Peanut, hazelnut, celery, soy, egg, milk, almond and sesame	Tetraplex PCR	*Arah2, cora1 gene, Mtd, Le1, 2S albumin, Pru1*	100 ppm	Tree nuts, soybean, sesame, milk, eggs, commercial food products	[101]
Peanut and hazelnut	Duplex PCR	*Cor a1 Ara h2*	50 pg in standard solution	Breakfast cereals, muesli snack, wafer chocolates, biscuits	[110]
Sesame/Hazelnut	Duplex RT-PCR	*Ses i 1/Cora1*	10 pg DNA sesame and hazelnut, 50 ppm in cookies	Commercial food products	[157]
Celery/White mustard	Duplex RT-PCR	*M6PR/MADS D protein*	50 ppm	Commercial food products	[158]
Pecan/Brazil nut	Duplex PCR	*Vicilin/Bere1*	1000 ppm	Commercial food products	[159]
MLPA					
Peanuts, cashews, pecans, pistachios, hazelnuts, sesame seeds, macadamia nuts, almonds, walnuts and brazil nuts.	LPA	*Arah2, anao3, Vicilin-gene, Bere1, Cor a gene*, CORA1.0401, 7S globulin mRNA, AMP2, extensin, sulfur-rich water-soluble seed protein	5 ppm	Tree nuts, soybean, sesame, milk, eggs, commercial food products	[104]

(continued)

Table 3
(continued)

Allergen	Method	Target gene	LOD	Food matrices tested	Reference
Sesame, soy, hazelnut, peanut, lupine, gluten, mustard, and celery.	LPA	*2S albumin, lectin (Le1), Cor a1, Arah2, ITS1, Glud1, SinA1, Apium graveolens*	10 ppm	Commercial food products	[105]
Lab on a chip					
Sesame/ celery	Lab on a Chip	*ITS*	1 ppm sesame/50 ppm celery	Plants, meat balls, soups	[160]

PCR methodology is an in vitro enzymatic synthesis of specific DNA sequences, which relies on the ability of *Taq* polymerase, an enzyme that catalyzes DNA-copying, to remain stable at high temperatures, and two carefully selected oligonucleotides that serve as primers for the reaction and hybridize to opposite strands that flank the region of interest in the target DNA. PCR relies in a repetitive series of thermal cycles (heating and cooling) involving template denaturation, primer annealing, and the extension of the annealed primers by DNA polymerase. This results in the exponential accumulation of a specific fragment which termini are defined by the 5′ ends of the primers. Thermal cycles are repeated 20–40 times. Because the primer extension products synthesized in one cycle can serve as a template in the next, the number of target DNA copies approximately doubles at every cycle amplifying the DNA of interest at a detectable level after 20–30 cycles.

The amplified product can be qualitatively visualized by staining after agarose gel electrophoresis, providing information on the size of the amplified product as is the case of the classical PCR reaction. The real-time PCR is a form of PCR where data are collected in "real time" as the reaction proceeds. Real-time PCR is a very sensitive technique, detecting down to a few molecules of target DNA. In contrast to classical PCR this method is based on fluorescence measurements to enable the visualization of PCR products during the amplified process. Real-time PCR has been the preferred approach for the quantitative analysis of specific DNA in a sample. In this technique, the reaction tube also contains a target-specific oligonucleotide probe together with a fluorescent reporter dye that has a quencher attached to it [80]. The detection of fluorescence is prevented by the proximity of the quencher to the dye. When the probe hybridizes to the amplified target DNA, the 5′ exonuclease activity of the polymerase cleaves the probe, thereby separating the quencher from the dye, which is displaced by the newly synthesized DNA strand. The newly synthesized DNA strand becomes soluble and the fluorescence of the free reporter dye can then be measured. An increase in fluorescence is proportional to the amount of target DNA present in the sample.

The advantage of real-time PCR over traditional PCR is the ability to quantify target DNA content in the sample. It provides a higher degree of specificity given by a fluorescent probe, which anneal in the sequence flanked by the two primers. It also reduces interferences due to the formation of primer dimers and nonspecific products [81]. Also, real-time PCR is less prone to contamination and is suitable for automation. Numerous assays based on real-time PCR have been developed and have proved effective for the detection of a wide range of traces of food allergens in raw materials and processed foods [82–98]. López-Calleja et al. [89] reported a real-time PCR based on the *Arah2* gene and *ITS* region for the detection of peanut with a LOD of 10 and 0.1 ppm, respectively. These same authors described a real-time PCR for the detection of hazelnut based on the *ITS1* region, which reached a detection limit of 0.1 ppm [90]. Also, de la Cruz et al. [100] reported a PCR assay based on *2S albumin gene* (*Ber e1*) for the detection of Brazil nut in commercial food products, achieving a limit of detection of 2.5 ppm. In addition to the conventional singleplex, PCR or real-time PCR reactions have the potential of simultaneously amplifying more than one analyte in a food matrix by using a multiplex format. This multiplex approach was recently demonstrated by Koppel et al. [101], who developed two tetraplex real-time PCR. In one multiplex reaction they detected simultaneously peanut, hazelnut, celery, and soy and in another they detected egg, milk, almond, and sesame with a LOD of 100 ppm. Also a multiplex PCR assay was developed by Hashimoto et al. [102] for the simultaneous detection of wheat, buckwheat, and peanut. This multiplex format has the advantages of saving time, costs and reducing probability of cross-contamination. However, it often decreases sensitivity of the assay, compared to singleplex PCR.

Although PCR-based methods require more expensive equipment than immune-based techniques, they have some key advantages over immunochemical methods [80]. Food processing can affect the conformation and solubility of proteins. Harsh extraction methods cannot typically be used since they could further affect antibody-binding epitopes. With DNA however, harsher extraction buffers can be used without affecting the detection of the target DNA. Amounts of DNA also tend to be more stable than protein levels, which can vary between various species or varieties. An additional advantage is that PCR-based tests are available for detection of DNA from a number of allergenic sources for which ELISA methods may not be available.

2.2.2 MLPA, Multiplex Ligation-Dependent Probe Amplification

A ligation-dependent probe amplification (LPA) is another DNA-based assay where adjacent ligation probes bind to the target and are ligated, resulting in ligation products of specific size for specific target DNA. The 5′ and 3′ ends of the ligation product contain a common sequence used as targets for a common set of primers, used for a PCR amplification of the ligation product. Further detection of the amplicons is carried out by capillary electrophoresis. This technique has been used successfully for the screening of multiple products within the same reaction [99, 103]. Ehlert et al. [104] described a multiplex ligation-dependent probe amplification (MLPA) method for the detection of different tree nuts (peanut, cashew, pecan, pistachio, hazelnut, macadamia nut, almond, walnut, and Brazil nut) and sesame seeds with a LOD of 5 ppm. Also, Mustorp et al. [105] developed a quantitative 10-plex competitive MLPA method for the detection of eight allergenic ingredients (sesame, soy, hazelnut, peanut, lupin, gluten, mustard, and celery) with a LOD of 10 ppm, depending on the allergenic ingredient. With allergen-MLPA, accurate quantitative results can be obtained. Although this DNA-based method does not detect the allergens as such, it shows many advantages, such as detecting a high number of targets simultaneously (multiplex format), providing quantitative specific, and sensitive results. Furthermore, this system is more flexible than real-time PCR, since it is modular and can therefore be easily adapted by removing or adding probe pairs for special purposes, as for example in those cases in which the number of targets (allergens) of interest increases.

2.2.3 DNA Biosensors

The detection of allergenic material in foods by using biosensor technology has been mainly limited to several antibody-based applications. However, biosensors have the potential to be developed also for DNA or PCR product detection. In this way, DNA-based biosensors, which are used for research rather than for routine analyses, are in increasing development. Sun et al. [106] developed an electrochemical DNA biosensor to detect peanut allergen Ara h1 in a peanut milk beverage with a LOD of 0.35 10–15 M. To this end, a 5′-SH and 3′-biotin dually labeled stem-loop probe was assembled on gold electrodes taking advantage of gold-thiol affinity. When the target was absent, the stem-probe was "closed," and after hybridizing with the target oligonucleotide, the conformation changed to "open." This change in stem-loop state modified the electron-transfer efficiency. Using a microfluidic-based platform (ImmuChip and ImmuSpeed, DiagnoSwiss S.A), Berti et al. [107] developed an enzyme-linked electrochemical genomagnetic assay to detect the presence of Cor a 1.04 allergen of hazelnut. The hybridization was performed on modified para magnetic micro-beads via sandwich hybridization with a capture probe and a biotinylated signaling probe. Quantitative allergen detection was determined based on enzymatic kinetics obtained after trapping the enzyme labeled biotinylated hybrid in a multichannel cartridge. Tortajada-Genaro et al. [108] developed a multiplexed DNA microarray method on a digital versatile disk (DVD) to simultaneously detect the presence of hazelnut, peanut, and soybean in foodstuffs. For that purpose, the surface of a DVD was printed with streptavidin and 5′-biotinylated probes that would hybridize with digoxin-labeled PCR products to be detected later on with a peroxidase-labeled digoxigenin antibody.

2.2.4 DNA Microarrays

The emerging micro technologies based on the use of microarrays have provided another possible tool for food allergen detection. A DNA Microarray also known as DNA chip or biochip is a very powerful tool for the simultaneous detection of multiple DNA sequences and multi-samples analysis. Microarrays based on oligonucleotides [109] or their analogues complementary to the DNA of several allergens have been developed [110], but few are commercially available. The specific probes are immobilized on a solid surface by different techniques and recognize the complementary fluorescently labeled PCR amplicons. Probe-target hybridization is usually detected and quantified by the detection of fluorophore, silver-, or chemiluminescence-labeled targets to determine the nucleic acid sequences present in the target. The resulting fluorescent spots are further read with a fluorescence scanner at the proper wavelength. The method is qualitative and useful for a rapid screening.

2.2.5 Commercial DNA-Based Test Kits

The majority of kits commercially available for routine food allergen analysis rely on immunological methods, while the number of companies offering PCR/real-time PCR kits (*R-Biopharm, 4labdiagnostics, Biotecon, Innosieve, Kogene, and Gen-ial GmbH*) is rather limited, probably because its use for the detection of food allergens is yet not as widely accepted. However, whenever ELISA kits are not available or not specific for the analysis of a particular specific allergenic ingredient, PCR-based kits become the method of election. These commercial DNA-based methods include both PCR and real-time PCR, which are used as qualitative and semiquantitative tests respectively allowing in many cases multiplexed analysis. All the kits have LOD values around or below 10 ppm of the allergenic food in the sample, although this value is matrix dependent. The quantitative analysis of PCR-based kits depends on the availability of reference materials and on the knowledge of the genomic sequences. Standard materials are provided together with the commercially available kits or are produced "in house." Among the different DNA-based commercial kits available at the moment, there are several real-time PCR kits provided by different suppliers for the detection of the following allergens: peanut, soy, lupine, almond, hazelnut, walnut, crustaceans, molluscs, sesame, celery, mustard, and gluten-containing cereals (wheat, rye, barley, and kamut), egg, fish, and milk (Table 4). However, up to date only one kit for peanuts provided by *Tepnel* has obtained the approval of full validated method by AOAC International. It should be noticed that the kits used for a collective group of allergens provide positive results across the different species belonging to the group. For example, the kit for fish is able to detect a large number of commercial fish species, and the kit for molluscs allows the detection of snails, mussels, and cephalopods. However, these kits are not designed to identify individual species.

Among the different DNA-based test kits, PCR kits are available in different formats, and real-time PCR kits are the most common. They generally contain an allergen reaction mix, an inhibition control (spike), a positive control, *Taq* polymerase and a fluorescence detection enhancer, which are sufficient for approximately 100 target DNA-specific reactions and 100 inhibition controls. The inhibition reactions help to minimize possible false-negative

Table 4
Commercial real-time PCR kits for detection of food allergens

	Company name					
	R-Biopharm	4labdiagnostics	Biotecon diagnistics	Innosieve diagnostics	Kogene	Gen-ial GmbH
Targets	Celery	Celery	Celery	Celery	Crustaceans	Celery
	Crustaceans	Gluten	Gluten	Mustard	Soy	Soy
	Fish	Crustaceans	Soy	Soy	Milk	Lupine
	Gluten	Lupine	Peanut	Hazelnut	Peanut	Mustard
	Lupine	Molluscs	Hazelnut	Walnut	Egg	Sesame
	Molluscs	Mustard		Wheat		Almond
	Milk	Sesame		Barley		Cashew
	Mustard	Soy		Rye		Hazelnut
	Sesame	Peanut				
	Soy	Hazelnut				
	Peanut	Almond				
	Hazelnut	Pistachio				
	Macadamia	Cashew				
	Almond	Walnut				
		Pecan				

test results caused by inhibition of the PCR process. The qualitative analysis of sample DNA can be performed with a detection limit of ten DNA copies. There are also end point PCR kits, in which PCR products are visualized by agarose gel electrophoresis. These kits include PCR master mixes, requiring only the addition of template and *Taq* polymerase. The master mixes are generally already colored with a gel-loading dye so that a later additional procedural step is eliminated. Spike and control DNAs are also included to ensure the reliability of the tests. Last, are the PCR–ELISA test kits that allow the detection of specific DNA targets by means of the PCR. Once the target DNA is amplified, it is subsequently detected via a labeled hybridization probe in an ELISA-like technique. The kit contains a PCR-binding buffer for both the rehydration of streptavidin and binding of the PCR products; a buffer for the denaturation of the PCR products, an initial wash buffer for both the removal of the denaturation buffer and unbound PCR products; a buffer for the hybridization of the DNA probes; a stringency buffer for the removal of unbound DNA probes and for stringency testing of the hybridization; a conjugate buffer for the dilution of the concentrated antibody conjugate; a second wash buffer for the removal of unbound antibody conjugate; and finally a substrate solution for the colorimetric reaction and a stop solution to arrest the reaction. The sample analysis is qualitative with a detection limit of 10–20 DNA copies.

3 New Challenges and Future

Although many important key questions in the area of food allergy still remain unanswered such as: what defines a major allergen? Why some individuals develop food allergies and others do not? Which are the environmental factors? Could the environmental factors be monitored through epigenetics or modified by changes in the microbiome? Can tolerance to food be induced? Why some foods are more likely to trigger allergies than others? Does the route and timing of exposure have any role on the sensitization? Within the last years the area of food allergen and food allergy as a whole has witnessed some important developments. The techniques listed and discussed above on analytical methods for determination of allergens in food products are an important but minor branch of a major and complex picture. With the availability of a great number of genomic sequences and NMR/crystallographic structural studies, it is now possible to trace the taxonomy and genetic relationships of a great number of common allergens and their progenitor plant or animal cells. As a consequence, a large number of techniques directed to the diagnosis of the disease have been suggested, among them in vitro cell-based techniques such as basophil/mast cell degranulation, DC-T cell activation, and protein microarray techniques [16]. In particular, the demonstration that passive sensitization using human mast cell (LAD2) reproduced in vitro the clinical reactivity to peanut in vivo [111] is an important landmark and opens an important precedent where cumbersome Skin Prick Tests and food challenges can potentially be replaced by in vitro cellular tests [16].

With the recent advances in microbiome and our incremental understanding of gut physiology, the whole area of food tolerance induced by the commensal bacteria and their epigenetic implication as modulator of the immune system is also going through a major revolution. Initial animal studies on the effect of food allergy on the gut microbial ecology have demonstrated that disease-associated microbiota may play an important role in food allergy [112].

Regarding treatment, the last few years have witnessed interesting new ideas on oral, subcutaneous, and epicutaneous desensitization using a plethora of methods such as anti IgE antibodies (omalizumab), herbal therapy, chimeric allergen-IgG, Fcε blockage, lymph node injection, and patch therapy among others [16, 113]. The demonstration that resolution of cows's milk and egg allergy in children can be accelerated by increasing dietary baked allergen intake [114] is on line with recent and well-publicized successes in peanut Oral Immune therapy (OIT) treatments [115]. Maybe, the most compelling and interesting recent findings related to food allergens and the development of food allergy are the demonstration that early introduction of peanuts significantly decreased the frequency of peanut allergy among high-risk children when compared with peanut avoidance at the age of 60 months [116]. Although these are still initial results and many aspects of the studies need to be worked out, these studies alter some preconceived ideas of our relationship with food allergens.

Acknowledgment

López-Calleja and de la Cruz Ares were supported by Ministerio de Economía y Competitividad of Spain (Grant No. AGL 2013-48018-R). Silvia de la Cruz is also recipient of a fellowship from the Ministerio de Educación, Cultura y Deporte of Spain (AP2010-0028).

References

1. Cianferon A, Spergel JM (2009) Food allergy: review, classification and diagnosis. Allergol Int 58:457–466
2. Lieberman JA, Sicherer SH (2010) The diagnosis of food allergy. Am J Rhinol Allergy 24:439–443
3. Burks AW, Tang M, Sicherer S, Muraro A, Eigenmann PA, Ebisawa M et al (2012) ICON: food allergy. J Allergy Clin Immunol 129:906–920
4. Rona R, Keil T, Summers C, Gislason D, Zuidmeer L, Sodergren E et al (2007) The prevalence of food allergy: a meta-analysis. J Allergy Clin Immunol 120:638–646
5. Zuidmeer L, Goldhahn K, Rona RJ, Gislason D, Madsen C, Summers C et al (2008) The prevalence of plant food allergies: a systematic review. J Allergy Clin Immunol 121:1210–1218
6. Madsen CB, Hattersley S, Buck J, Gendel SM, Houben GF, Hourihane JO et al (2009) Approaches to risk assessment in food allergy: report from a workshop developing a framework for assessing the risk from allergenic foods. Food Chem Toxicol 47:480–489
7. Kanny G, Moneret-Vautrin DA, Flabbee J, Beaudouin E, Morisset M, Thevenin F (2001) Population study of food allergy in France. J Allergy Clin Immunol 108:133–140
8. Sastre J (2010) Molecular diagnosis in allergy. Clin Exp Allergy 40:1442–1460
9. Gadermaier G, Hauser M, Egger M, Ferrara R, Briza P, Souza Santos K et al (2011) Sensitization prevalence, antibody cross-reactivity and immunogenic peptide profile of Api g 2, the non-specific lipid transfer protein 1 of celery. PLoS One 6:24150
10. Boyce J, Assa'ad A, Burks A, Jones S, Sampson H, Wood R et al (2011) Guidelines for the diagnosis and management of food allergy in the United States: summary of the NIAID-sponsored expert panel report. J Allergy Clin Immunol 126:S1–S58
11. Taylor SL, Nordlee JA, Niemann LM, Lambrecht DM (2009) Allergen immunoassays – considerations for use of naturally incurred standards. Anal Bioanal Chem 395:83–92
12. Taylor S, Moneret-Vautrin D, Crevel R, Sheffield D, Morisset M, Dumont P et al (2010) Threshold dose for peanut: risk characterization based upon diagnostic oral challenge of a series of 286 peanut allergic individuals. Food Chem Toxicol 48:814–819
13. Sicherer S, Sampson H (2010) Food allergy. J Allergy Clin Immunol 125:116–125
14. Kauffman HF, Tamm M, Timmerman JAB, Borger P (2006) House dust mite major allergens Der p 1 and Der p 5 activate human airway-derived epithelial cells by protease-dependent and protease-independent mechanisms. Clin Mol Allergy 4:5–5
15. Trompette A, Divanovic S, Visintin A, Blanchard C, Hegde RS, Madan R et al (2009) Allergenicity resulting from functional mimicry of a Toll-like receptor complex protein. Nature 457:585–588
16. Alcocer MJC, de la Cruz S, López-Calleja I (2016) Recent advances in food allergy. Braz J Food Technol 19:e2016047
17. Metcalfe DD, Astwood JD, Townsend R, Sampson HA, Taylor SL, Fuchs RL (1996) Assessment of the allergenic potential of

foods derived from genetically engineered crop plants. Crit Rev Food Sci Nutr 36:S165–S186

18. Cochrane S, Salt LJ, Wantling E, Rogers A, Coutts J, Ballmer-Weber BK et al (2012) Development of a standardized low-dose double-blind placebo-controlled challenge vehicle for the EuroPrevall project. Allergy 67:17–113
19. Bindslev-Jensen C, Briggd D, Osterballe M (2002) Can we determine a threshold level for allergenic foods by statistical analysis of published data in the literature? Allergy 57:741–746
20. Codex Alimentarius (1999) Codex general standard for the labelling of pre-packaged foods. FAO/WHO, Geneva
21. Gendel SM (2012) Comparison of international food allergen labeling regulations. Regul Toxicol Pharmacol 63:279–285
22. Hefle SL, Nordlee JA, Taylor SL (1996) Allergenic foods. Crit Rev Food Sci Nutr 36:S69–S89
23. Reus KE, Houben GF, Stam M, Dubois AE (2000) Food additives as a cause of medical symptoms: relationship shown between sulfites and asthma and anaphylaxis; results of a literature review. Ned Tijdschr Geneeskd 144:1836–1839
24. Alvarez PA, Boye JI (2012) Food production and processing considerations of allergenic food ingredients: a review. J Allergy 2012:746125
25. Bremer MGEG, Smits NGE, Haasnoot W (2009) Biosensor immunoassays for traces of hazelnut protein in olive oil. Anal Bioanal Chem 395:119–126
26. Pollet J, Delport F, Janssen KPF, Tran DT, Wouters J, Verbiest T et al (2011) Fast and accurate peanut allergen detection with nanobead enhanced optical fiber SPR biosensor. Talanta 83:1436–1441
27. Trashin S, Cucu T, Devreese B, Adriaens A, De Meulenaer B (2011) Development of a highly sensitive and robust Cor a 9 specific enzyme-linked immunosorbent assay for the detection of hazelnut traces. Anal Chim Acta 708:116–122
28. Kerbach S, Alldrick AJ, Crevel RWR, Dömötör L, DunnGalvin A, Mills CEN et al (2009) Managing food allergens in the food supply chain – viewed from different stakeholder perspectives. Qual Assur Saf Crop 1:50–60
29. Lockley AK, Bardsley RG (2000) DNA-based methods for food authentication. Trends Food Sci Technol 11:67–77
30. Mafra I, Ferreira IMPLVO, Oliveira MBPP (2008) Food authentication by PCR-based methods. Eur Food Res Technol 227:649–665
31. Rice JA, Lupo AJ (2014) Immunodiagnostics in food allergen testing. In: Siragakis G, Kizis D (eds) Food allergen testing: molecular, immunochemical and chromatographic techniques. John Wiley & Sons, New York, NY, pp 13–28
32. Ćirković-Veličković T, Gavrović-Jankulović M (2014) Methods for allergen identification and quantification in food matrices. In: Ćirković-Veličković T, Gavrović-Jankulović M (eds) Food allergens, food microbiology and food safety. Springer, New York, NY, pp 77–93
33. Smith KA, Nelson PN, Warren P, Astley SJ, Murray PG, Greenman J (2004) Demystified... recombinant antibodies. J Clin Pathol 57:912–917
34. Szeto K, Latulippe DR, Ozer A, Pagano JM, White BS, Shalloway D et al (2013) RAPID-SELEX for RNA aptamers. PLoS One 8:e82667
35. Toh SY, Citartan M, Gopinath SCB, TangTH (2015) Aptamers as a replacement for antibodies in enzyme-linked immunosorbent assay. Biosens Bioelectron 64:392–403
36. Sathe SK, Teuber SS, Roux KH (2005) Effects of food processing on the stability of food allergens. Biotechnol Adv 23:423–429
37. Paschke A (2009) Aspects of food processing and its effect on allergen structure. Mol Nutr Food Res 53:959–962
38. Diaz-Amigo C (2010) Antibody-based detection methods: from theory to practice. In: Popping B, Diaz-Amigo C, Hoenicke K (eds) Molecular biological and immunological techniques and applications for food chemists. John Wiley & Sons, New York, NY, pp 223–245
39. Lee P, Taylor SL (2011) Fish, crustaceans, and mollusks. In: van Hengel AJ (ed) Food allergens. Analysis instrumentation and methods. Taylor and Francis Group, LLC, Oxfordshire, pp 177–205
40. van Hengel AJ (2007) Food allergen detection methods and the challenge to protect food-allergic consumers. Anal Bioanal Chem 389:111–118
41. Thompson M, Ellison SLR, Wood R (2002) Harmonized guidelines for single-laboratory validation of methods of analysis (IUPAC technical report). Pure Appl Chem 74:835–855
42. Schubert-Ullrich P, Rudolf J, Ansari P, Galler B, Führer M, Molinelli A et al (2009)

Commercialized rapid immunoanalytical tests for determination of allergenic food proteins: an overview. Anal Bioanal Chem 395:69–81
43. Haasnoot W, Smits N, Kemmers-Voncken A, Bremer M (2004) Fast biosensor immunoassays for the detection of cows' milk in the milk of ewes and goats. J Dairy Res 71:322–329
44. Warriner K, Reddy SM, Namvar A, Neethirajan S (2014) Developments in nanoparticles for use in biosensors to assess food safety and quality. Trends Food Sci Technol 40:183–199
45. Billakanti JM, Fee CJ, Lane FR, Kash AS, Fredericks R (2010) Simultaneous, quantitative detection of five whey proteins in multiple samples by surface plasmon resonance. Int Dairy J 20:96–105
46. Rebe Raz S, Liu H, Norde W, Bremer MGEG (2010) Food allergens profiling with an imaging surface plasmon resonance-based biosensor. Anal Chem 82:8485–8491
47. Yman IM, Eriksson A, Johansson MA, Hellens K-E (2006) Food allergen detection with biosensor immunoassays. J AOAC Int 89:856–861
48. Godoy-Navajas J, Aguilar Caballos MP, Gómez-Hens A (2011) Heterogeneous immunoassay for soy protein determination using nile blue-doped silica nanoparticles as labels and front-surface long-wavelength fluorimetry. Anal Chim Acta 701:194–199
49. Wang W, Han J, Wu Y, Yuan F, Chen Y, Ge Y (2011) Simultaneous detection of eight food allergens using optical thin film biosensor chips. J Agric Food Chem 59:6889–6894
50. Cao Q, Zhao H, Yang Y, He Y, Ding N, Wang J, Wu Z, Xiang K, Wang G (2011) Electrochemical immunosensor for casein based on gold nanoparticles and poly(L-arginine)/multi-walled carbon nanotubes composite film functionalized interface. Biosens Bioelectron 26:3469–3474
51. Eissa S, Tlili C, L'Hocine L, Zourob M (2012) Electrochemical immunosensor for the milk allergen β-lactoglobulin based on electrografting of organic film on graphene modified screen-printed carbon electrodes. Biosens Bioelectron 38:308–313
52. Yang C, Gu B, Xu C, Xu X (2011) Self-assembled ZnO quantum dot bioconjugates for direct electrochemical determination of allergen. J Electroanal Chem 660:97–100
53. Jiang D, Ji J, An L, Sun X, Zhang Y, Zhang G, Tang L (2013) Mast cell-based electrochemical biosensor for quantification of the major shrimp allergen Pen a 1 (tropomyosin). Biosens Bioelectron 50:150–156
54. Huang Y, Bell MC, Suni II (2008) Impedance biosensor for peanut protein Ara h 1. Anal Chem 80:9157–9161
55. Huang Y, Suni II (2008) Degenerate Si as an electrode material for electrochemical biosensors. J Electrochem Soc 155:J350–J354
56. Singh R, Sharma PP, Baltus RE, Suni II (2010) Nanopore immunosensor for peanut protein Ara h 1. Sens Actuat B Chem 145:98–103
57. Xiulan S, Yinzhi Z, Jingdong S, Liyan S, He Q, Weijuan Z (2010) A quartz crystal microbalance-based Immunosensor for shrimp allergen determination in food. Eur Food Res Technol 231:563–570
58. Chu PT, Lin CS, Chen WJ, Chen CF, Wen HW (2012) Detection of gliadin in foods using a quartz crystal microbalance biosensor that incorporates gold nanoparticles. J Agric Food Chem 60:6483–6492
59. Picariello G, Mamone G, Addeo F, Ferranti P (2011) The frontiers of mass spectrometry-based techniques in food allergenomics. J Chromatogr A 1218:7386–7398
60. Cifuentes A (2013) Foodomics: principles and applications. In: Cifuentes A (ed) Foodomics: advanced mass spectrometry in modern food science and nutrition. John Wiley & Sons, Inc., New York, pp 1–13
61. Kirsch S, Fourdrilis S, Dobson R, Scippo ML, Maghuin-Rogister G, De Pauw E (2009) Quantitative methods for food allergens: a review. Anal Bioanal Chem 395:57–67
62. Christofakis M, Xila A (2014) Immunodiagnostics in food allergen testing. In: Siragakis G, Kizis D (eds) Food allergen testing: molecular, immunochemical and chromatographic techniques. John Wiley & Sons, New York, NY, pp 50–65
63. Monaci L, Visconti A (2009) Mass spectrometry-based proteomics methods for analysis of food allergens. Trends Anal Chem 28:581–591
64. Gallardo JM, Carrera M, Ortea I (2013) Proteomics in food science. In: Cifuentes A (ed) Foodomics: advanced mass spectrometry in modern food science and nutrition. John Wiley & Sons, Inc., New York, pp 125–165
65. Catherman AD, Skinner OS, Kelleher NL (2014) Top down proteomics: facts and perspectives. Biochem Biophys Res Commun 445:683–693
66. Mattarozzi M, Bignardi C, Elviri L, Careri M (2012) Rapid shotgun proteomic liquid chromatography – electrospray ionization – tandem mass spectrometry-based method for the lupin (*Lupinus albus* L.) multi-allergen deter-

mination in foods. J Agric Food Chem 60:5841–5846

67. Pedreschi R, Nørgaard J, Maquet A (2012) Current challenges in detecting food allergens by shotgun and targeted proteomic approaches: a case study on traces of peanut allergens in baked cookies. Nutrients 4:132–150
68. Meissner F, Mann M (2014) Quantitative shotgun proteomics: considerations for a high-quality workflow in immunology. Nat Immunol 15:112–117
69. Monaci L, Losito I, Palmisano F, Visconti A (2010) Identification of allergenic milk proteins markers in fined white wines by capillary liquid chromatography-electrospray ionization-tandem mass spectrometry. J Chromatogr A 1217:4300–4305
70. Fæste CK, Rønning HT, Christians U, Granum PE (2011) Liquid chromatography and mass spectrometry in food allergen detection. J Food Prot 74:316–345
71. Fanali C, Dugo L, Dugo P, Mondello L (2013) Capillary-liquid chromatography (CLC) and nano-LC in food analysis. Trends Anal Chem 52:226–238
72. Weber D, Raymond P, Ben-Rejeb S, Lau B (2006) Development of a liquid chromatography-tandem mass spectrometry method using capillary liquid chromatography and nanoelectrospray ionization-quadrupole time-of-flight hybrid mass spectrometer for the detection of milk allergens. J Agric Food Chem 54:1604–1610
73. Monaci L, Losito I, Palmisano F, Visconti A (2011) Reliable detection of milk allergens in food using a high-resolution, stand-alone mass spectrometer. J AOAC Int 94:1034–1042
74. Heick J, Fischer M, Kerbach S, Tamm U, Popping B (2011) Application of a liquid chromatography tandem mass spectrometry method for the simultaneous detection of seven allergenic foods in flour and bread and comparison of the method with commercially available ELISA test kits. J AOAC Int 94:1060–1068
75. Chassaigne H, Nørgaard JV, van Hengel AJ (2007) Proteomics-based approach to detect and identify major allergens in processed peanuts by capillary LC-Q-TOF (MS/MS). J Agric Food Chem 55:4461–4473
76. Di Bernardo G, Del Gaudio S, Galderisi U, Cascino A, Cipollaro M (2007) Comparative evaluation of different DNA extraction procedures from food samples. Biotechnol Prog 23:297–301
77. Di Bernardo G, Galderisi U, Cipollaro M, Cascino A (2005) Methods to improve the yield and quality of DNA from dried and processed figs. Biotechnol Prog 21:546–549
78. Kirsh S, Fourdrilis S, Dobson R, Scippo ML, Maghuin-Rogister G, De Pauw E (2009) Quantitative methods for food allergens: a review. Anal Bioanal Chem 395:57–67
79. López-Calleja IM, González I, Fajardo V, Martín I, Hernández PE, García T et al (2007) Quantitative detection of goats' milk in sheep's milk by real-time PCR. Food Control 18:1466–1473
80. Poms RE, Klein CL, Anklam E (2004) Methods for allergen analysis in food: a review. Food Addit Contam 21:1–31
81. Brzezinski JL (2006) Detection of cashew nut DNA in spiked baked goods using a real-time polymerase chain reaction method. J AOAC Int 89:1035–1038
82. Brezna B, Kuchta T (2008) A novel real-time polymerase chain reaction method for the detection of pecan nuts in food. Eur Food Res Technol 226:373–377
83. Brezna B, Dudánová H, Kuchta T (2008) A novel real-time polymerase chain reaction method for the qualitative detection of pistachio in food. Eur Food Res Technol 228:197–203
84. Brezna B, Dudásová H, Kuchta T (2010) A novel real-time polymerase chain reaction method for the detection of Brazil nuts in food. J AOAC Int 93:197–201
85. Brezna B, Hudecova L, Kuchta T (2006) A novel real-time polymerase chain reaction (PCR) method for the detection of walnuts in food. Eur Food Res Technol 223:373–377
86. Brezna B, Piknova L, Kuchta T (2009) A novel real-time polymerase chain reaction method for the detection of macadamia nuts in food. Eur Food Res Technol 229:397–401
87. López-Calleja IM, de la Cruz S, González I, García T, Martin R (2014) Survey of undeclared allergenic pistachio *(Pistacia vera)* in commercial foods by hydrolysis probe real-time PCR. Food Control 39:49–55
88. López-Calleja IM, de la Cruz S, González I, García T, Martin R (2015) Market analysis of food products for detection of allergenic walnut (*Juglans regia*) and pecan (*Carya illinoinensis*) by real-time PCR. Food Chem 177:111–119
89. López-Calleja IM, de la Cruz S, Pegels N, González I, García T, Martin R (2013) Development of a real time PCR assay for detection of allergenic trace amounts of peanut *(Arachis hypogaea)* in processed foods. Food Control 30:480–490
90. López-Calleja IM, de la Cruz S, Pegels N, González I, García T, Martin R (2013) High

resolution TaqMan real-time PCR approach to detect hazelnut DNA encoding for ITS rDNA in foods. Food Chem 141:1872–1880

91. Pafundo S, Gullì M, Marmiroli N (2009) SYBR GreenER real-time PCR to detect almond in traces in processed food. Food Chem 116:811–815

92. Platteau C, De Loose M, De Meulenaer B, Taverniers I (2011) Detection of allergenic ingredients using real-time PCR: a case study on hazelnut (*Corylus avellana*) and soy (*Glicine max*). J Agric Food Chem 59:10803–10814

93. Scaravell E, Brohee M, Marchelli R, Van Henge A (2008) Development of three real-time PCR assays to detect peanut allergen residue in processed food products. Eur Food Res Technol 227:857–869

94. Hupfer C, Waiblinger HU, Busch U (2007) Development and validation of a real-time PCR detection method for celery in food. Eur Food Res Technol 225:329–335

95. Mujico JR, Lombardia M, Carmen MM, Mendez E, Albar JP (2011) A highly sensitive real-time PCR system for quantification of wheat contamination in gluten-free food for celiac patients. Food Chem 128:795–801

96. Hirao T, Imai S, Sawada H, Shiomi N, Hachimura S, Kato H (2005) PCR method for detecting trace amounts of buckwheat (Fagopyrum sp.). Food Biosci Biotechnol Biochem 69:724–731

97. Demmel A, Hupfer C, Ilg Hampe E, Busch U, Engel KH (2008) Development of a real-time PCR for the detection of lupine DNA (*Lupinus* species) in foods. J Agric Food Chem 56:4328–4332

98. Ehlert A, Hupfer C, Demmel A, Engel KH, Busch U (2008) Detection of cashew nut in foods by a specific real-time PCR method. Food Anal Methods 1:136–143

99. Ehlert A, Moreano F, Busch U, Engel KH (2008) Development of a modular system for detection of genetically modified organisms in food based on ligation-dependent probe amplification. Eur Food Res Technol 227:805–812

100. de la Cruz S, López-Calleja IM, Alcocer MJC, González I, Martín R, García T (2013) Taqman real-time PCR assay for detection of traces of Brazil nut (*Bertholletia excelsa*) in food products. Food Control 33:105–113

101. Koppel R, Dvorak V, Zimmerli F, Breitenmoser A, Eugster A, Waiblinger HU (2010) Two tetraplex real-time PCR for the detection and quantification of DNA from eight allergens in food. Eur Food Res Technol 230:367e374

102. Hashimoto H, Makabe Y, Hasegawa Y, Sajiki J, Miyamoto F (2007) Detection of allergenic substances in foods by a multiplex PCR method. J Food Hyg Soc Jpn 48:132–138

103. Moreano F, Ehlert A, Busch U, Engel KH (2006) Ligation-dependent probe amplification for the simultaneous event-specific detection and relative quantification of DNA from two genetically modified organisms. Eur Food Res Technol 222:479–485

104. Ehlert A, Demmel A, Hupfer C, Busch U, Engel KH (2009) Simultaneous detection of DNA from 10 food allergens by ligation-dependent probe amplication. Food Addit Contam 26:409–418

105. Mustorp SL, Dromtorp SM, Holck AL (2011) Multiplex, quantitative, ligation-dependent probe amplification for determination of allergens in food. J Agric Food Chem 59:5231–5239

106. Sun X, Guan L, Shan X, Zhang Y, Li Z (2012) Electrochemical detection of peanut allergen Ara h 1 using a sensitive DNA biosensor based on stem–loop probe. J Agric Food Chem 60:10979–10984

107. Berti F, Laschi S, Palchetti I, Rossier JS, Reymond F, Mascini M, Marrazza G (2009) Microfluidic-based electrochemical genosensor coupled to magnetic beads for hybridization detection. Talanta 77:971–978

108. Tortajada-Genaro LA, Santiago-Felipe S, Morais S, Gabaldón JA, Puchades R, Maquieira Á (2012) Multiplex DNA detection of food allergens on a digital versatile disk. J Agric Food Chem 60:36–43

109. Bettazzi F, Lucarelli F, Palchetti I, Berti F, Marrazza G, Mascini M (2008) Disposable electrochemical DNA-array for PCR amplified detection of hazelnut allergens in foodstuffs. Anal Chim Acta 614:93–102

110. Rossi S, Scaravelli E, Germini A, Corradini R, Fogher C, Marchelli R (2006) A PNA-array platform for the detection of hidden allergens in foodstuffs. Eur Food Res Technol 223:1–6

111. Santos AFG, Toit D, Douiri A, Radulovic S, Stephens A, Turcanu V et al (2015) Distinct parameters of the basophil activation test reflect the severity and threshold of allergic reactions to peanut. J Allergy Clin Immunol 135:179–186

112. Prescott S, Allen KJ (2011) Food allergy: Riding the second wave of the allergy epidemic. Pediatr Allergy Immunol 22:155–160

113. Sicherer SH, Sampson HA (2014) Food allergy: epidemiology, pathogenesis, diagnosis, and treatment. J Allergy Clin Immunol 133:291–307

114. Leonard SA, Sampson HA, Sicherer SH, Noone S, Moshier EL, Godbold J et al (2012) Dietary baked egg accelerates resolution of egg allergy in children. J Allergy Clin Immunol 130:473–480
115. Anagnostou K, Islam S, King Y, Foley L, Pasea L, Bond S et al (2014) Assessing the efficacy of oral immunotherapy for the desensitisation of peanut allergy in children (STOP II): a phase 2 randomised controlled trial. Lancet 383:1297–1304
116. Du Toit G, Roberts G, Sayre PH, Bahnson HT, Radulovic S, Santos AF et al (2015) Randomized trial of peanut consumption in infants at risk for peanut allergy. N Engl J Med 372:803–813
117. James D, Schmidt AM (2004) Use of an intron region of a chloroplast tRNA gene (trnL) as a target for PCR identtification of specific food crops including sources of potencial allergens. Food Res Int 37:395–402
118. Watanabe S, Akiyama H, Maleki S, Yamakawa H, Iijima K, Yamazaki F et al (2006) A specific qualitative detection method for peanut (*Arachis hypogaea*) in foods using polymerase chain reaction. J Food Biochem 30:215–233
119. Hird H, Lloyd J, Goodier R, Brown J, Reece P (2003) Detection of peanut using real-time polymerase chain reaction. Eur Food Res Technol 217:265–268
120. Stephan O, Vieths S (2004) Development of a real-time PCR and a sandwich ELISA for detection of potentially allergenic trace amounts of peanut (*Arachis hypogaea*) in processed foods. J Agric Food Chem 52:3754–3760
121. Scaravelli E, Brohee M, Marchelli R, van Hengel A (2008) Development of three real-time PCR assays to detect peanut allergen residue in processed food products. Eur Food Res Technol 227:857–869
122. López-Calleja IM, de la Cruz S, Pegels N, González I, Martín R, García T (2014) Sensitive and specific detection of almond (*Prunus dulcis*) in commercial food products by real-time PCR. LWT Food Sci Technol 56:31–39
123. Holzhauser T, Stephan O, Vieths S (2002) Detection of potentially allergenic hazelnut (*Corylus avellana*) residues in food: a comparative study with DNA PCR-ELISA and protein sandwich-ELISA. J Agric Food Chem 50:5808–5815
124. Germini A, Scaravelli E, Lesignoli F, Sforza S, Corradini R, Marchelli R (2005) Polymerase chain reaction coupled with peptide nucleic acid high-performance liquid chromatography for the sensitive detection of traces of potentially allergenic hazelnut in foodstuffs. Eur Food Res Technol 220:619–624
125. Holzhauser T, Wangorsch A, Vieths S (2000) Polymerase chain reaction (PCR) for detection of potentially allergenic hazelnut residues in complex food matrixes. Eur Food Res Technol 211:360–365
126. Herman L, Block JD, Viane R (2003) Detection of hazelnut DNA traces in chocolate by PCR. Int J Food Sci Technol 38:633–640
127. Arlorio M, Cereti E, Coïsson JD, Travaglia F, Martelli A (2007) Detection of hazelnut (*Corylus* spp.) in processed foods using real-time PCR. Food Control 18:140–148
128. Piknová L, Pangallo D, Kuchta T (2008) A novel real-time polymerase chain reaction (PCR) method for the detection of hazelnuts in food. Eur Food Res Technol 226:1155–1158
129. D'Andrea M, Coission JD, Travaglia F, Garino C, Arlorlo M (2009) Development and validation of a SYBR-Green I real-time PCR protocol to detect hazelnut (*Corylus avellana* L.) in foods through calibration via plasmid reference standard. J Agric Food Chem 57:11201–11208
130. Piknová L, Kuchta T (2007) Detection of cashew nuts in food by real-time polymerase chain reaction. J Food Nutr Res 46:101–104
131. Yano T, Sakai Y, Uchida K, Nakao Y, Ishihata K, Nakano S, Yamada T, Sakai S, Urisu A, Akiyama H, Maitani T (2007) Detection of walnut residues in processed foods by polymerase chain reaction. Biosci Biotechnol Biochem 71:1793–1796
132. Wang H, Yuan F, Wu Y, Yang H, Xu B, Liu Z, Chen Y (2009) Detection of allergen walnut component in food by an improved real-time PCR method. J Food Prot 72:2433–2435
133. Janská V, Piknová L, Kuchta T (2011) Relative quantification of walnuts and hazelnuts in bakery products using real-time polymerase chain reaction. Eur Food Res Technol 232:1057–1060
134. Janská V, Piknová L, Kuchta T (2012) Semi-quantitative estimation of the walnut content in fillings of bakery products using real-time polymerase chain reaction with internal standard material. Eur Food Res Technol 235:1033–1038
135. Barbieri G, Frigeri G (2006) Identification of hidden allergens: detection of pistachio traces in mortadella. Food Addit Contam 23:1260–1264
136. Brežná B, Dudášová H, Kuchta T (2008) A novel real-time polymerase chain reaction method for the qualitative detection of pistachio in food. Eur Food Res Technol 228:197–203

137. Röder M, Filbert H, Holzhauser T (2010) A novel, sensitive and specific real-time PCR for the detection of traces of allergenic Brazil nut (*Bertholletia excelsa*) in processed foods. Anal Bioanal Chem 398:2279–2288
138. Brzezinski JL (2007) Detection of sesame seed DNA in foods using real-time PCR. J Food Prot 70:1033–1036
139. Schöringhumer K, Cichna-Markl M (2007) Development of a real-time PCR method to detect potentially allergenic sesame (*Sesamum indicum*) in food. J Agric Food Chem 55:10540–10547
140. Mustorp S, Engdahl-Axelsson C, Svensson U, Holck A (2008) Detection of celery (*Apium graveolens*), mustard (*Sinapis alba*, *Brassica juncea*, *Brassica nigra*) and sesame (*Sesamum indicum*) in food by real-time PCR. Eur Food Res Technol 226:771–778
141. Meyer R, Chardonnens F, Hübner P, Lüthy J (1996) Polymerase chain reaction (PCR) in the quality and safety assurance of food: detection of soya in processed meat products. Z Für Lebensm Unters Forsch 203:339–344
142. Torp AM, Olesen A, Sten E, Stahl Skov P, Bindslev-Jensen U, Poulsen LK et al (2006) Specific, semi-quantitative detection of the soybean allergen Gly m Bd 30 K DNA by PCR. Food Control 17:30–36
143. Yamakawa H, Akiyama H, Endo Y, Miyatake K, Sakata K, Sakai S et al (2007) Specific detection of soybean residues in processed foods by the polymerase chain reaction. Biosci Biotechnol Biochem 71:269–272
144. Gryson N, Messens K, Dewettinck K (2008) PCR detection of soy ingredients in bread. Eur Food Res Technol 227:345–351
145. Soares S, Mafra I, Amaral JS, Oliveira MBPP (2010) A PCR assay to detect trace amounts of soybean in meat sausages. Int J Food Sci Technol 45:2581–2588
146. Dovicovicova L, Olexova L, Pangallo D, Siekel P, Kuchta T (2004) Polymerase chain reaction (PCR) for the detection of celery (*Apium graveolens*) in food. Eur Food Res Technol 218:493–495
147. Stephan O, Weisz N, Vieths S, Weiser T, Rabe B, Vatterott W (2004) Protein quantification, sandwich ELISA, and real-time PCR used to monitor industrial cleaning procedures for contamination with peanut and celery allergens. J AOAC Int 87:1448–1457
148. Palle-Reisch M, Wolny M, Cichna-Markl M, Hochegger R (2013) Development and validation of a real-time PCR method for the simultaneous detection of black mustard (*Brassica nigra*) and brown mustard (*Brassica juncea*) in food. Food Chem 138:348–355
149. Köppel E, Stadler M, Lüthy J, Hübner P (1998) Detection of wheat contamination in oats by polymerase chain reaction (PCR) and enzyme-linked immunosorbent assay (ELISA). Z für Leb Forsch A 206:399–403
150. Yamakawa H, Akiyama H, Endo Y, Miyatake K, Sakata K, Sakai S, Toyoda M, Urisu A (2007) Specific detection of wheat residues in processed foods by polymerase chain reaction. Biosci Biotechnol Biochem 71:2561–2564
151. Sandberg M, Lundberg L, Ferm M, Malmheden Yman I (2003) Real time PCR for the detection and discrimination of cereal contamination in gluten free foods. Eur Food Res Technol 217:344–349
152. Hernández M, Esteve T, Pla M (2005) Real-time polymerase chain reaction based assays for quantitative detection of barley, rice, sunflower, and wheat. J Agric Food Chem 53:7003–7009
153. Dahinden I, von Büren M, Lüthy J (2001) A quantitative competitive PCR system to detect contamination of wheat, barley or rye in gluten-free food for coeliac patients. Eur Food Res Technol 212:228–233
154. Aranishi F, Okimoto T (2004) PCR-based detection of allergenic mackerel ingredients in seafood. J Genet 83:193–195
155. Choi KY, Hong KW (2007) Genomic DNA sequence of mackerel parvalbumin and a PCR test for rapid detection of allergenic mackerel ingredients in food. Food Sci Biotechnol 16:67–70
156. Brzezinski JL (2005) Detection of crustacean DNA and species identification using a PCR-restriction fragment length polymorphism method. J Food Prot 68:1866–1873
157. Schöringhumer K, Redl G, Cichna-Markl M (2009) Development and validation of a duplex real-time PCR method to simultaneously detect potentially allergenic sesame and hazelnut in food. J Agric Food Chem 57:2126–2134
158. Fuchs M, Cichna-Markl M, Hochegger R (2013) Development and validation of a duplex real-time PCR method for the simultaneous detection of celery and white mustard in food. Food Chem 141:229–235
159. Hubalkova Z, Rencova E (2011) One-step multiplex PCR method for the determination of pecan and Brazil nut allergens in food products. J Sci Food Agric 91:2407–2411
160. Coïsson JD, Cereti E, Garino C, D'Andrea M, Recupero M, Restani P et al (2010) Microchip capillary electrophoresis (Lab-on-chip®) improves detection of celery (*Apium graveolens* L.) and sesame (*Sesamum indicum* L.) in foods. Food Res Int 43:1237–1243

Index

Jing Lin and Marcos Alcocer (eds.), *Food Allergens: Methods and Protocols*, Methods in Molecular Biology, vol. 1592, DOI 10.1007/978-1-4939-6925-8, © Springer Science+Business Media LLC 2017

V

W

www.ingramcontent.com/pod-product-compliance
Lightning Source LLC
Chambersburg PA
CBHW080734150926
51501CB00005B/164
* 9 7 8 1 4 9 3 9 6 9 2 3 4 *